IMMEDIATE care of the acutely ill and injured

IMMEDIATE care of the acutely ill and injured

Edited by
Hugh E. Stephenson, Jr.
A.B., B.S., M.D., F.A.C.S.

Professor of Surgery, University of Missouri
School of Medicine, Columbia, Missouri

The C. V. Mosby Company
SAINT LOUIS   1974

Library of Congress Cataloging in Publication Data

Stephenson, Hugh E
    Immediate care of the acutely ill and injured.

    1. Medical emergencies. 2. Care of the sick.
I. Title. [DNLM: 1. Emergencies. 2. Emergency
health services. WB100 S834i 1974]
RC87.S793 616'.025 73-14584
ISBN 0-8016-4782-7

E/M/M 9 8 7 6 5 4 3 2 1

Contributors

John P. Adams, B.S., M.D., F.A.C.S.
Professor and Chairman, Department of Orthopaedic Surgery, George Washington
University Medical Center, Washington, D. C.

John T. Bonner, M.D.
Assistant Professor of Surgery (Neurosurgery), Neurological Surgery, Fresno, California;
formerly Assistant Professor of Surgery (Neurosurgery), University of Missouri,
Columbia, Missouri

Elwyn L. Cady, Jr., J.D., B.S. (Medicine)
Medicolegal Consultant of the Independence, Kansas City, and St. Louis, Missouri Bars,
Kansas City, Missouri

Richard O. Coe, Jr., M.D.
Ophthalmology, Mission, Kansas

Marshall B. Conrad, M.D., F.A.C.S.
Assistant Professor of Orthopaedic Surgery, Washington University School of Medicine;
Chairman, St. Louis Regional Committee on Trauma, American College of Surgeons,
St. Louis, Missouri

Jefferson C. Davis, M.D., Colonel, USAF, MC
Chief, Aerospace Medical Branch, USAF School of Aerospace Medicine,
Brooks AFB, Texas

Jean-René Dupont, M.D., F.A.C.S.
Department of Surgery, Ferguson Medical Group and Missouri Delta Community
Hospital, Sikeston, Missouri

Charles F. Frey, M.D., F.A.C.S.

Associate Professor of Surgery, University of Michigan School of Medicine,
Ann Arbor, Michigan

Wesley Furste, M.D., F.A.C.S.

Senior Attending Staff, Department of Surgery, Riverside Methodist Hospital,
Columbus, Ohio

George R. Gay, M.D.

Chief, Heroin Section and Director, Drug Detoxification, Rehabilitation and Aftercare
Project, Haight-Ashbury Free Medical Clinic, San Francisco, California

†Russell E. Hanlon, M.D.

Formerly Assistant Professor of Obstetrics and Gynecology, University of Missouri School
of Medicine, Columbia, Missouri

John H. Henzel, M.D.

Assistant Professor of Surgery, University of Missouri School of Medicine,
Columbia, Missouri

Walter Ford Keitzer, M.D.

Professor of Surgery, University of Missouri School of Medicine, Columbia, Missouri

James M. Landeen, M.D.

Assistant Professor of Surgery (Otolaryngology), Laurel, Mississippi; formerly
Assistant Professor of Surgery (Otolaryngology), University of Missouri,
Columbia, Missouri

Edgar L. Lichti, Ph.D.

Assistant Professor of Surgery, University of Missouri School of Medicine,
Columbia, Missouri

Richard H. Martin, M.D.

Professor of Medicine and Physiology; Director, Division of Cardiology,
University of Missouri School of Medicine, Columbia, Missouri

William V. Miller, M.D.

Director, Missouri-Illinois Red Cross Blood Program, St. Louis, Missouri;
Associate Professor of Pathology; Medical Director, Central Kentucky Blood Center,
University of Lexington School of Medicine, Lexington, Kentucky

Franklin L. Mitchell, B.S., M.D., F.A.C.S.

Associate Professor of Surgery; Director, Emergency Medical Services, University of
Missouri School of Medicine, Columbia, Missouri

†Deceased.

Walter Kirt Nichols, M.D.

Assistant Professor of Surgery, University of Missouri School of Medicine,
Columbia, Missouri

Georgia B. Nolph, M.D.

Assistant Professor of Community Health and Medical Practice, University of Missouri
School of Medicine, Columbia, Missouri

Gilbert J. Ross, Jr., M.D., F.A.C.S.

Professor of Surgery (Urology), University of Missouri School of Medicine,
Columbia, Missouri

Hugh E. Stephenson, Sr., D.D.S.

Columbia, Missouri

Hugh E. Stephenson, Jr., A.B., B.S., M.D., F.A.C.S.

Professor of Surgery, University of Missouri School of Medicine,
Columbia, Missouri

Boyd E. Terry, M.D., F.A.C.S.

Assistant Professor of Surgery, University of Missouri School of Medicine,
Columbia, Missouri

Gerard J. Van Leeuwen, M.D.

Professor and Chairman, Department of Pediatrics, University of Nebraska School of
Medicine, Omaha, Nebraska

Fred A. Wappel, A.B., Trainer Certified

Athletic Trainer, Intercollegiate Athletics and Instructor in Physical Education, University
of Missouri, Columbia, Missouri

James M. A. Weiss, M.D.

Professor and Chairman, Department of Psychiatry, University of Missouri School of
Medicine, Columbia, Missouri

Earl J. Wipfler, Jr., B.S., M.D., F.A.C.S.

General Surgery, St. Charles, Missouri

With the editorial assistance of

Robert S. Kimpton, A.B., B.S., M.Ed.

Journalistic Consultant, Columbia, Missouri

DEDICATED TO

*Students whose interest and enthusiasm
in this subject during the past 20 years have
stimulated the writing of this book.*

Foreword

Change seems to be characteristic of the twentieth century. It may well be that people in each period have similar beliefs but historically we seem to have more direct evidence of change, such as the technological burst; the swing to urban living; the communications revolution as seen in telephone, radio, television, and satellite; transportation by railroad, motor car, airplane, and rocket. Congestion, speed, and use of mechanical devices have resulted in increased illness and injury.

The near defeat of contagion by scientific public health methods has also brought into prominence the increasing losses from stress and injury. The public has been taught to believe that good health is their right and they have concurred enthusiastically with the medical tenet that immediate care is a part of good treatment. Has the medical profession responded adequately?

Specialization, even in ever narrowing fields, has largely replaced general practice. The hospital, formerly a place to go to die, has become the primary physician to the majority in large cities. Outside of regular office hours the physician is not generally available in his office and does not make house calls. The disposition of the immediate care of the acutely ill and injured thereby becomes an unsettled problem.

While this load grows constantly, the medical profession, at least until quite recently, has shown little interest in the field. For more than 60 years the American Red Cross has been engaged in teaching first aid to laymen. Except in wartime this has rarely been widely popular. The Boy Scouts, Camp Fire Girls, Bureau of Mines, and public schools have also worked on this to a limited extent. Forty years ago an occasional medical school in this country and Canada conducted such a course for the first-year medical student. It seemed only fair, when he went home for his first Christmas vacation and his acquaintances called him "Doc," that he might know as much about first aid as a well-trained Boy Scout.

Dr. Stephenson recognized the need for such a course nearly 20 years ago and started one as an optional elective, which soon involved nearly 100% of the class. This has had sluggish adoption by medical schools in general. Dr. Stephenson circulated two medical school questionnaires on the subject and the majority of schools now seem to pay some attention to immediate care.

The circulation of these questionnaires was a major influence in adoption of such courses. Also the wide recommendation of mouth-to-mouth artificial respiration and, beginning in 1960, the acceptance of external cardiac compression brought home forcibly the great number of unnecessary deaths occurring each year from heart attacks and motor vehicle accidents because of lack of knowledge and training on the part of physicians and laymen in their use. In the past 10 years the brush fire of interest in immediate care has become a conflagration extending not only to doctors, but to nurses, ambulance personnel, and police and fire departments.

I have been interested in the field since World War I. To my knowledge no book covering immediate care has been written previously for the medical student. Dr. Stephenson has had this in mind for a number of years. It has come to fruition admirably as a result of his long period of dedicated teaching of this subject. He has gathered contributors who cover their subjects in similar fashion. His editing has succeeded in allowing few repetitions and making the book read like the composition of a single author. The coverage is broad and is up to the minute.

Quite uniformly, the text is limited to *immediate* care; otherwise, the size of the book would have been impractical. Into whatever specialty the medical student enters, this material is basic to knowledge of his immediate care of a patient. He will put it to good use subconsciously when he may not even appreciate that he is doing so. This includes those who enter a life of teaching and research.

We are approaching the point where the medical profession will be adequately prepared to respond to the changes required in the quality of immediate care. This volume goes far toward filling the need of the medical and paramedical professions for learning and having ready reference assistance in the problems of immediate care.

Robert H. Kennedy, M.D., F.A.C.S.

Preface

This book provides a "why and how" for immediate care and management of acutely ill and injured persons by utilizing a rational approach based on anatomic and physiologic considerations. Despite adequate definitive care in hospitals and clinics, the eventual outcome of a medical emergency is frequently determined by the care rendered immediately following the initial insult to the patient. The quality of immediate care is a major determinant of the degree of permanent disability.

The major impetus for this book stems from a belief in the increasing urgency to provide students with formal instruction in the pathophysiology and management of one of the major health problems of our time. The need for adequate emergency care is obvious when we consider that the principal cause of death until age 39 in the United States is trauma. For the population as a whole, accidents rank behind only cardiovascular disease and cancer as a leading cause of death. During the past decade 450,000 persons have died from accidents on our highways.

Of even greater impact, however, is the realization that the principal health problem is the high incidence of sudden cardiac death occurring outside of the hospital. It is estimated that as many as 365,000 such deaths occur each year in the United States. It is no longer debatable that large numbers of these victims, mostly with malignant cardiac arrhythmias, can be saved.

How effectively are students being trained for the delivery of emergency care efforts? In an effort to determine curriculum commitments by the medical schools to the teaching of emergency care for the acutely ill and injured, I conducted two national surveys at 5-year intervals in my role as State Trauma Chairman of the American College of Surgeons Trauma Committee. It seems quite apparent that medical school curriculum committees, mindful of or committed to this current trend, are accelerating efforts to revise and reshape curriculum content to include formalized instruction in the management of emergency care, including that of the trauma victim. Slightly more than half of all of the medical schools now provide such formal instruction. Whereas the teaching of emergency medical care of the acutely ill and injured patient has too often in the past been relegated to an insignificant role in the undergraduate medical curriculum, there now appears to be a trend toward a sophisticated and organized presentation to the student.

With regard specifically to the matter of trauma, the spectrum of instruction is becoming increasingly broad to provide the necessary exposure to the ecologic patterns of injury, to the pathogenesis of injury, and to the psychologic and economic ramifications of injury. The Trauma Committee has expressed strong recommendations for an increased tempo of instruction in the care of the injured patient as an integral part of the medical curriculum. From their survey it is apparent that a wide variety of approaches is currently in use. These vary from elective courses for freshman and sophomore students in emergency care to specific surgical and medical clerkship periods devoted to the subject. Student assignment to the emergency unit of the hospital is commonly employed. The potential benefits of effectively administered emergency care are greater than at any previous time. It is high time that curriculum priorities recognize this potential.

Nurses and paramedical personnel also have a growing role in the delivery of immediate care. The emergency room personnel, perhaps more than any others, must work well as a team. So it is hoped, and intended, that this book will be used by these people as well as by medical students.

In an effort not to overlap with other areas of the medical curriculum, we have avoided inclusion of material concerning definitive care beyond the immediate or emergency stage or concerning emergencies of a medical and surgical nature occurring primarily within the hospital.

Medical students interested in the subject of immediate care of the acutely ill and injured have been the major stimulus to the writing of this book and to them I am grateful. Over a period of 20 years the subject has been presented to the freshmen or sophomore class, either as an elective or required course. Several medical students at the University of Missouri have served as journalistic consultants during the writing of the book, and I am indebted to them for their help. They were Glenn H. Bock, Eric Jan Carlson, Donald Clayton Patterson, Linda Pauline Boch, John W. Williams, Jr., John Dale Yeast, Donna Conard, Sanford J. Greenberg, David G. Hof, Martha J. Holt, John J. Krautman, and James E. Remkus.

Several years of contact with Dr. Robert H. Kennedy while at Bellevue and University Hospital in New York City served as an initial stimulus to my interest in this field. Dr. Kennedy has been a source of continued personal encouragement and enthusiastic support in efforts to initiate or accentuate the teaching of emergency care in the medical schools of the United States. Like so many others whom he has influenced, I, too, am grateful. His legacy to the Trauma Committee of the American College of Surgeons can hardly be fully appreciated. Dr. Wilbur P. McDonald, as Regional Chairman of the Trauma Committee, has always strongly supported our efforts on trauma here at the University of Missouri.

Through a long gestational period this book has changed form as new trends and developments emerged in emergency medical care. I am grateful to the contributors, whose efforts have been outstanding. Mr. Robert S. Kimpton has struggled with the manuscript and its many revisions. His suggestions and contributions to the book over a period of 10 years are greatly appreciated. The friendly prodding and continued assistance of my secretary, Miss Ruth McCown, who finally brought the book to fruition, are appreciated.

A special thanks should go to the faculty members of the medical schools of this country and Canada who kindly cooperated in both of our surveys of the teaching of emergency care in the medical schools. Drs. Oscar P. Hampton, Jr., Curtis P. Artz, J. Cuthbert Owens, and a host of others on the Trauma Committee of the American College of Surgeons have given their support and encouragement. These studies added much insight into the various approaches being used and the subject matter being presented.

Finally, I wish to thank my wife, Sally, as well as Ted and Ann, for their patience, tolerance, and sharing of many weekends and evenings with this effort.

Hugh E. Stephenson, Jr.

Contents

■ part one

Evaluation of immediate care priorities

chapter 1

Examination and evaluation of the patient requiring immediate aid

Initial evaluation is the crux of successful immediate care. How capable, reliable, knowledgeable, and observant are the initial evaluation efforts? The first person capable of rendering immediate aid to the acutely ill and injured victim obviously has a major responsibility—these initial efforts may not only be lifesaving but may well determine the degree and extent of any future disability.

Unlike the careful, methodic, and all-inclusive examination one would perform under well-controlled situations—for example in the office or hospital examination room—the evaluation of the patient at the scene of an accident, in a near-drowning situation, or under other such chaotic conditions requires a much quicker appraisal of the nature of the victim's problem and, indeed, may be a most demanding situation even for the most experienced practitioner. Frequently, without any medical equipment and with an uncooperative or even comatose patient, the physician may lack even the bare essentials desirable for the usual rendering of medical care. The medical history may be impossible to obtain. Any knowledge of previous illnesses or prior treatment may be lacking. The disruptive influence of a crowd or the sense of panic experienced by the patient or the family adds to the difficulties of making calm and objective decisions. Nevertheless, the need for lifesaving measures may be obvious.

First attention is directed to the victim's cardiorespiratory system. Is the patient breathing? Are palpable pulses present? Are the pupils dilated? The priority of maintaining adequate tissue perfusion to the vital organs of the body, and most importantly the brain, tops the list. The usually emphasized "ABCD's" (airway, breathing, cardiac massage, and definitive therapy) of emergency care may vary somewhat in that external cardiac massage may need be the first in the order of activities, given almost simultaneously with artificial ventilation efforts. In an emergency situation one usually assumes an optimistic view as to the probability of successful cardiopulmonary resuscitation. Obvious exceptions exist and will be discussed in Chapter 10.

When the patient's pulse is still present but when he is in a comatose or unconscious state, one quickly makes a judgment regarding need for artificial ventilation. Are respiratory efforts labored? Is the patient cyanotic? Is there evidence of acute hypoxia, asphyxia, and cyanosis? Is obstruction of the airway by the patient's tongue, vomitus, or

3

hemorrhage a possibility? Obviously, immediate measures are indicated to remove any upper airway obstruction and to keep the patient's head and neck in the proper position for maintaining an adequate airway. Regardless of the elective method of artificial ventilation, whether it be mouth-to-mouth, expired air ventilation, or bag-compression ventilation, delay cannot be tolerated.

The establishment of an adequate airway and the maintenance of artificial ventilation and assisted circulation by external cardiac compression is extremely basic to present-day immediate care needs and should be a part of the armamentarium of even the freshman medical student. These techniques are outlined in detail elsewhere in the book and are referred to throughout much of the text.

The presence of blood on the patient's body and clothing may present a dismaying sight. Control of hemorrhage and the prevention of exsanguination require prompt and decisive efforts. Necessary clothing should be removed in order to identify the area of hemorrhage. Most sources of external bleeding can be quickly controlled or stopped by direct application of pressure over the bleeding area; only infrequently will a tourniquet be required. The assessment of internal hemorrhage is, of course, much more difficult. Active intraabdominal or intrathoracic bleeding represents one of the few indications for unusually rapid transportation to the hospital.

One should make a quick assessment of the state of consciousness of the patient. Does the patient respond to stimuli? What is the response to verbal stimulation? If he is responsive to pain but not to verbal stimulation the patient is often regarded as being in a "stupor." If the patient is unresponsive to both verbal and painful stimuli, then a status of "coma" is commonly designated. Not only is the immediate appraisal of the state of unconsciousness important, but one should also make frequent and serial notations because of their bearing on future diagnostic efforts when definitive care is reached. Similarly, one should note the patient's "affect." Does it appear appropriate to the situation? Is the patient hallucinating and out of touch with reality?

Throughout the initial evaluation and establishment of immediate priorities of care one should display an attitude of confidence, reassurance, and optimism. Other individuals immediately available should be properly utilized to seek aid and to call for an ambulance, if available. Traffic may need to be controlled until the police arrive.

Concurrently with the examination and evaluation of the patient, a history of events leading to the emergency may be elicited from family, friends, or bystanders. When time is available one should make careful note of the circumstances surrounding the event, since a definitive description of the emergency may be unavailable to physicans in the emergency room or hospital at a later date.

Some patients carry emergency medical tags signifying their predisposition to allergic reactions or to such conditions as diabetes or the presence of a particular cardiac problem, including an implanted pacemaker.

The person giving immediate care must be cognizant of not only the things that need doing but also of the many "don't's" of immediate care. The mistakes of commission as well as omission will be emphasized throughout the text. For example, serious harm may be done by the well-intentioned person providing emergency care at the time of a burn, an eye injury, or an injury to the hand. Unfortunately, improper emergency measures may seriously jeopardize future definitive care in such situations.

Although one is prone to focus attention on the obvious, one should conscientiously "touch all bases" so as not to overlook the less obvious but equally important conditions amenable to immediate care. While it may not be feasible to completely disrobe the patient in order to fully examine him, one can observe precautions. For example, as outlined in detail in Chapter 26, special pains must be taken to avoid movement of the patient with back and neck injuries, since he may possibly have associated damage to the spinal cord. Any areas of deformity, tenderness, or swelling should be particularly noted. Pressure over the scalp, rib cage, and cervical spine is important, as is pressure over the anterior superior iliac spine and pubic symphysis. As discussed in Chapter 21, one needs to immediately tamponade an open chest wound. One should pay particular attention to the highly important principle of immediate and proper splinting of fractures, which has been very properly discussed by Dr. Conrad (Chapter 14). Open wounds should be protected and covered with sterile dressings prior to transportation of the patient to the hospital.

Once again, it should be emphasized how important comparative observations can be relative to the patient's vital signs. For example, once the patient arrives in the emergency room it is most significant if there has been a recent increase in the pulse rate along with a change in the skin to a cool clammy condition and a decreased alertness of the patient.

One's ability to examine and evaluate the patient requiring immediate care is largely dependent upon awareness of the many pathophysiologic changes encountered in emergency care of patients. Many portions of this book are devoted to a logical extension of this chapter as it involves specific emergency type problems largely outside of the hospital.

chapter 2

Initial priorities in the management of the patient with multiple injuries

Because of the involvement of a wide number of organ systems, the injured patient can present as an emergency fraught with much frustration, confusion, and feelings of inadequacy on the part of the examiner. By observing established principles of diagnosis and management, many of the pitfalls presented by the patient with multiple injuries can be avoided.

DETERMINATION OF LIFE-THREATENING SITUATION

Upon being faced with the responsibility of giving immediate care to an injured victim, one can often assume that more than one organ system is involved. The first question to be answered is whether or not a life-threatening situation is present.

1. If the patient appears to be well oxygenated, is breathing without evidence of obstruction, and is conscious, a likelihood of any major respiratory problems is diminished.
2. If the patient's peripheral pulses are full and regular, if the skin is warm and dry, and if there are no outward signs of major blood loss, then the likelihood of an exsanguinating hemorrhage is diminished.
3. If the patient is able to communicate the lack of any neck or back distress, if there is no numbness or tingling in the hands or feet, and if the patient is able to move all extremities without difficulty, then there is certainly a reduced likelihood of any injury to the spinal cord.
4. If the patient is conscious and relatively alert, he will be able to point to any obvious fracture site because of pain and tenderness.

SPECIFIC PRIORITIES

Obviously any effective management of the patient with multiple injuries is predicated on an adequate system of priorities. Usually these priorities are centered upon the necessity of establishing airway adequacy, recognition of and effective efforts to slow or stop exsanguinating hemorrhage with resultant hypovolemic shock, and, of course, the immediate institution of cardiopulmonary resuscitation techniques should circulatory arrest have occurred. Each of these priorities is a subject of detailed discussion in subsequent chapters.

Needless to say, the ability to maintain an adequate airway under even the most adverse situations and to allow for adequate respiratory exchange is a skill in which one should be well versed from the very start. Similarly, an adequate ability to artificially maintain the circulation by closed-chest resuscitation should be a part of the armamentarium of all personnel.

OBTAINING AN ADEQUATE HISTORY

Once the patient arrives at the emergency room of the hospital, there are a number of definitive examinations that can obviously be carried out at once. At the scene of the accident evaluation will be much more difficult. Because of the above mentioned priorities it is important to realize that evaluation and treatment may need to go hand in hand. In addition to a careful attention to the all-important priorities, one should attempt to obtain as much of a reconstruction of the accident as possible. Were there witnesses? If so, they should be questioned closely in order to obtain valuable leads as to the nature of the impact, velocity on impact, and such further points as will help to evaluate what anatomic areas may have received the brunt of the force applied. For example, if one of the victims has been thrown against the steering wheel, the possibility of intrathoracic trauma including flail chest, hemothorax, pneumothorax, and cardiac tamponade will need be entertained. Was there a period of temporary unconsciousness? Did the victim walk about?

BLOOD LOSS

One should make an absolute effort to estimate blood loss, not only at the scene of the accident but also during the trip to the hospital and in the emergency room. One should not hesitate to remove as much of the victim's clothing as may be required for immediate assessment of the necessary priorities.

VITAL SIGNS

It will be helpful to establish baselines regarding all vital signs so that when the patient arrives in the emergency room any deviation from usually accepted norms can be evaluated. This will be the subject of Chapter 5.

The suspicion of a rupture of the spleen or trauma to the intraabdominal viscera should always be present if there has been any likelihood of a blow to or penetration of the abdomen. When the patient is seen in the emergency room, it is helpful to know what the abdominal findings were immediately after the accident.

Before moving the patient to the ambulance, one generally will have time to inspect the head for any evidence of obvious injury to the skull or evidence of bleeding from the ears or nose. Is there any asymmetry of the pupils?

PREVENTION OF ASPIRATION

One can take certain preventative measures at the scene of the accident or on the way to the emergency room that might be of a lifesaving nature. For example, many patients will vomit shortly after an accident, regardless of the seriousness of the accident. To prevent aspiration of vomitus, the patient should be positioned so that his head is turned to the side. Any standard ambulance will provide an adequate suction apparatus to use. Few situations permit giving the patient liquids by mouth.

TRIAGE OF THE INJURED

The initial management of injury to a number of patients deserves some special consideration.

In cases of disaster such as tornadoes, fires, airplane crashes, or any accident that involves a number of persons, the concept of *triage* becomes important. Triage is simply another name for a sorting out of casualties in order that the maximum effect can be achieved in the saving of lives and the prevention of crippling injuries by establishing proper treatment priorities based on the initial examination. Because of the need for hospitals to have a disaster plan, many persons have participated in a simulated hospital disaster program during which they have served as victims, stretcher bearers, aides, or various types of assistants.

During these disaster drills one is exposed to the various aspects of a disaster preparedness plan. These include an adequate notification system for all personnel and a continuous communication line using telephones, walkie-talkies, and other means of communication. Traffic control, equipment distribution, and the various logistics of transportation are all a part of the exercise.

At each sorting location it is essential that an adequate written record be maintained of any pertinent observations and any subsequent treatment rendered. Since the clinical picture may vary considerably in a short period of time, it is most important for the physician treating the patient to have a complete account of all findings.

Sorting of casualties occurs at several places along the line. Basically, *triage is an establishment of proper priorities* regarding each patient and the needs for his effective care. Effective triage allows for the immediage attention of patients with airway insufficiency problems, hemorrhage, and cardiorespiratory collapse. Every effort is made to avoid diversion to less urgent problems and to center on the life-threatening ones.

SUMMARY

By recognizing broad general principles in the management of the injured person, a sizable percentage of patients will reach the hospital where definitive care can be administered. It is estimated that approximately 20% of the traffic fatalities in the United States could be averted if proper attention were given at the scene of the accident to the maintenance of the airway, control of hemorrhage, and recognition of the potential presence of severe neurologic injury. Much of this book will be devoted to these key considerations.

chapter 3

The unconscious patient: a rational approach for diagnosis

A consideration of the unconscious patient excites one's attention as much as or more than any other topic in the area of immediate care and first aid. When suddenly faced with an unconscious patient, how does one proceed, particularly in view of the multitude of possibilities as to the etiology of the unconsciousness?

In my lectures I usually select a patient who, along with some special prompting, may provide an ideal "unconscious patient." One of the best such "patients" is a 65-year-old physician who has had a bilateral below-knee amputation for vascular insufficiency. After properly "preparing" the patient with an intravenous vasopressor, placing clotted blood in the external auditory canal, bandaging a simulated laceration of the scalp, dilating the pupils with 10% phenylephrine (Neo-Synephrine), and adding a strong odor of ethyl alcohol, one of the members of the class is instructed to go to the emergency room and help a resident bring up the "victim" who has just been admitted to the emergency room. Upon arrival in the classroom the patient's controlled respirations are of a Cheyne-Stokes nature, and he can barely be aroused. The patient has an emergency medical identification tag around his neck indicating that he is a diabetic.

At this point one of the members of the class volunteers to examine the patient and, with the help of the rest of the class, the whole gamut of possible explanations of unconsciousness is explored. During a recent lecture on the unconscious patient, the doctor mentioned was brought in on a stretcher with a prosthesis on one leg while the other leg stump was exposed. It was a source of much good-natured amusement to the class when one of their number affirmed that there were good peripheral pulses over the prosthesis!

Upon one occasion, a student became quite agitated, believing that the patient's condition was rapidly deteriorating in the classroom. In addition, several students have admitted to being somewhat irritated that such a severely ill patient should be used for teaching purposes in the classroom.

Such a demonstration provides an excellent opportunity to show the uninitiated medical student the importance of careful observation simply by using one's sense of sight, touch, hearing, and even smell.

It is not surprising that medical students react to a discussion of the unconscious patient with considerable interest. Not only does the evaluation of the unconscious patient present an unusual challenge in the delegating of the immediate priorities, but a denouement of the etiologic possibilities brings forth the best of diagnostic acumen.

Often without any history relating to the patient, one is required to make the best possible use of one's observatory capacities, including one's sense of smell. It is with the undiagnosed, unconscious patient that the real "medical detective" emerges. Comatose patients are found in all types of situations with innumerable unknowns. The duration of their unconscious state may be unknown. They are found by complete strangers, police, or individuals with only fragmentary knowledge of the patient. Positive revealing physical signs may be virtually absent or misleading.

Unfortunately, medical personnel are seldom schooled in the diagnosis and management of the unconscious patient. Little wonder that each year personnel in emergency rooms inadvertently release alcoholics who subsequently die a few hours later on the streets or in jail from an undiagnosed head injury. Unfortunately, too many unconscious patients are initially given poor or inadequate treatment by bystanders, ambulance attendants, or emergency-room personnel. The unconscious patient may be shaken, doused with cold water, or given smelling salts or have various liquids including alcohol poured into his mouth. On reaching the emergency room, further examination of the patient by ill-advised flexion or positioning of the head and neck may convert a simple cervical fracture into one associated with quadriplegia.

Keeping in mind the don't's of caring for the unconscious patient, one should turn first to the problem usually requiring immediate attention: the matter of the airway and adequate ventilation. While this aspect is covered in detail in Chapters 10 and 12, emphasis is again given to the need to maintain an open airway—whether this requires manual maintenance of an extended head in relationship to the neck, an oral airway, an endotracheal airway, or occasionally a tracheostomy. Oral-pharyngeal suctioning may be urgently required. Whenever doubt exists about the adequacy of ventilation, mouth-to-mouth breathing should be instituted.

Obvious hemorrhage should be controlled by the means outlined in Chapter 23.

If clinical features of shock are evident—such as a faint thready pulse, cool moist skin, and hypotension—initial efforts should be directed toward improved tissue perfusion. After an intravenous route is established, 5% dextrose and water to which 10 mg of phenylephrine (Neo-Synephrine) has been added can be used to provide some mild support in raising the level of blood pressure.

Once the initial priorities have been met, attention is turned to a more thorough examination in order to accurately pinpoint the reason for unconsciousness. The patient must be disrobed. The respiratory excursions are observed. Are they thoracic or abdominal in origin? Do the ala nasi move excessively? Are accessory muscles of respiration in play? How regular are the excursions?

There is often significance in noting the various types of respiration. For example, Cheyne-Stokes respirations are deep and somewhat labored excursions alternating with periods of absent respiration (apnea). While Cheyne-Stokes respirations often indicate a poor prognosis such as is associated with severe head injuries or brain damage, this is not always true.

Patients in diabetic coma may present with respiratory activity increased in both depth and rate. Although many laboratory procedures will require sophisticated techniques and a certain amount of time, one can usually get an immediate urinalysis leading one to suspect diabetic acidosis. A hemoglobin and white cell count can give almost immediate worthwhile information.

The tendency of one cheek to puff out each time the patient exhales is indicative of partial facial paralysis.

The *color* of the skin and mucous membranes is a significant observation. If the patient is obviously pale, the possibility of blood loss anemia or shock is suggested. A plethoric red appearance may mean either a hypertensive encephalopathy or a cerebrovascular accident or both (or even a state of septic shock). Drug reactions or a febrile illness will give the skin a reddish color, as will a sunburn. The tell-tale bright cherry red color of carbon monoxide poisoning should immediately prompt one to institute resuscitation measures as outlined in Chapter 26.

Localized discolorations are also important, since they suggest blunt trauma. Icteric sclera prompts one to think of hepatic failure. Most importantly, generalized cyanosis must be detected early so that means for adequate tissue perfusion may be employed.

Examination of the eyes may be especially revealing in the unconscious patient. Are the eyes sunken within the orbits, indicating marked dehydration or severe wasting? Pupillary inequality (anisocoria) suggests a subdural hematoma on the side opposite the dilated pupil. Bilaterally dilated pupils may mean barbiturate intoxication. Dilated pupils may also be seen in the highly emotional patient and in the patient with glaucoma or with fever. A constricted pupil is often present in old age, after pilocarpine injection, or with Horner's syndrome.

Bilaterally dilated pupils may indicate severe brain damage. Completely dilated pupils are present when cerebral circulation has ceased. Failure of the pupils to respond to light is especially ominous. Pinpoint pupils classically suggest morphine or a similar drug intoxication. Don't forget the possibility of a glass eye!

Look at the eyegrounds. Papilledema of the fundus generally indicates brain tumor or subarachnoid hemorrhage or even hypertensive encephalopathy. Marked arteriovenous nicking supports the likelihood of cerebral arteriosclerosis. The luetic Argyll Robertson pupil accommodates but not to light. The patient with epilepsy may have fixed and staring eyes. Cotton wool exudates are seen with uremic coma.

Are there *breath odors* that should be noted? Perhaps the odor of alcohol is the most frequently encountered, but again caution is urged lest the observation serve as a red herring. Diabetic acidosis may produce a fruity odor such as from overripe apples. The foul, uriniferous odor of uremia may be present, in which instance the patient may also present with "uremic frost" about the upper lip and face. Some instances of poisoning are associated with characteristic odors, for example, the garlicky odor of phosphorus poisoning. If one knows the odor of bitter almonds or peach kernels, one may recognize prussic acid (hydrocyanic acid) poisoning.

The matter of *terminology* may prove disturbing but is important, particularly as one records any changing levels of consciousness or responsiveness to the environment, providing one notes the mode of stimulation along with the subsequent response.

Syncope refers to a brief loss of consciousness. Other terms including drowsiness, stupor, lethargy, coma, and semicoma have been used to describe varying levels of unconsciousness; however, their usage has varied among physicians and today it may be preferable to note merely the means of stimulation and the manner of response.

What is the depth of consciousness? Can the patient be aroused? Stimuli likely to arouse patients in a semicomatose state may be provided by pressure on the supraorbital nerve at its foramen. Rubbing the knuckles on the sternum with pressure may arouse the patient, or even a simple pinprick may do the job.

There are many ways of grouping unconscious patients. Some authors prefer to group them according to signs and symptoms. One possible grouping would include a broad categorization under central nervous system pathology:

1. Cerebral strokes caused by embolism, hemorrhage, or thrombosis
2. Intracranial tumor
3. Subarachnoid hemorrhage
4. Cerebral anemia. This would include the patient who is briefly unconscious from fainting caused by general cerebral anemia of a temporary nature. Also included in this group would be unconscious states accompanying shock, cardiac output failure, arrhythmias, and general morbid states.
5. Cerebral edema most commonly resulting from hypertensive encephalopathy
6. Head injuries most commonly associated with intercranial hematomas, concussions, and the like
7. Psychogenic factors, psychosis and hysteria being the most common
8. Poisonings from alcohol, narcotics, and other drugs
9. Metabolic disorders, including a broad group of unconscious states caused by uremia, hepatic failure, hypoglycemia, and diabetic acidosis
10. Infections including meningitis, encephalitis, and septic shock

Persons subject to recurrent medical emergencies may wear medical *wristbands* or *necklaces* and pertinent information may be found in their pocketbooks or among their clothing. Diabetic, hemophiliac, or cardiac patients or those subject to convulsive episodes often carry some sort of medallion. Some patients may have certain drug sensitivities. Pills found in the possession of the patient must be properly identified since the patient may be on steroid therapy.

A note of warning: Do not touch the unconscious patient at the scene of an accident until the possibility of electrocution is excluded. Many would-be rescuers have themselves been electrocuted.

Touch the patient. Pinch the skin. Is there dehydration? Is the skin warm and dry, suggesting heat stroke? A cold, clammy skin—indicative of peripheral vasoconstriction—often means shock or impending shock, including insulin shock and blood loss or hemorrhagic shock. Palpation of abdominal viscera may give clues. A posterior penetrating abdominal aortic aneurysm as a cause of intraabdominal hemorrhage and shock may be detected. More rarely, an enlarged spleen or liver will indicate hepatic failure or some hematologic disorder.

Feel the pulse. Palpate large vessels. Is it a bounding pulse, a weak thready pulse, or a paradoxic pulse?

Look for needle marks indicating an intravenous injection.

Listen. In addition to the stertorous stridor of respirations, less obvious auditory clues may be in the offing. With the stethoscope one should carefully auscultate the heart, noting any abnormalities in rate or rhythm. Occasionally a markedly slow heartbeat may lead one to suspect digitalis intoxication, and, of course, syncope resulting from heart block may be detected. The heart may be beating so fast that the tachycardia prevents an output sufficient to provide the necessary brain perfusion to maintain cerebration. Listen carefully to the lungs for any area of obviously absent breath sounds or rales. The possibility of unconsciousness on the basis of inadequate ventilation may be detected by findings suggestive of bronchial obstruction.

Sighing respirations may make one suspect "unconsciousness" of a psychosomatic nature. Respirations are generally slow in the uremic patient, the diabetic individual, the patient with morphine intoxication, the acute alcoholic individual, and the patient with intracranial bleeding.

Throughout the examination, maintain a watch on the vital signs. When possible, turn the patient's head to the side in order to prevent aspiration if he vomits. Save the specimen of the vomitus for analysis. Has involuntary defecation or urination occurred? Is there drainage from any body orifice? Blood from the ear alerts one to the possibility of basal skull fracture. Clear fluid drainage from the nose may indicate fracture of the cribriform plate.

Check for any apparent stiffness or rigidity of the patient's neck as a possible indication of meningeal irritation.

Obviously, the many aspects of diagnosis and management of the unconscious patient go beyond the problems of immediate care with which this text is concerned. Until definitive care is given, the unconscious patient should be watched closely and, of course, should never be left alone. Tracheal suctioning may be required. Oxygen administration may be indicated on the way to the hospital in the ambulance.

If marked hyperthemia or temperature elevation is present, one should immediately make efforts to reduce the temperature. This can be accomplished by rubbing ice over the surface of the body, sponging the patient, or using alcohol soaks. When the patient reaches the hospital a cooled oxygen tent, tapwater enemas, or a hypothermic blanket can be applied. Even though the etiology of the patient's hyperthermia may not be known, one should not delay in trying to control excessive temperature elevation. In the emergency room, the use of icepacks, sponging, or, subsequently, hypothermic blankets may be necessary.

If there is strong evidence that unconsciousness is based on poisoning or drug overdosage, then measures outlines in Chapter 30 should be followed.

Even though the patient is unable to communicate, much valuable history may be neglected if all details of the patient's state prior to unconsciousness are not exploited. The family may possibly be able to provide much of this information. The ambulance attendant should be questioned as to the circumstances surrounding the patient when first seen by him.

Unlike many other medical situations, the patient in coma may need certain types of treatment even before a diagnosis is made. It should not be difficult to note that throughout much of this book there is repeated emphasis upon the establishment of an adequate airway and ventilation along with the need for an accurate assessment of circulatory status.

Finally, there may be more than one reason for the unconscious state of the patient. As a result of a systemic disturbance of one type or another, the patient may have suddenly lost consciousness and in falling may have hit his head with sufficient force to cause a significant intracranial hemorrhage. Throughout the duration of the patient's unconscious state, changes are taking place, and the importance of continually monitoring the patient's vital signs should be obvious.

Although, once again, this book is concerned chiefly with the immediate and urgent needs of the acutely ill and injured patient, some brief mention can be made of more definitive diagnostic and therapeutic measures for the unconscious patient, such as, in many instances, the need for a spinal tap. It should not, of course, be an indiscriminate diagnostic procedure but one made with a great deal of judgment on the basis of careful neurologic studies and, oftentimes, only after consultation with a neurologist and neurosurgeon if they are available. Subsequently, the unconscious patient may have skull films ordered, but generally this is not in the urgent category. Electroencephalography may also be ordered.

It must again be emphasized that aspects of the management of the unconscious patient often cannot always await definitive diagnosis. Attention to airway obstruction or respiratory difficulties obviously requires immediate priority.

chapter 4

Immediate treatment for shock

As is true with many major emergencies, the immediate treatment of the patient in shock may be multifaceted. If the causative factors still persist—such as continuing hemorrhage—efforts must be directed toward achieving hemostasis or control of hemorrhage. To avoid duplication these efforts will not be discussed here but are detailed elsewhere. The shock victim may, of course, have received multiple injuries, and considerations mentioned in Chapter 2 are paramount. As with all emergencies, the patency of the airway and the adequacy of ventilation are of the first priority. Because of the reduced oxygen-carrying potential of the blood caused by reduced blood volume, oxygen should be administered if it is available. If one is satisfied that there has been no head injury, the patient should be kept in a supine or flat position or, better still, with his lower extremities moderately elevated. The patient should not be allowed to stand or sit. In order to reduce further soft tissue injury and to control pain, fractures should be splinted as soon as it is feasible and before transportation of the victim to the hospital.

DEFINITION

What is shock? While shock, with its various aspects of circulatory derangement, may be considered a wastebasket term, there are certain features common to all forms. More than anything else, certainly, shock represents a defective or low perfusion rate of blood through the tissues. This inadequate oxygenation of tissues, regardless of its cause, sets up a cyclic reaction leading to generalized metabolic acidosis, decreased cardiac output, increasing hypotension, and further reduction of tissue perfusion, to start another cycle. Effective immediate care dictates that this chain reaction be broken at the earliest possible time before irreversible changes have taken place.

A number of pathologic states may produce the shock picture, such as electric shock, septicemic shock, cardiogenic shock, burn shock, or shock from the loss of blood.

DIAGNOSTIC DIFFICULTIES

What clinical features are common to most shock states? Early in the evolution of the shock state one will be impressed by the evidence of peripheral vasoconstriction, as evidenced by cool, moist, and clammy skin; a pale face; a subjective feeling of faintness and weakness; and an inability to remain in the upright or erect position. Usually the pulse is fast and less full than normal. If considerable blood loss is the etiologic factor, the patient will generally show signs of obvious apprehension and not infrequently he is

15

thirsty and requests water. As a shock state increases in severity, mental sluggishness, increased restlessness, and further increase in the pulse rate will occur. Nausea may be present at an early stage. Respirations will increase in rate and in depth as the shock state progresses, often to the state of gasping air hunger. Quite often the pupils will be dilated.

The blood pressure readings may be deceptively normal. Because of compensatory mechanisms, including increased peripheral vasoconstriction and increased cardiac output caused by sympathetic hyperactivity, a fall in blood pressure may not occur for some period of time. The amount of blood loss likely to produce a shock state may vary with the age of the patient, the preexisting health state of the patient, and associated pain factors. Generally speaking, most individuals will show signs of peripheral vasoconstriction with cool, moist skin and an increased pulse rate if much more than 500 ml of blood is lost very rapidly. Profound shock states will be present if more than a third of the blood has been lost. "Irreversible" shock is seen if profound blood loss is allowed to persist for more than a brief period of time.

Estimating the amount of blood loss at the scene of an accident is a difficult task even for the experienced physician. Even so, some approximation of the amount of blood visibly lost by the patient will be of help to those supplying definitive care in the hospital.

The amount of blood lost within the internal body cavity or in the soft tissue of the body is a factor considerably more difficult to assess, but consideration of this possibility is not one to be overlooked. For example, it is not uncommon for a patient with a fractured hip to lose more than 1,000 ml of blood into the soft tissues about the site of the fracture. Injuries of the thigh are notorious in harboring or sequestering huge quantities of blood in a hematoma.

This chapter does not delve to any great extent into the pathophysiology of shock but confines its discussion mainly to the immediate problem of hemorragic or blood-loss shock. Other examples or etiologic factors are either touched on elsewhere in the book or are beyond the scope of this presentation. These include shock of a neurogenic nature, psychogenic shock, septic shock resulting from infection, cardiogenic shock, metabolic shock, and anaphylactic shock as an allergic reaction.

RESTORATION OF BLOOD VOLUME

Several years ago a well-known professor of surgery in a Canadian school would talk to the medical students about hemorrhagic shock. Because of his conviction that whole blood was the preferable replacement for lost blood rather than a crystalloid or colloid solution, he would dramatically state that the treatment of hemorrhagic shock is with *blood* and with that he would throw a unit of blood against the blackboard, causing a considerable splash! At least no one in that class ever forgot the treatment for hemorrhagic shock!

Of paramount importance in the treatment of shock is the restoration of the circulating blood volume in order that adequate tissue oxygenation may occur and so that irreversible damage to particularly susceptible organs such as the brain, kidney, and myocardium may be prevented. With evidence of a massive hemorrhage, emergency room physicians are alert to the need for establishing a rapid and secure intravenous route. If the veins are too much collapsed, a cutdown over one of the veins of an extremity will be required and either a needle or, preferably, a catheter may be inserted into the vein. The establishment of an intravenous route at the scene of the accident may be a lifesaving effort and should be done whenever possible. In such cases administration of lactated Ringer's solution or a solution of normal saline can be started. Ideally, a plasma expander should be immediately administered. Low molecular weight dextran not only serves to enlarge the vascular space but is extremely helpful in preventing the blood from clotting. In the shock state there is frequently a sludging of blood in the peripheral circulation, which leads to intravascular thrombosis. If plasma is available it is preferred to one of the artificial plasma expanders.

At the same time that an intravenous route is being established, blood should be drawn for immediate typing and cross-matching. In many instances the urgency of the situation is so great, however, that uncross-matched blood from a universal donor (O, Rh negative) must be administered.

CONTROL OF PAIN DURING SHOCK

Much can be done to relieve the patient's pain without the use of drugs. Reassurance is vital. Tell the patient that you understand his situation and that he will receive the best possible care. Keep him informed of plans for his rescue, immediate comfort, and eventual professional aid. Proper positioning of and support for injured extremities can greatly decrease pain in these areas. *Ask* the patient: "Is this more comfortable or would that be better?" Let him know that you care. Slit or loosen tight clothing or shoes in any way that will increase comfort.

The difficulties with the indiscriminate use of pain medication are several. The patient's respirations are already depressed and use of narcotics may further aggravate the situation. Particularly are narcotics contraindicated when there is a possibility of intraabdominal injury, since these agents will, in many instances, almost completely block the symptoms of abdominal muscle guarding, peritoneal irritation, and other signs of an acute surgical abdomen. Furthermore, the administration of narcotics by either intramuscular or subcutaneous injection at a time when there is marked peripheral vascular constriction will not be followed by an early uptake of the narcotic, and its desired effect will not only be delayed but perhaps compounded by a second narcotic injection given subsequently.

A more detailed discussion of the control of pain is presented in Chapter 6.

Should any fluids be given by mouth? Sometimes well-intentioned bystanders may offer the patient water and occasionally coffee, tea, or other fluids. Generally speaking, nothing should be given to the patient by mouth until it is clearly evident that no operative procedures will be indicated. This is a decision that should be made by the individual responsible for definitive care of the patient.

chapter 5

Monitoring of vital signs in the emergency situation

Edgar L. Lichti

From the onset of immediate care of the injured or acutely ill individual, careful and meaningful observations must be made continuously until such time as more definitive treatment is available. How does one adequately monitor the crucial physiologic functions of the patient? Under most emergency conditions sophisticated electronic and mechanical devices are not available. Instead one must rely on one's own clinical observations.

OBJECTIVES

What does one hope to achieve by effective monitoring? By periodic and almost constant attention to the patient's vital signs one hopes to receive early warning of impending catastrophe. For example, cardiac arrest or cardiovascular collapse may be preceded by changes in the pulse rate and rhythm. Internal hemorrhage may be suspected when the patient has a rising pulse rate, thirst, apprehension, and cool, moist skin, even though the blood pressure remains at near normal levels. Respiratory obstruction, similiarly, may be detected earlier by close observation of the respiratory rate, excursion pattern, color of mucous membranes, and sensorium.

As both ambulance care and equipment are being rapidly upgraded and as emergency rooms provide increasingly sophisticated immediate care, monitoring methods are changing. For example, at the University of Missouri Medical Center the emergency medical service provides ambulances equipped with electrocardiographic equipment, the readings of which can be transmitted via radio telephone to personnel in the emergency room and to the heart station where immediate interpretation and subsequent advice can be rendered. The value of attempting to stabilize the cardiac status prior to transportation of the patient is, of course, well documented. Continuous pulse and blood pressure monitoring can be initiated and continued throughout the patient's removal to the hospital.

In spite of mechanical devices, "eyeball observations" have no substitute, and one needs to continually improve his knowledge of what to look for and his ability to observe.

Basically, as mentioned, monitoring refers to qualitative and quantitative observations, over a period of time, of the physiologic functions in a clinical context. More specifically it refers to the cardiovascular, respiratory, renal, and central nervous systems as well as observation of the electrolytic balance. Single observations of these systems, especially taken out of context, are of limited value in the evaluation of the therapeutic needs of the patient. Multiple observations naturally add a dimension of time and help to predict trends.

Urine output, for example, needs to be monitored via the indwelling catheter. Not only does it provide proof of the adequacy of renal blood flow but, under some conditions, gives support to any decision regarding requirements for the use of intravenous fluids or osmotic diuretics.

Similarly, the monitoring of the patient's central venous pressure is a means of acquiring much-needed information that may mirror blood volume deficiency or excess. Although not always immediately available, its overall inportance has prompted its inclusion in this chapter. A central venous catheter may be placed through a number of routes, each with certain advantages. Presently the subclavian or internal jugular vein approaches are most commonly employed, although any vein approach may be used in an emergency, providing it does in fact tap the central venous pool. In addition to providing readings of the central venous pressure, the catheter may be utilized for obtaining repeated venous pH and gas tensions as well as for fluid infusions. While there are pitfalls in the interpretations of central venous pressures, one generally uses them as a guide to prevent overloading of patients with blood or certain intravenous fluids at a time when adequate estimation of blood loss is difficult. More accurately, central venous pressure is an index of the function of the right ventricle and the ability of the heart to handle returning blood volume at any given time. False readings may reflect a mechanical obstruction of the returning venous blood that results from such factors as a pericardial collection of blood or fluid resulting in cardiac tamponade. Compression of the mediastinal structures can likewise give false elevations. Return flow may be slowed partially or obstructed by high intrathoracic pressures from a pneumothorax or from improperly employed artificial respirators.

Although gas tension determinations are generally considered in the definitive treatment, mention is made here because of their increasing availability in the emergency room. More and more reliance is placed on a monitoring of the gas tensions and blood pH in the severly traumatized patient. These measurements provide sensitive indication of respiratory and metabolic abnormalities. Repeatedly, these indicators have warned of serious problems before significant changes in pulse, blood pressure, electrocardiogram, venous pressure, or skin perfusion indicators. Blood pH and gas tension changes are particularly helpful when serial readings are performed. Abnormalities, if corrected promptly, may prevent serious cardiovascular complications. Cardiac arrest, for example, is rare in the injured patient with a normal pH in the central venous blood.

Oxygen and carbon dioxide tensions are primary indices of ventilation and reflect pulmonary gas exchange. Venous oxygen tension values may serve to reflect the relationship between metabolic requirements for oxygen and oxygen transport by the circulating blood.

Monitoring requirements vary from patient to patient. The acutely ill individual with a sunstroke requires continuous temperature readings. Many acutely injured patients likewise need a careful monitoring of their heat regulatory mechanism.

USE OF ULTRASONIC MONITORING OF ACUTE VASCULAR DEFICIENCIES

Because of our conviction that the Doppler ultrasonic flowmeter will play an increasing role in the evaluation of the critically injured patient, we are including the following material in order to introduce the reader to the potential of ultrasonic monitoring.

The surgeon has long desired a more adequate, readily available, relatively inexpensive means of determining blood flow in the critically injured patient. The routine physical modes of visualization and palpation during examination are gross and may be ineffectual. As an adjunct in the determination of vascular patency and continuity, arteriography is not without associated morbidity nor does it in many cases allow delineation of microcirculation in the digits. Mercury strain gauge plethysmography, though extremely useful in the evaluation of digital flow, requires extraneous equipment (that is, a recorder) in order to evaluate vascular patency. The ultrasonic flowmeter is an instrument that can transcutaneously provide an assessment of vascular injury, atraumatically, in the emergency room. It is a noninvasive device.

The principle involves changes in sound pitch as the distance between the sound and the listener is varied. The Doppler ultrasonic flowmeter consists of an oscillator, a transducer containing two piezoelectric crystals of matched oscillatory characteristics, a detector sensitive to frequencies in the audible range, an amplifier to amplify the output of the detector so that the signal may be presented in audio or video form, and a speaker or oscilloscope for the presentation of the signal. A frequency shift (f_d) or change in pitch is noted when the output of the piezoelectric crystal, being oscillated at its natural frequency, encounters intravascular particulate matter in motion from which it is backscattered. The backscattered ultrasound will have a slightly different frequency than the original because of a gain or loss in energy that is directly proportional to the velocity of the blood flow. Turbulence or laminarity of flow may also be noted with the Doppler as change in direction of flow is noted in a variation of f_d; multiplicity of f_d is indicative of turbulence in a vessel.

The clinical use of the Doppler is analogous to the use of the stethoscope. Continued use allows the development of expertise with the instrument. In a normal vessel two and sometimes three sounds are heard during each cardiac cycle. The first sound is that of ventricular contraction, which causes blood to be ejected from the heart in systole. This is normally a crisp, rapid sound. At the end of systole there is a slight reversal of flow in the vasculature, which is followed by the sound of arterial contraction in diastole causing a surge of forward flow. If the vasculature is in good physical condition, the overshoot of the second sound is followed by another period of reverse flow with a surge of forward flow again caused by arterial contraction resulting from the elasticity of the arterial wall. The sound of continual flow is noted in diastole since only the f_d is heard without discrimination as to the positive or negative sign. If the vessel monitored with the Doppler probe contains a distal occlusion, there is a loss of continuous flow sounds noted in diastole; as the operator approaches the occlusion with the probe a "water-hammer effect" may be noted. When the probe is directly over the occlusion no flow sounds are noted, though some sounds denoting wall motion of the vessel may be heard. "Leaks," such as the sound of blood running from a transected vessel into an interfacial plane and causing a pseudoaneurysm, may be detected. The size of the pseudoaneurysm may be denoted because of its pulsatile nature. The following case reports illustrate a few of the uses that may be made of the Doppler to aid in the diagnosis of vascular injury.

Case 1. A 17-year-old white female was seen in the emergency room by the orthopedic surgeon following an automobile accident. Tentative diagnosis of left femoral fracture was made and the Doppler was utilized to ascertain that the vasculature in the leg was normal. Ankle pressures taken with the Doppler were approximately 50 mm Hg bilaterally, while the arm pressure of the patient was 150 mm Hg. These findings were indicative of aortic coarctation, and on this basis arteriography was rapidly obtained that demonstrated a lesion in the descending aorta, with the tamponade causing coarctation of the vessel. Repair of the lesion was made using cardiopulmonary bypass for patient maintenance. Though surgery was successful, the patient died as a result of extensive lung lacerations caused by the automobile accident, which lowered her blood oxygenation capacity to an ineffectual level.

Case 2. A 23-year-old male suffered a sharp transverse laceration of the right wrist, dividing all the flexor tendons. The median and ulnar nerves and the radial and ulnar arteries were also divided. The right hand, on physical examination, was cool, somewhat pale, and pulseless. Doppler and mercury strain gauge plethysmography studies indicated that an adequate blood supply to the hand was being carried by the interosseous artery. The radial and ulnar arteries were ligated, since it was believed that to repair the vessels, if repair was at all possible, would not have contributed to the final result.

Brachial angiography taken 8 days postoperatively confirmed the findings of the Doppler at operation. Blood flow to the hand was via the posterior interosseous artery. Subsequently the patient had a functional hand. The radial pulse was palpable but Doppler and arteriographic findings demonstrated retrograde flow in the segment. Color of the hand was normal and the patient exhibited no cold intolerance.

Case 3. A 49-year-old painter who had suffered a distal tibial fracture was seen in the emergency room. Following closed reduction, Doppler examination revealed diminished blood flow in the anterior tibial artery. Increased superficial (subcutaneous) venous flow was noted in the area of the fracture, indicating that there was compromise of the deep venous passages. Following this examination a fasciotomy was performed and the vasculature, both arterial and venous, returned to its normal flow state.

Case 4. A 21-year-old university student with an open fracture of the left humerus was admitted to the emergency room about 3 hours following a motorcycle accident. The ipsilateral hand was pale and cold, with no pulses palpable in the radial or ulnar artery. Doppler examination disclosed that collateral vessels were functional in the forearm, but these were small and provided the hand with little or no flow. A "water hammer" was noted in the area of the axillary artery, and flow through the circumflex vessels at the humerus was nonexistent. At operation it was noted that thrombotic occusion of the axillary artery was 1 cm proximal to the circumflex humeral vessels where the distal segment of the humerus had impacted high into the axilla.

chapter 6

Control of pain

John H. Henzel

"Pain is always a sinister gift which diminishes man, and the strict duty of the doctor is to endeavor to supress it, if he can. . . ." Had LeRiche included the trauma victim in his classic statement about the physician's duty toward pain relief, he would have admonished clinicians to suppress pain only when accurately indicated, at a stage when selective administration of a specific agent would not mask or confuse existing symptoms or further depress already obtunded vital functions.

Unfortunately, physicians inexperienced in the initial care of trauma victims still equate extensive injury with pain, despite the fact that experience has shown that most victims of major trauma do not complain of pain during the early period following injury.

VARIABLES AFFECTING PERCEPTION AND EXPRESSION OF PAIN

Individual awareness of and response to pain is tremendously variable and is not necessarily related to the severity of the trauma. Reaction to real pain and the degree to which an individual's mental and physical behavior and performance are affected are influenced by such factors as mental alertness, emotional stability, personal stoicism, and, in the case of the conscious trauma victim, anxiety about the extent and potential sequelae of his injury. In healthy, uninjured persons, such painful experiences as an abscessed tooth or migraine headache may either be ignored or be totally incapacitating, depending upon coexisting psychologic-environmental variables. The abscessed tooth that throbs unbearably while the afflicted individual is at work may be almost ignored throughout an exciting football game.

Variables such as age, fatigue, and intelligence also influence perception and expression of pain. In addition, drugs and diseases affecting mental alertness and performance also modify response to injury and pain, a fact that is occasionally forgotten or overlooked in the tense atmosphere of the emergency room. A number of trauma victims, particularly older persons, are taking drugs that may have been primarily responsible for the accident and that may have then altered the patient's response to injury. Specific problems arise in the trauma victim who is receiving anticoagulants, digitalis preparations, and antihypertensive drugs. In evaluating any injured patient's clinical behavior relative to apparent pain, one should be alert to the possibility that a tranquilizer or antihistamine depressed the level of mental alertness prior to the accident and may be partially or totally responsible for obtunding both the level of consciousness and vital functions following injury. The well-known effects of alcohol are usually apparent. However, since it is often necessary to reexamine trauma victims repeatedly over a number of hours in deciding for or against surgical intervention, it is prudent to submit a specimen of blood for baseline alcohol and barbiturate levels whenever one suspects that either of these agents may be contributing to the overall clinical picture. The effects of drug addiction can mimic pain, and the examining physician must also consider hard drug habituation or withdrawal in the inappropriately hyperactive or "wild" youthful victim. Finally, it is important to remain alert for the rare trauma victim whose abnormal conscious behavior is related to diabetic coma, adrenal insufficiency, or anticoagulant-related intracranial hematoma.

In the acutely injured patient, restlessness, groaning, or requests for relief (clinical behavior suggestive of pain) may be manifestations of something other than pain. The physician who evaluates or treats trauma victims must be familar with those factors that can mimic or mask pain and avoid administration of an analgesic until he knows the exact etiology of the pain.

ACCURATE INTERPRETATION OF CLINICAL BEHAVIOR

As the conscious trauma victim is being examined, an attempt should be made to alleviate anxiety by calmly informing him of the nature of his injury and describing insofar as possible the needed form of therapy. If the patient understands what has occurred and what to anticipate and is able to establish confidence in the examining physician, apparent need for analgesia will either decrease markedly or be eliminated. While conversation may be difficult or impossible in an occasional situation in which seconds may make the difference between saving and losing a patient, in the long run the frequency with which trauma victims are afforded accurate diagnosis and efficient, safe management will be increased if one constantly remembers that *pain is a symptom complex that is occasionally controlled by little more than simple communication with the patient.* If the actual presence and intensity of pain are to be accurately evaluated, it is particularly essential that one pay attention to seemingly insignificant, often minimized, and frequently ignored parameters of patient comfort. Two case histories will illustrate this point.

Case 1. A 21-year-old injured male is lying on his left side and groaning loudly with his legs drawn up. Examination discloses a through-and-through gunshot wound of the right thorax about 2 inches directly lateral to the nipple. While intravenous fluids are being started, the junior surgical resident arrives on the scene and confirms the suspicion of alcohol on the patient's breath. He ascertains from the accompanying police officer that the youth was shot as he left a tavern after 2 hours of beer drinking with his friends. After examining the patient's thorax and abdomen, the surgical resident initiates nasal oxygen and inserts a chest tube and bladder catheter. After 1,050 ml of urine has filled the collection bag and while air from the pneumothorax is bubbling into the closed chest thoracostomy bottle, the injured youth stops moaning, relaxes, and appears surprisingly comfortable.

In this situation, clinical behavior suggestive of pain was, in actuality, the result of hypoxia related to pneumothorax and distended bladder in a semiinebriated patient. Had morphine been administered hypoxia would have been aggravated, the level of consciousness further obtunded, and discovery of the full bladder delayed. As a result of accurate interpretation and precise nontoxic treatment, the patient was able to be discharged after 3 days.

Case 2. In the emergency room on a snowy November night, a disheveled middle-aged male is rolling from side to side and moaning in apparent delirium. Examination discloses shivering and pallor, a 2-cm superficial laceration through the right eyebrow, and a closed fracture-deformity of the right lower extremity. It is ascertained that after the victim was struck by a slow-moving motorcycle while crossing the street against a green light, he had laid on the pavement in near-freezing rain for some 15 minutes while waiting for the ambulance to arrive. While wet clothing is being removed and the fracture immobilized, the patient's wife arrives. After learning that he is conscious, she produces a pair of glasses, concerned that her husband is "nearly blind without them." A half hour later, a calm, perfectly coherent, and surprisingly alert patient bemoans the pitfall of a shirtsleeve sprint across a busy street against a red light for a cup of coffee on a very cold day.

In this instance, environmental exposure, visual disadvantage, and fracture pain intensified by uncontrollable shivering combined to produce a clinical picture suggestive of severe pain. After wet clothing had been removed, warm covers supplied, and the patient's glasses made available, the relatively minor extent of injury became apparent. Appropriate x-rays ruled out additional trauma other than the closed tibial fracture, and the extent of total treatment amounted to suture of the supraorbital laceration, a long leg cast, and 24 hours of in-hospital observation.

While restlessness, moaning, and excess motor activity may be erroneously interpreted as severe pain by the novice treating his first accident victim, such clinical behavior raises the *possibility of cerebral trauma or developing hypoxia.* While the novice requests a syringe of morphine, his experienced colleague is firmly assuring the patient while simultaneously examining him for evidence of cerebral damage, occult hemorrhage, or pneumothorax, for example.

NARCOTIC OBTUNDATION OF SUBCLINICAL PATHOPHYSIOLOGY

Three principal reasons underlie the rationale for avoiding unnecessary analgesia in the acutely injured patient:

1. Drug idiosyncrasy may superimpose unnecessary and confusing symptoms on an already complex clinical situation. Undesirable drug side effects such as retching, excitement, fever, or allergic reaction will cloud those clinical parameters on which the physician must depend for early accurate diagnosis and precise therapy.
2. Not only may the pain threshold be increased but the patient's ability to express concern about new or more intense symptoms may be blunted.
3. Perhaps most importantly, nonapparent and unsuspected subclinical depression of vital functions may unknowingly be further depressed at a time when compensatory factors are already straining maximally to maintain homeostasis.

It is in the third area that we have greatest concern, and only in recent years has clinical use of diagnostic methods previously confined to the experimental laboratory allowed us to detect and monitor subclinical, premorbid derangements in cardio-vascular-respiratory physiology.

During World War II, physicians noticed that certain clinical behavior suggestive of pain actually resulted from altering so-called vital functions. Restlessness, excitement, and hyperactivity were recognized as manifestations of acute head injury, and the eponym "traumatic wet lung" was affixed to characteristic x-ray changes that accompanied the progressive asphyxia that resulted from certain types of thoracic trauma. However, accurate understanding of the exact changes, their prognostic significance, and the methods for reversing these changes had to await understanding and delineation of shock at the microcirculatory level and of respiratory gas mechanics (relative to acid-base equilibrium) at the cellular and subcellular level. During the past 5 years, however, trauma units have begun to use central venous pressure monitoring, sequential arterial blood gas analyses, pyuvate-lactate determinations, radioisotope-computer assessment of intra- and extravascular fluid dynamics, cardiac output determination, pulmonary-peripheral resistance, and arteriovenous shunting during resuscitation and treatment of the severely injured patient. Ten years ago, the effect of 10 mg of intravenous morphine was barely evident to the experienced clinician, principally because the earliest changes of respiratory depression or oligemic acidosis are subclinical. Today sophisticated methodology readily documents the hypoxemia, hypercapnia, acidosis, and altered microcirculatory dynamics that occur in the face of narcotic overdosage.

Contraindicated or excessive narcotic administration does nullify or derange compensatory life-preserving processes. Knowing how narcotic administration can jeopardize already tenuous physiologic homeostasis in the trauma victim, physicians who treat these patients should be alert to three specific situations in which erroneous interpretation of clinical behavior may precipitate a vicious circle of diagnostic-therapeutic misadventure.

The first relates to trauma-precipitated changes in respiratory mechanics. Significant reduction in vital capacity is associated with such injuries as fractured ribs, pneumothorax, and peritoneal contamination by blood, bile, urine, or gastrointestinal content. Somewhat similarly, pulmonary contusion, massive fat embolization, and fluid overload atelectasis also result in varying combinations of hypoxia, hypercapnia, and acidosis. In each of these situations, irritability and restlessness related to and resulting from hypoxemia may erroneously be interpreted as pain. Administration of an analgesic further diminishes respiratory effort and hence compounds the overall situation.

A second, not uncommon pitfall is the interpretation of hyperventilation in a hypotensive, poorly responsive trauma victim as pain, when the increased respiratory rate is actually a necessary physiologic compensation for a developing metabolic acidosis. Administration of a narcotic may diminish or abolish this necessary compensation and thereby accentuate the acidosis.

The third pitfall constitutes an example of a situation in which partial knowledge precipitates well-meaning, partially correct, but dangerous therapy. When one interprets tachypnea and restlessness as being partially related to hypoxia in extensive thoracic cage trauma, both oxygen and a narcotic are administered. Hypoxia may be corrected, but coexisting hypercapnia is compounded as the respiratory rate is therapeutically diminished.

ADMINISTRATION OF INDICATED ANALGESIA

The actual indications for administration of an analgesic to victims of major trauma are rare and specific. Experienced trauma surgeons administer narcotics only when real and severe pain is present (usually after its cause has been determined), when there must be a delay before the completely evaluated and stable trauma victim can receive definitive treatment, and when a conscious trauma victim's clinical response to painful stimuli precludes definitive or accurate evaluation. There are no occasions when analgesia should be adminsitered to a transportable trauma victim at the scene of an accident and few if any instances in which the patient should receive a narcotic in the emergency ward prior to being evaluated by the physician who will be responsible for his care.

Since there is neither time nor place for indecision in managing the acutely injured person and since trauma respects neither age nor degree of health, it is best to adopt one drug for use in trauma, become familiar with its dosage and specific pharmacologic properties, and learn how to use it. Morphine sulfate has stood the test of time, and for one reason or another, most persons learn and retain the dosage and side effects of this narcotic. For these reasons and because of personal preference, discussion will be limited to this drug.

Morphine relieves pain either by elevating the perception threshold of such stimuli or by altering the patient's response to painful stimuli. In the latter action, this drug remains superior to other narcotics and as a result is uniquely applicable to the trauma victim, in whom profound responses (more profound than apparent stimuli warrant) may mask morbid injury or exaggerate minimal trauma. It is important that the route of administration be standardized and that the dosage be individualized. Undesirable side effects attributed to a specific drug are all too frequently caused by lack of attention to the individual need of the patient.

ROUTE OF ADMINISTRATION

Considering that all agents administered by the intramuscular or subcutaneous route require a period of time for absorption and that ideally the physician should be able to observe the effects of the analgesia, the intravenous route is the preferred method of administration. Direct injection into the bloodstream avoids the risks associated with inconstant absorption and minimizes considerations associated with using this route in the trauma victim. First, the drug should be given in markedly reduced dosages; second, the physician who administers the narcotic should remain in attendance to observe the immediate effects.

The frequent occurrence of cardiovascular shock is another reason for administering morphine intravenously to a trauma victim. Whether hypotension is present, impending, or a possible eventuality, the intravenous route assures controlled regulation of observable and effective therapy. Morphine should never be given via the subcutaneous or intramuscular route to patients in shock. During World War II it was observed that a number of the soldiers who received morphine on the battlefield experienced narcotic overload (respiratory depression in particular) once they reached the aid station and received definitive care. Morphine sequestered in the periphery while the patient was in shock would suddenly be absorbed into the circulation all at once as administered blood or colloid returned blood pressure toward normal. Clinically, ineffectiveness secondary to lack of absorption (because of peripheral vascular collapse) may precipitate a second or third "shot for relief of pain." Toxic overdosage then results when the peripheral circulation suddenly becomes effective and several doses are absorbed at once. This potential danger, particularly in a cold environment, exists in any acutely injured patient and should constantly be borne in mind.

INDIVIDUALIZED DOSAGE

The ultimate determination of dosage depends upon the patient's metabolic activity, which varies with age. Basal levels of metabolism are increased by pain and anxiety and decreased by debilitating diseases. Negroes and Orientals have lower basal metabolic levels, and these persons tolerate depressant drugs less well, thereby requiring smaller doses than other patients.

Although therapeutic levels of morphine affect cardiovascular dynamics minimally, excessive amounts will depress both respiration and vascular responses to oligemia. A safe dosage of morphine for the average adult is 0.05 to 0.1 mg per kilogram of body weight, diluted to a 10- to 20-ml volume. Injection through a 25-gauge needle will slow administration and thereby overcome a natural tendency for rapid injection. One should allow a minimum of 2 to 3 minutes for administering the total calculated amount and should then wait 10 to 15 minutes before giving additional drug. Experience with slow intravenous administration of diluted morphine sulfate, repeated if necessary, will produce desired analgesia with minimal risk of diagnostic error, therapeutic complications, or iatrogenic catastrophe. Drugs to relieve pain and restlessness are never given when one is evaluating possible acute head injury. In those few instances in which convulsions or hyperactivity of neurologic injury are too intense to allow accurate evaluation of suspected coexisting injury, 1 ml of paraldehyde may be diluted to a 10 ml total volume and administered intravenously.

chapter 7

Metabolic response to trauma

Walter Ford Keitzer
Walter Kirt Nichols

Acute trauma calls into play a number of homeostatic mechanisms perfected from eons of biologic evolution. Our role in caring for the acutely injured patient is to aid and support these vital mechanisms and not to block, overload, or reverse them.

One should remember that trauma has been a part of all life and that many trauma victims survived long before the invention of the hollow needle. We do not mean to advocate therapeutic nihilism in regard to trauma; instead, we suggest that we can learn much by understanding how the organism can survive without support and by knowing the limits of its inherent mechanisms.

The very mechanism important to survival in uncomplicated trauma can turn upon the organism and become the principal mediator of one of the organ system failures. For example, the intense sympathetic-mediated vasoconstriction that aids in hemostasis, maintains cardiac output, and redistributes the cardiac output to vital cardiac and cerebral circulation is also the mechanism that can set the stage in the microcirculation for the development of irreversible shock or acute renal failure.

We need to recognize the fact that overzealous or inappropriate therapeutic efforts can compound the problem and convert a vital defense mechanism to one lethal to the patient. As in the example cited previously, it took many years to recognize the antisurvival effect of norepinephrine as a therapeutic agent for shock.

Our purpose in this chapter will be to outline the principal alterations in the metabolic balance associated with any trauma, to define the associated mechanism, and to discuss the therapeutic implications.

VARIOUS IMBALANCES

Trauma initiates several alterations of the metabolic balance. Principally these involve the balance of water, of protein (the chief constituent of protoplasm), of sodium (the chief cation of the extracellular fluid), and of potassium (the chief cation of the intracellular fluid). The degree of alteration of these constituents can be a measure of the magnitude of the trauma. These elements represent the "visible" part of complex metabolic mechanisms for establishing homeostasis and survival of the injured organism. The purpose of these alterations is not only to promote survival but also to reorient the body's metabolic priorities for initiation of wound healing.

ALTERATIONS IN WATER AND ELECTROLYTE BALANCE

One of the most fundamental responses of the injured organism is the tendency to maintain and conserve energy in the circulatory system, the principal function of which is to deliver to the tissue sufficient hydraulic energy to maintain function: kinetic energy of flow to transport nutrients, wastes, and humoral agents to and from tissues, and potential energy to direct the fluids of the blood through the nutrient and nonnutrient circuits of the microcirculation. In order for the heart to produce sufficient hydraulic energy, it must have sufficient mass to act upon, which means the blood volume must be maintained. This tendency to maintain volume is one of the strongest responses of the injured organism.

MAINTAINING BLOOD VOLUME

The blood volume is a part of the extracellular fluid (ECF) space, and changes in the ECF tend to parallel changes in the blood volume. Changes in the ECF are intimately related to the metabolic balance of sodium, potassium, and body water. Under ordinary conditions the volume of the ECF is largely a function of the total amount of sodium present. External losses, and thus the balance of sodium and water, are controlled primarily by the kidney. Trauma initiates two principal mechanisms that cause almost complete reabsorption of sodium and maximum reabsorption of water in the kidney and thus maintain the ECF volume. These mechanisms are the antidiuretic hormone (ADH) effect and the aldosterone effect. (We prefer using the term *effect,* since volume regulation is not entirely the result of diurectic hormone nor is sodium conservation a result of aldosterone alone. Although these hormones are the principal mediators of these mechanisms, both are more complex than can be explained by the physiologic action of each hormone alone.)

In addition to renal conservation of water and sodium by the ADH and aldosterone effects, trauma initiates a general redistribution of body water from intracellular fluid (ICF) to the compartments of the ECF in response to ECF losses. Trauma can cause a loss of blood volume not only through hemorrhage but also by sequestration of extracellular fluid into the so-called third space. Sequestered ECF, although not fluid lost from the body, is fluid that is no longer functional in the sense of supporting or replacing blood volume. For all practical purposes the ionic content of sequestered fluid is the same as that of the ECF. Examples of sequestered fluid include vast accumulation of fluid in the gastrointestinal tract secondary to ileus associated with trauma, fluids in edematous regions of traumatized tissue, or transudates associated with pleural or peritoneal irritation. In disease states other then trauma, fluid from the ECF can also be lost from the body during vomiting, diarrhea, or fistulization.*

The contraction of the ECF, resulting either from sequestration or fistulization, is rapidly corrected by redistribution of ICF to ECF. At the same time the intravascular compartment of the ECF is rapidly replaced by movement of interstitial fluid across the capillary membranes to reestablish the blood volume. Water entering the ECF from the ICF is termed endogenous water. This water is sodium free but rich in potassium and amino acids. Endogenous water is derived not only from intracellular water but also from catabolism of fat, carbohydrate, and protein. The largest source is fat; approximately

---

*Any abnormal loss of isotonic fluids from the gastrointestinal tract through intubation or fistulas.

1,050 ml per kilogram of fat is utilized as opposed to about 575 ml from each kilogram of protein. In general, approximately 750 ml of endogenous water is obtained from each kilogram of lean body mass metabolized. The rest of the water is obtained from reduction of cell volume without loss of cell integrity.

Following injury a large amount of albumin is liberated by the liver into the intravascular compartment. This raises or maintains the oncotic pressure of the intravascular fluid (with an associated decrease in hydrostatic pressure at the capillary level), and there is a positive movement of water from the interstitial space to the intravascular space of the ECF. Thus the primacy of the blood volume is maintained.

Dilution of blood volume

The redistribution of body water is characterized by dilution. The dilution of the greatest magnitude is in the blood volume by reduction of erythrocyte concentration. Since endogenous water is sodium free, there is a strong tendency to dilute the ECF sodium concentration. Thus in the trauma patient, one characteristically sees a drop in hematocrit and serum sodium concentration. The change in hematocrit is always greater than the decrease in serum sodium. On the average the hematocrit will change 3% for each unit of blood lost from the body. This equilibration begins immediately after trauma and is fairly well established in a matter of a few hours. On the other hand, the maximum decrease in serum sodium is not seen for several days. The addition of exogenous blood and sodium will influence the final concentrations; however, even with adequate replacement of blood by transfusion and isotonic replacement of sodium one should still anticipate some degree of dilution. Thus after an injury or operation one can expect a continued drop in hematocrit, which does not necessarily mean continued blood loss.

Independent of hemodynamic factors controlling the filtration rate, there will be a reduction in water and sodium excretion from the ADH and aldosterone effects despite adequate exogenous water and sodium loading. In fact, with excessive loads of water and sodium, dilution of the red cell mass and extracellular sodium can be greater than that which is usually seen or that which would be anticipated. On the other hand, severely deficient isotonic replacement (by decreasing renal blood flow) will be associated with a further reduction of the excretion of the water and sodium. This combination of hemodynamic and hormonal mechanisms in the kidney, even in the face of such restriction, may still accomplish complete protection of the ECF volume, and one may still expect to see the tendency toward dilution.

Changes in electrolytes

Following trauma, the various volume shifts of body water are accompanied by changes in the electrolyte concentrations in the ICF and ECF. One might expect osmotic gradients to develop; however, the rapid fluid shifts will minimize the osmotic gradients. The tonicity of the ICF is maintained by movement of potassium ions from the cell into the ECF where they are rapidly excreted by the kidney. During the initial period following trauma, 60 to 80 mEq of potassium will be released into the ECF by endogenous water transfer. Cell destruction in traumatized tissue and lysis of red cells in accumulated blood is another rich source of potassium to the ECF. One should remember that normal potassium concentration is 4 mEq/liter in the ECF, and the total potassium content of the ECF will normally be 60 to 68 mEq. Thus it is easy to see how the serum potassium concentration can rise rapidly when renal excretion of potassium is impaired. The renal reduction of free water results in a urine osmolality of about 750 mOsm/kg and the reduction of sodium excretion in the urine results in a urine concentration of less than 10 mEq/liter. Thus the osmolality of extracellular fluid is maintained by conservation of sodium. If the glomerular filtration rate is lowered by severe reduction of circulating blood volume, excretion of urea will be impaired and the resulting azotemia can increase the osmolality to a degree greater than one would expect from the serum sodium concentration. As a general rule the ADH effect following trauma tends to be stronger than the aldosterone effect, thus the body tends to maintain volume at the expense of tonicity. Nevertheless, the osmolality through all compartments will be equal. Thus if one sees extracellular hypotonicity, one can be sure there is an accompanying intracellular hypotonicity.

Diuretic phase

Beginning 1 to 5 days following trauma, the positive water and sodium balance reverses. This reversal is characterized by a diuresis of dilute urine containing increasing amounts of sodium. The negative potassium balance that characterizes the immediate posttraumatic period is rapidly reversed during the diuretic phase. If the patient was potassium depleted prior to injury by medication or other disease processes, serious problems with hypokalemia can occur late in the diuretic phase or after it. The time of onset of the diuretic phase is, in part, a function of the magnitude of the trauma. In general the onset is not delayed by sepsis or starvation, but a continued blood-volume deficit can delay the onset. The volume of the diuresis depends upon the magnitude of the expansion of the ECF resulting from internal fluid shifts and upon the magnitude of the water and salt loading given in the posttraumatic period. Although some of the fluid from the ECF will replace the transferred ICF, much of the expansion of the ECF is caused by endogenous water resulting from proteolysis. Replacement of this water in the ICF occurs with the onset of anabolism late in the posttraumatic period when there is an established positive nitrogen balance. One should avoid exogenous fluid loading during the posttraumatic period because of the great risk of overloading ECF compartments of the lung and brain.

During the diuretic phase not only is the volume expansion of the extracellular compartment returned to normal but also the sequestered fluid from the ECF now becomes functional. If renal blood flow and glomerular filtration rate are impaired because of heart failure or previous renal disease, there is a high risk of translocation of the returning sequestered fluid to the ECF in the lungs and brain. Usually this fluid becomes evident as subcutaneous edema, most evident under the skin of the back in the recumbent patient. If significant overloading of the ECF occurred in the posttraumatic period in order to replace the sequestered fluid into the "third space," the reabsorption of the sequestered fluid into the functional ECF can pose serious problems. This is especially true if one gives additional exogenous fluids. As a result of increased use of extracellular volume replacement in the posttraumatic period, the incidence of renal failure secondary to inadequate renal perfusion from a contracted ECF volume has significantly decreased in recent years. Simultaneously, there appears to be an associated increase in incidence of pulmonary problems, the so-called posttraumatic pulmonary insufficiency syndrome. The latter problem seems to occur most frequently during the period in which one would expect the diuretic phase. .

ALTERATIONS IN PROTEIN, CARBOHYDRATE, AND FAT

In injuries that cause alterations in the balance of water, sodium, and potassium, the metabolic response is directed toward maintaining the volume of the extracellular fluid space. Of no less importance than the volume homeostatic mechanisms is the metabolic alteration of protein, carbohydrate, and fat that follows trauma. This catabolism is the principal source of energy to maintain metabolism following injury. In most situations involving acute trauma, the added complication of chronic nutritional depletion does not need to be considered, and discussion will follow alterations caused by trauma in healthy individuals.

Supplying caloric needs

Acute starvation is one of the initiating factors of the metabolic alterations following injury. Indeed, many of the initial metabolic changes in water, electrolytes, and metabolic nutritional stores can be detected following a 24-hour fast in an uninjured person. The average person will burn about 2,000 calories per day, and this will be balanced with a nutrient intake equivalent to 2,000 calories. Most trauma of any significance will be associated with a total cessation of oral caloric intake. After trauma the caloric need will increase the basal metabolic requirements; however, the total energy requirements may remain unchanged since muscular activity is reduced to a minimum. The increase in basal metabolic requirement is usually only a moderate 10% to 15% in uncomplicated trauma but may rise to levels as high as 200% following extensive full-thickness burns.

Certain complications of trauma can markedly alter the metabolic caloric requirement. Sepsis and associated fever are obvious causes of increased caloric expenditure. Pulmonary problems cause increased caloric expenditures not only through increased muscular activity associated with labored respirations but also through metabolic effects of anoxia and associated temperature elevations. Following extensive burns there is a marked increase in evaporative water loss from the body. Most of the energy utilized as latent heat of vaporization is derived from the metabolic heat of the body. This is the probable reason for greatly elevated energy expenditures in extensive burns.

Following trauma, the initial energy requirements are obtained by oxidation of body glycogen stores. In the normal adult these stores are probably not greater than 200 gm, thus limiting this source of energy to a total of 800 calories. After glycogen stores are rapidly expended, further energy sources are in fat and protein, although there is little utilization of protein as compared to fat.

Proteolysis

Obligatory proteolysis for caloric needs is one of the characteristic metabolic responses to injury. As protein is broken down, between 10 and 20 gm of nitrogen per day is excreted in the urine following significant trauma. Each gram of nitrogen in the urine represents a utilization of 30 gm of muscle mass. Although there is no loss of muscle cell integrity, this negative nitrogen balance represents a loss of 300 to 600 gm of muscle weight per day, and only 250 calories are provided during excretion of 10 gm of nitrogen per day. Therefore, protein is not a good source of body energy.

Although negative nitrogen balance is a somewhat unavoidable response to injury, any measure that can be taken to minimize nitrogen loss is of considerable value in supporting homeostatic defense mechanisms. Intravenous infusion of 100 gm of glucose per day will decrease the negative nitrogen balance approximately 50%. Unfortunately, infusion of an equal amount of additional glucose will not show an equal reduction in negative nitrogen balance. In fact the glucose infusion is more effective in reducing the negative nitrogen balance of starvation than that seen following trauma, where much of the excreted nitrogen comes from the breakdown of protein content of translocated fluids and blood retained in body cavities and tissues. The breakdown of this protein is a necessary part of wound healing, and it will not be altered by exogenous or endogenous sources of calories.

Fat catabolism

The principal source of energy to the body after injury lies in the breakdown of fat. Despite extensive catabolism of protein for energy sources, much of the weight loss following injury can be attributed to loss of body fat. One gram of fat provides 9 calories of energy. During starvation, 75 to 150 gm of fat are burned per day; after injury three or four times this amount of fat may be utilized for energy requirements, which can account for production of 2,000 to 4,500 calories per day. For each kilogram of fat utilized the body gains 1,050 ml of endogenous water. As stated before, endogenous water obtained from the catabolism of fat is an important source of water for expansion of the ECF. Because of the ADH effect and resultant water retention, the net weight loss by the body is minimized.

Exogenous caloric supply

As one can see from the previous material, endogenous energy sources in order of importance are fat, protein, and carbohydrate. In managing the acutely injured patient one might like to administer foodstuffs in the same order of importance and efficiency as utilized by the body from its endogenous sources; but, for all practicable purposes, the availability of exogenous energy sources is reversed. Glucose remains the most available and important material for intravenous support. Other carbohydrates such as fructose and sorbitol can be used. Blood, plasma, and serum albumin are the only practical forms of protein for intravenous and serum albumin are the only practical forms of protein for intravenous use. The use of protein hydrolysates has limited value in the management of acutely injured patients. Emulsified fats have been used in the past but they carry a risk to the patient, and if they are used, they can be used only in limited amounts. For this reason fat sources for intravenous use have no practical value in the acute situation.

Hormonal relationships

The mechanism for mobilizing the body's sources of energy appears to be related principally to the hormones of the adrenal gland: both the adrenocortical hormones and the catecholamines of the adrenal medulla. Epinephrine and norepinephrine from the adrenal medulla (along with other sources of catecholamines) appear to be involved in the mechanism for the rapid glycogenolysis that follows trauma. There is evidence that beta function of the sympathetic system is important for the mobilization of fat. The initial part of the negative nitrogen balance following injury can be imitated by injection of cortisone or other glucocorticoids in normal persons. Importance of adrenocortical hormones in the vital defense mechanisms following trauma is clearly evidenced by the response of the adrenalectomized organism to stress without hormone substitution. The adrenalectomized animal cannot respond with volume protection mechanisms or with energy mobilization mechanisms. Since the mobilization of adrenocortical hormones comes from the stimulus of ACTH, hypophysectomized animals respond in an identical manner to stress.

FACTORS INITIATING THE METABOLIC RESPONSE TO INJURY

Initiating factors in the metabolic response to trauma fall into two groups: endogenous and exogenous.

The most important and principal endogenous factor in inducing the neurohumoral mechanism that controls metabolic response is volume reduction. As noted before, volume reduction can occur in its most obvious form during hemorrhage or in the more subtle sequestration of extracellular fluid. No matter what the mechanism for reducing the functional volume of the ECF, receptors (both peripheral and within the central nervous system) act through the neurohypophysis to trigger both the ADH and aldosterone effects.

Exogenous factors are pain, sepsis, and pharmacologic agents. Pain, as well as emotional stimuli, can act through the neurohypophysis to initiate the metabolic responses described previously. Pain is the universal accompaniment of trauma, and it is one of the important factors in activating the homeostatic mechanisms.

Wound infection and sepsis are included here as an exogenous factor for initiating metabolic response. More importantly, these are probably a principal factor in the continuing homeostatic defense mechanisms as a complication of trauma. Infection acts not only through pain from the tissues involved but also through toxins elaborated from organisms causing the infection or sepsis. In general infection has to be controlled before catabolism associated with the metabolic alterations can be reversed.

Drugs can be an important contributing factor not only to the induction of the metabolic response but to the magnitude and duration of the response. Ether and cyclopropane are potent stimulators of the catecholamine sources in the body. A number of vasodepressors such as reserpine and chlorpromazine can induce volume reduction mechanisms by blocking the catecholamines and by direct vasodilation, causing hypotension. A number of diuretics are well known for depleting the body of sodium or potassium or both, thus limiting the normal volume regulatory mechanisms. Certain central nervous system drugs can inhibit the normal response to the neurohypophysis in controlling volume.

chapter 8

Rescue and extrication

Franklin L. Mitchell

EXTRICATION FROM AN AUTOMOBILE

Automobile crashes resulting in serious injury do not always allow easy access to the injured person. Basic rescue and extrication equipment must be available in every ambulance, and the emergency medical technician must be well trained in the use of the equipment. The institution of lifesaving procedures is too critical to await the arrival of special rescue teams or equipment.

Minimal Recommended Ambulance Extrication Equipment*
1. Wrench, 12 inches, open end
2. Screwdriver, 12 inches, regular blade
3. Screwdriver, 12 inches, Phillips type
4. Hacksaw, twelve-wire carbide blades
5. Pliers, 10 inches, visegrip
6. Hammer, 5 pounds, 15-inch handle
7. Fire-ax butt, 15-inch handle
8. Wrecking bar, 24 inches
9. Crowbar, 51 inches
10. Bolt cutter, 1 ¼-inch jaw
11. Portable power jack and spreader tool
12. Shovel, 49 inches, with pointed blade
13. Double action tin snips, 8 inches
14. Manila ropes two, 50 feet long, ¾-inch diameter
15. Rated chain with grab hook and running hook, 15 feet long
16. Fire extinguishers
17. Optional equipment:
    a. Power winch, front-mounted
    b. Power saw

In extrication maneuvers always bear in mind the following: *save the life, prevent further injury,* and *do not move the patient until he is stabilized.* Rescue and extrication procedures follow a logical sequence of events.

Achieve access to the patient. The emergency medical technician will need to enter the wrecked vehicle in order to maintain an airway or stop bleeding before extrication begins. If easy access is not apparent, entry through the rear window is frequently possible, otherwise forcing of doors or roof removal becomes necessary. *Never return a vehicle to*

---

*List prepared by the American College of Surgeons.

the upright position to gain access. Additional injury to the victim will undoubtedly result.

Initiate emergency medical care. Begin medical treatment as soon as access is achieved. Priorities of care are mentioned earlier in this section. Stay with the victim while others proceed with extrication maneuvers. If extrication is prolonged, intravenous fluids may be initiated at this time.

Disengage automobile from patient. Peel the automobile from around the victim gently. With the listed equipment, steering wheels can be cut away, brake pedals divided, dashboards elevated, seats forced backward, doors popped open, and sheet metal skinned off. Never use the power saw unless firefighting equipment is present.

Stabilize the patient. Prevent additional injury. Before removing the patient from the vehicle, splint fractures, apply a short backboard, and dress wounds. Any *unconscious* patient is assumed to have a spine injury until proved otherwise.

Remove patient from vehicle. Make the portal of exit large enough to allow removal of the victim under your complete control. Apply long splints immediately after extrication if not previously possible. Do not remove the patient from the backboard.

GENERAL RESCUE AND EXTRICATION

Entrapments of a simple nature are handled in the same manner as automobile entrapments. As entrapments become higher above the ground, deeper below the ground, or under heavier material, specialists in rescue technique are essential. Usually fire departments are prepared for heavier rescue needs. Ambulance services, emergency rooms, and central dispatches should keep a ready list of who is capable of the various types of rescue work in their area.

Dr. J. D. Farrington has described some extrication techniques relating exclusively to automobile accidents. Briefly stated the important principles are as follows:
1. Elimination of possible hazards to rescue personnel and on-lookers, such as live wires and gasoline spills
2. Penetration of the vehicle by rescue personnel to attend to life-threatening conditions such as airway obstruction and hemorrhage and to reassure the victim
3. Application of splints or a spine board if necessary
4. Removal of any part of the vehicle pinning the victim and preventing safe extrication
5. Finally, removal of the victim properly splinted and bandaged for safe transport to a medical facility

These principles apply whether the victim is trapped in an automobile wreck, buried in a cave-in, or trapped in a collapsed building. Many jurisdictions have trained rescue personnel available, usually in the fire service. Where such service is not available, ambulance attendants must have some rescue capabilities and must carry certain minimum equipment for extrication. All too frequently in rural and suburban localities the victims must await the arrival of the tow truck before being released from the wrecked vehicle; such a delay may well prove fatal. Adequate training in this phase of emergency care is very important since overturned vehicles are still being righted with victims in them or victims are being improperly removed from a cave-in or collapsed building. Such improper handling is very likely to aggravate already serious injuries unnecessarily and can be prevented with proper training and supervision by the medical profession.

chapter 9

Continuance of immediate care during transportation

Franklin L. Mitchell

Medical care begins at the site of an accident or sudden illness. The emergency medical care that the patient receives before he arrives in the emergency room may irreversibly influence his morbidity or mortality. Just as a physician has an obligation to monitor and improve the quality of the medical care given in his hospital, it seems no less important that he be knowledgeable of the ambulance and personnel who transport his critically ill or injured patient. Ambulance service must be considered an integral part of the total medical care of the patient. Studies of emergency care reveal that 20% of persons killed in automobile crashes could have been saved if adequately trained ambulance service had been available. Recent work with trained mobile coronary care units has shown a significant reduction in deaths from myocardial infarctions. Increasing emphasis is being given to the prehospital medical care of the patients with excellent results.

The ambulance and its personnel should be thought of as an extension of the emergency room. The personnel need to be at least as well trained as the personnel who work in the emergency room. The equipment should complement the skills of the ambulance personnel. Medical students and physicians have an obligation to understand and improve the quality of their ambulance services.

GENERAL CONSIDERATIONS

Ambulance service guidelines include the following:
1. Two *trained* technicians on every ambulance call
2. Equipment to complement ability of technicians
3. Patient compartment space sufficient for resuscitation
4. Maximum of *two critically ill patients* in the ambulance
5. Two-way voice radio communication with hospital emergency room
6. Central dispatch for the area
7. No exceeding of posted speed limits
8. Written record of patient condition and treatment
9. No patient moved before emergency medical care given

The general priorities of emergency room medical care are followed in prehospital emergency treatment.
1. Save the life

2. Prevent additional injury

3. Transport the patient

Basic emergency medical care requires that any life-threatening condition be corrected at the site and controlled during transportation. First consideration must be always given to those conditions threatening the patient's life (for example, airway obstruction, hemorrhage, shock).

Second priority is given to those conditions that may increase morbidity during movement or transportation. Injuries or illnesses that may be compounded by movement must be stabilized before transportation is begun (for example, spine injuries, fracture, patient position). Only the removal of the patient from a hostile environment, such as a burning car, takes precedence over these procedures.

AMBULANCE PERSONNEL

Ambulance personnel work independent of physician supervision most of the time. They make immediate decisions that may affect the ultimate outcome for the patient. They must be considered members of the medical team if effective medical care is to be achieved. An exchange of ideas must occur between emergency room physicians, medical students, nurses, and ambulance personnel if continued excellence is to be achieved.

National emphasis is being given to the paramedical profession of emergency medical technicians. A National Registry of Emergency Medical Technicians was established in 1971. The following is the topic outline of a suggested 81-hour basic training program for emergency medical technicians. This program was developed by the Department of Transportation, National Highway Traffic Safety Administration, American Academy of Orthopedic Surgeons, American College of Surgeons, International Rescue and First Aid Association, and the National Research Council.

Curriculum	Hours
Responsibilities and equipment of emergency medical technicians	3
Airway obstruction and pulmonary arrest	3
Mechanical aids to breathing and pulmonary resuscitation	3
Cardiac arrest	3
Bleeding, shock—practice airway and cardiac resuscitation	3
Practice and test of above	3
Wounds and dressings	3
Fractures—upper extremity	3
Fractures—lower extremity	3
Injuries—head, face, neck, spine	3
Injuries—eye, chest, abdomen, pelvis	3
Practice and test of above	5
Medical emergencies—poisons, bites, heart attack, stroke, asthma	3
Medical emergencies—acute abdomen, infectious diseases, emotionally disturbed, alcoholic, epileptic, unconscious patient	3
Childbirth	3
Lifting and moving patients	3
Practice and test of above	3
Environmental emergencies—burns, heat, drowning, gas poisoning	3
Extrication from automobiles	3
Defensive driving—records—communications	3
Ambulance call procedures	3

	Hours
Situational review	3
Final testing—practical and written	3
In-hospital experience—operating room, emergency room, delivery room, intensive care unit	10

This is the minimum background training ambulance personnel should have. Do your ambulance personnel have this background?

EQUIPMENT

The American College of Surgeons has established a guideline list of essential equipment for ambulances. This is a basic and minimum list.

1. Portable suction apparatus
2. Hand operated bag-mask ventilation unit
3. Oropharyngeal airways
4. Mouth-to-mouth artificial ventilation airways
5. Portable oxygen equipment with transparent masks
6. Mouth gags
7. Intravenous fluids with administration kits
8. Universal dressings—10 X 36 inches
9. Sterile gauze pads—4 X 4 inches
10. Soft roller, self-adhering bandages—6 inches X 5 yards
11. Roll of aluminum foil—18 X 25 inches, sterile
12. Plain adhesive tape—3 inches
13. Two sterile burn sheets
14. Hinged half-ring lower extremity traction splint
15. Padded boards—4½ feet X 3 inches
16. Padded boards—15 X 3 inches
17. Inflatable plastic splints
18. Short and long spine boards
19. Triangular bandages
20. Large size safety pins
21. Shears for bandages
22. Sterile obstetric kit
23. Poison kit—syrup of ipecac and activated charcoal
24. Blood pressure manometer, cuff, and stethoscope

Trained emergency medical technicians may well use additional equipment, especially if they are hospital based or linked by radio to the emergency room. This equipment would include:

1. Drug injection kit
2. Electrocardiograph—defibrillator
3. Cricothyrotome set
4. Pleural decompression set

Ambulances should carry a kit for physician use, which would include the following:

1. Tracheal intubation set
2. Venous cutdown set
3. Minor surgery kit

4. Tracheostomy set

5. Urinary catheters

THE AMBULANCE

The ambulance should be envisioned as a four-wheel emergency room that could substitute for a treatment room in the emergency department. This room must have adequate space for the patient, emergency medical technician, emergency equipment, supply storage, and working area. There must be sufficient head room to effectively give cardiac resuscitation and administer intravenous fluids by gravity flow. (An unforgettable sight is the arrival of a hearse-type ambulance with the intravenous fluids being held out the window by the attendant.) The minimal workable internal dimensions of the patient compartment are:

1. Minimum height—54 inches

2. Minimum width—72 inches

3. Minimum length—110 inches

Most modern ambulances are of the van type design or camper body–truck chassis configuration. Both meet these criteria for space.

Adequate power is needed to operate the medical equipment. Power for speed is unnecessary. Very rarely will exceeding the speed limit favorably influence the patient's outcome. Much more commonly, the ambulance becomes involved in another accident, with additional injury or death resulting. Adequately trained technicians will have stabilized their patient and do not require excessive speed. A speeding ambulance indicates a sick patient with an untrained attendant.

COMMUNICATIONS

Too often an ambulance carrying a medical emergency victim arrives unannounced at the hospital. The staff is performing routine duties and the physicians are not immediately available. Unnecessary loss of valuable time occurs.

Two-way radio communication between the ambulance and emergency room of each hospital is essential for effective and efficient medical care. The ambulance personnel will alert the emergency room regarding the condition of the patient being transported. If necessary the emergency room physician can give advice in the care of the patient to the emergency medical technicians.

Advanced ambulance services are sending electrocardiographs and other vital signs by radio telemetry to the hospital emergency room. Not only is the emergency room physician alerted as to the problem, but he can direct that additional appropriate medications or treatment be given by the ambulance personnel.

Ideally, each community should have a central dispatch for all emergency requests and responses. This provides coordination of fire, law enforcement, and health facilities.

part two

Immediate care of cardiopulmonary inadequacies

chapter 10

Cardiopulmonary resuscitation

Few if any advances have so dramatically altered the area of emergency medical care as the advent and widespread application of mouth-to-mouth ventilation and closed-chest augmentation of the circulation. Sudden, unexpected death, in terms of absolute loss of life, poses the greatest single medical problem today. It is the most common mode of death in the adult population. The actual incidence of sudden death may represent almost 30% of all natural deaths. It is estimated that ventricular fibrillation in structurally good hearts occurs over 900 times a day in the United States in victims outside a hospital. Approximately 70% of deaths from arteriosclerotic heart disease occur in persons who die outside a hospital or who are dead on arrival. Advancements and refinements in cardiopulmonary resuscitation should significantly reduce these deaths.

Within recent years the training of firemen, policemen, lifeguards and other rescue workers in the application of cardiopulmonary resuscitation techniques has accelerated. Likewise, training in the basics of resuscitation techniques has been extended into the high schools of the nation and among the lay public. Certainly it seems logical that medical personnel should be exposed as early as possible to a period of sophisticated training in all of the ramifications of effective cardiopulmonary resuscitation. Unfortunately, there are some medical workers who are completely lacking in the knowledge of even basic rescuscitation techniques.

This chapter is intended to provide information for basic life support of the patient until transportation to an advanced life support station can be accomplished.

It should be repeatedly emphasized that the crux of successful resuscitation centers on a realization that time is of the essence in successful resuscitation in that the irreversible cerebral damage may occur as early as 3½ to 4 minutes after sudden cessation of cerebral circulation. Immediate application of mouth-to-mouth artificial ventilation and closed-chest compression for circulatory augmentation, if applied properly, may maintain life for a lengthy period of time, allowing for further definitive measures to be applied, leading to eventual successful resuscitation of the patient.

Medical personnel are likely to encounter patients requiring resuscitation efforts under a variety of circumstances and always at most unexpected moments. Since these personnel are in the proximity of high-risk patients, it behooves them to develop confidence and ability in the application of resuscitation techniques.

43

RECOGNITION OF CARDIAC ARREST

How does one recognize or diagnose cardiac arrest? Admittedly, the term, to some, has a rather wastebasket connotation. Nevertheless, until a better name is suggested for sudden, unexplained, and unexpected cessation of cardiac activity, the term *cardiac arrest* will continue to be used. Regardless of the cause, failure of the heart action to maintain an adequate cerebral circulation indicates a need for immediate assistance.

Obviously, one must have considerable insight into the differential diagnosis between a medical emergency such as fainting or a grand mal attack on the one hand and a cardiac arrest on the other. Although it is unlikely that much harm would necessarily be done in the case of a mistaken diagnosis and the subsequent use of closed-chest resuscitation, the potential dangers of resuscitative techniques are sufficiently serious as to warrant some discussion in the use of resuscitative techniques.

In general, if there is no carotid or femoral blood pressure, if the pupils are dilated, and if all respiratory action has ceased or is inadequate, one may assume that cardiac output is inadequate to maintain cerebral function. The statement is well phrased when mention is made that "though the patient is 100% dead one does not need to prove that he is 200% dead." The burden of proof in such situations is on the individual who says that cardiopulmonary function is adequate to maintain life.

Spontaneous respirations cease very rapidly after cerebral circulation fails, usually within 20 to 40 seconds. A brief convulsive episode may occasionally be seen. A few agonal respiratory efforts may be noted.

The color of the patient's skin is of uncertain diagnostic value, and, of course, it is especially difficult to detect cyanosis in the dark-skinned individual. Palpation over one of the large arteries of the body such as the carotid or femoral fails to reveal any activity. The pupils usually begin to dilate and within 30 to 45 seconds will be completely dilated, with few exceptions. (People who have just had morphine or individuals with poor dilation mechanisms may not dilate readily, and of course there is the case of the individual with the glass eye!) Therefore, if there is no pulse and if the pupils are dilated, there is very little reason to suspect any effective cardiac output. More patients lose their chance for total recovery during this crucial period between arrest and diagnosis than at any other time in the resuscitative period. It must be remembered that in almost every case of cardiac arrest there is a period during which reversibility and resuscitation are possible. To allow this short period to pass because of indecision, because of the use of various ineffective stimulants, or because of a frantic search to locate a consultant is certain to add disaster to an already serious tragedy.

Cases are well known in which the time limit has not been well observed or in which early resuscitative efforts were totally inadequate. The prolongation of life in a decerebrate state represents one of the most serious of events, not to mention the sociologic and economic ramifications.

More refined methods of diagnosing cardiac arrest seldom have much application in the emergency occurring outside of the hospital. If the situation occurs outside of the hospital—or even outside of the recovery room or operating room—certainly it is a wasted effort to attempt a funduscopic examination. Blood pressure determinations may take valuable time. A precordial auscultation is suggested if immediately applicable. An electrocardiogram prior to the institution of cardiopulmonary resuscitation is, for obvious reasons, contraindicated in a great majority of instances simply because the patient cannot safely experience the luxury of this much delay.

A degree of optimism should be a part of every resuscitator's outlook. A large number of patients fail to be resuscitated because of half-hearted attempts, efforts that after all are generally ineffective. It should be recalled, on the other hand, that nearly every heart can be restored to a regular rhythm if proper resuscitative techniques are used and if a proper diagnosis of the underlying mechanism of arrest is made.

Once the patient arrives at the hospital emergency room, efforts should be made to determine the exact state of the myocardium—that is, whether the heart is in asystole or whether ventricular fibrillation is present. Throughout the transport of the patient it is most vital that, as a sign of adequate oxygenation and ventilation, the pupils be maintained in a constricted state and that a palpable pulse be maintained.

CAUSES OF CARDIAC ARREST

When we refer to the term *cardiac arrest* we are speaking of the sudden, superficially unexplained, and unexpected cessation of an effective cardiac output. Sudden cessation of an adequate cardiac output to maintain consciousness or adequate cerebral oxygenation may be caused by the absence of all cardiac activity, which is cardiac asystole. The same inadequate cardiac output may result from the sudden onset of ventricular fibrillation, which represents a wild, uncoordinated, and disorganized myocardial contraction resulting in the complete absence of any cardiac output. A third condition may occasionally prevail: the heart may be beating feebly but at such a depressed rate or with such an ineffective stroke volume that the net result is very much the same as with cardiac asystole or ventricular fibrillation. In any event, all three conditions require immediate efforts to artificially establish circulation in order that irreversible brain damage may not occur.

Although statistically the great bulk of potential cardiac resuscitation will be in the patient with myocardial occlusion, frequent arrests do occur in victims of near-drowning and accidental electrocution. Such possibilities present themselves in numerous everyday situations. Coming into contact with faulty electrical wiring is not uncommon. Victims of lightning shock, anaphylactic shock, chest injuries, certain poisonings, and hemorrhagic shock may require cardiopulmonary resuscitation.

It is now generally recognized that the majority of deaths from acute myocardial infarction occur within 24 hours of the onset of symptoms. At least 50% of these deaths occur within the first hour after the onset of difficulty. As mentioned, ventricular fibrillation is commonly associated with the early stages of an acute myocardial infarction. Following an acute myocardial infarction, it is reassuring to know that the instance of ventricular fibrillation is not necessarily related to the size of the infarct. The electric stability of the heart can be a fragile affair. Areas of anoxic changes in the myocardium may trigger electric discharges sufficient to throw the heart into fibrillation.

Vagal reflex patterns may have an important role. When the cardioinhibitory nerve is stimulated, one will commonly notice an effect upon the cardiac conduction mechanism involving a depression of the sinus node, depression of the atrioventricular node, and impairment of atrioventricular conduction, resulting in auricular or ventricular slowing or, as a matter of fact, standstill in all degrees of atrioventricular heart block. Clinically there is evidence to support the view that the sensitivity of the heart is more affected by vagal stimulation under hypercapnic states or in patients with an increased serum potassium level or hyperpotassemia. Hypercapnia simply refers to an increase in carbon dioxide often associated with respiratory acidosis. These factors are particularly reflected in the increased frequency with which sudden cardiac arrest, most frequently ventricular asystole, is seen in the burned patient. Severely burned patients have an increased potassium level in their serum as a result of tissue breakdown. Patients with obstructive jaundice (from a stone in the common duct or a cancer of the ampulla of Vater or head of the pancreas) may be very sensitive to vagal influences.

Those persons who have studied neuroanatomy will understand why pressure on the eyeball often results in a slowing of the patient's radial pulse. In many instances the bradycardia associated with operations about the eye, particularly involving the rectus muscles, may involve a certain risk of cardiac arrest. The efferent limb of the reflex arc consists of the vagus nerve, whereas the trigeminal nerve constitutes the afferent limb. This reflex, which we may call the oculocardiac reflex, results from stimulation of the first division of the trigeminal nerve (ophthalmic). While there is pressure on the globe or when the extraocular muscles are stretched, electrocardiographic tracings will often reflect abnormalities supporting the role of the vagus nerve in the production of various cardiac arrhythmias.

Mention should again be made of sudden cardiac arrest following severe anaphylactic reactions in such instances as the injection of penicillin, local anesthetic agents, vaccines, and various types of sera. Systemic reactions following stings by bees, hornets, wasps, and yellowjackets may, as is generally well known, cause severe anaphylactic reactions in certain individuals.

Still another explanation for sudden cardiac arrest in a sizable percentage of patients is that caused by a block in the conductive system of the heart. *Stokes-Adams disease* is a term applied to many of the conditions characterized by sudden failure of the ventricles to contract. It may be associated with markedly slowed idioventricular beats, ventricular tachycardia, or ventricular fibrillation. Patients with Stokes-Adams disease may suddenly have an attack without any warning. Within the last decade a large percentage of diagnosed Stokes-Adams cases have been managed successfully with long-term implantation of electric cardiac pacemakers.

There are many other diseases and conditions associated with a high instance of cardiac arrest. For example, cardiac arrest following carotid sinus pressure may occur.

Factors that mechanically block an effective cardiac output may produce the same ultimate damage as that which results from a sudden cardiac arrest. A pericardial tamponade is such an example. The pericardial sac becomes quickly distended and may interfere with the cardiac input and, to a degree, with the output of the heart. This condition may be caused by penetrating wounds of the heart or contusions in such accidents as a steering wheel injury. The relief of the cardiac tamponade is urgent. Air emboli forming a large bolus in the outflow tract of the right ventricle or between the right atrium and right ventricle may effectively block cardiac output, as will a large pulmonary artery embolus.

IMMEDIATE RESUSCITATIVE MEASURES

Once it is determined that the patient's respiratory activity and circulation is absent or even markedly depressed, immediate application of resuscitative techniques is indicated.

The first step of emergency resuscitation usually calls for assurance that the airway is open and for prompt artificial ventilation by mouth-to-mouth or mouth-to-nose techniques. The simple maneuver of maximum backward tilt of the head will often be ample for achieving an open airway. By placing one's hand beneath the patient's neck and the other hand on his forehead, one can lift the neck with one hand and tilt the head backward by pressure with the other hand. In such a fashion the neck is extended and the tongue is lifted away from the back of the throat, relieving any anatomic obstruction of the airway produced by the tongue lying against the back of the throat.

Which should one start first: closed-chest resuscitative efforts or artificial ventilation? Physicians may debate the merits of each as a priority. The truth of the matter generally involves an almost simultaneous beginning of both aspects of resuscitation. The most crucial point in question is that of cerebral circulation. The first priority involves artificial augmentation of the circulation with oxygenated blood. Obviously the circulating blood, if unoxygenated, will have limited value. Likewise a well-ventilated lung will have no value to the patient unless the circulation is moving. Again, it should be repeated for emphasis that one effort without the other is virtually worthless. Unfortunately in the excitement of an emergency this apparently obvious fact is frequently overlooked. In rare situations of marked cardiopulmonary collapse while the heart is still beating, the patient will be revived by artificial ventilation alone.

Method of artificial ventilation

Beginning almost simultaneously with closed-chest compression, one attempts to expire oxygen into the patient's lungs to achieve artificial respiration. A variety of expired air techniques is available, but perhaps the simplest and most readily available is mouth-to-mouth respiration. Either mouth-to-nose artificial respiration or mouth-to-tube ventilation can also be easily accomplished outside of the hospital. In each instance, the factor of prime importance is that of airway patency. Herein lies the greatest pitfall in artificial ventilation. The ease with which the airway is partially or completely obstructed in the unconscious patient is well known to the physician. With the head overextended on the neck and the chin elevated, the likelihood of a patent airway is generally assured.

By simply filling one's own lungs with air and expiring forcefully into the patient's opened mouth with the head and chin in the prescribed position, one can see an expansion of the chest wall over the lungs. The elasticity of the lungs and chest wall will adequately expel the air, along with some ventilatory aspects of the accompanying closed-chest procedure itself. In cases of drowning it is even possible to begin mouth-to-mouth resuscitation while towing the victim back to shore. The few seconds saved in this way may be just enough to prevent irreparable damage to the brain. After about three to five lung inflations, one should feel briefly for the pulse. The wrist pulse, although useful in the conscious victim, is often very difficult to find in the unconscious victim in need of resuscitation. It is therefore better when resuscitating an unconscious victim to use the artery in the neck by feeling with two fingers for the carotid artery. This is located on either side below the jaw to the side of the windpipe.

If there is a pulse but still no adequate breathing, continue mouth-to-mouth resuscitation and get someone to go for help. Blow forcefully into an adult and gently into a child's airway. Watch the chest. When the chest rises, take your mouth off of the patient's mouth and let him exhale by himself. When the patient has finished exhaling blow in the next deep breath and repeat in succession every 3 to 5 seconds.

With mouth-to-mouth resuscitation your hand is free to prevent air from going into the stomach by pressing between the breast bone and the navel. Avoid aspiration of gastric contents by turning the victim's head and shoulders to one side. Timing and rhythm are secondary; volume is most important. If you cannot get the air into the lungs through the mouth, blow into the nose. Close his lips and get a wide contact with your mouth around his nose. Blow in until the lungs expand. With mouth-to-nose breathing, exhalation is often blocked. If this is the case be sure the air can escape through the mouth. Again, repeat the cycle every 3 to 5 seconds.

If the first attempts at inflating the lungs don't move the chest in spite of the backward tilt of the head, check for swallowed objects or vomitus in the throat. The general rule is if there is vomitus or other foreign matter on the face, wipe the mouth and throat clean and begin mouth-to-mouth resuscitation. If the face is clean, start mouth-to-mouth resuscitation and clear the throat only to remove an obstruction. It may be possible to remove an object in the upper part of the throat with your fingers, but extreme caution must be used to avoid pushing the object deeper into the throat. If you cannot remove the obstruction, don't panic. Attempt to get air through the mouth or nose by blowing more forcefully. Once the throat is clear continue mouth-to-mouth resuscitation. If the child is quite small one may cover both the nose and mouth with one's mouth. With babies do not blow but puff gently to avoid damaging the lungs. Their rate of inflation should be twenty to thirty times a minute. The backward tilting of the infant's neck should be only moderate, since the neck of an infant is so pliable that airway obstruction may be produced. An object in the throat of an infant may be dislodged by holding the patient briefly head down and striking him between the shoulder blades.

Technique of closed-chest cardiac resuscitation

With the patient in the supine or flat position, preferably on a hard, nonyielding surface, efforts are directed to compress the heart between the sternum and the thoracic vertebrae. By so doing, enough cardiac output is achieved to maintain adequate cerebral circulation as well as adequate blood flow to the myocardium and to other vital tissues (up to 35% of normal). The technique involves intermittent pressure on the lower third of the sternum with the minimum possible pressure to the adjacent rib cage. This can be accomplished by using the base of the palm. Ideally, one should be directly over the victim with the elbows rigidly extended and with the pressure exerted from the shoulders downward. Pressure directed at an angle to the chest wall is more likely to produce complications such as rib fractures and soft tissue injuries. In the middle-aged or older patient one usually starts off with an intermittent depression of the sternum that gradually increases in depth as the sternum and rib cage become slightly more mobile and elastic. Too vigorous initial compression is often a tendency of the uninitiated.

One should position himself at either side of the patient. The heel of one hand is placed over the lower half of the patient's sternum and the heel of the other hand is placed on top of the first hand. (One should avoid placing the hand over the lower tip of the sternum.) The sternum should then be downwardly displaced toward the spine for 1½ to 2 inches. It should be held down for a fraction of a second and then rapidly released. Contact with the chest is maintained during relaxation. A rate of 60 to 80 impressions per minute is probably ideal in most cases, but in children the rate should probably be raised to 100 to 120 impressions per minute. In compressing the sternum one should use the weight of one's entire body rather than just the strength of the arms in order to avoid undue fatigue. One should be careful to keep one's fingers raised so as to avoid pressure on the rib cage.

If the patient is a child the principle is the same, but much less pressure should be used. In small children the force of the heel of one hand is sufficient. With babies, moderate pressure should be applied with the tips of the fingers only to the center of the breast bone. One must not press too hard, since it is easy to bruise the baby's myocardium. An infant's sternum is depressed ½ to ¾ inch. Young children require ¾ to 1½ inches. It is also possible to encircle the chest of small infants with one's hands and compress the midsternum with both thumbs.

How does one gauge the effectiveness of closed-chest compression? If by one's closed-chest compression efforts one is able to maintain a blood pressure above 60 to 70 mm Hg (if a blood pressure cuff and a person to use it are available), or if an easily palpable pulse is present and if the pupils are maintained in a constricted state, then one can generally assume that cardiac output is adequate to sustain life. If the patient also appears well oxygenated, then one should assume that pulmonary resuscitative efforts are also adequate.

Combining closed-chest and mouth-to-mouth techniques

How does one combine external cardiac compression with intermittent positive pressure artificial ventilation? If one is alone with the patient, probably the best combination is that of alternating two mouth-to-mouth lung inflations with fifteen sternal compressions at about a 1-second interval. With only one rescuer, chest compressions should be given at a more rapid rate, that is, eighty per minute. Two full lung inflations are delivered in rapid succession, within a period of 5 or 6 seconds, without allowing full exhalation between breaths. If a second person is available to apply artificial respiration, the worker supplying ventilation should interpose one deep lung inflation after every fifth sternal compression. Sometimes it may be difficult to do this; if so, one should briefly stop at the end of every fifteen sternal compressions and give two quick lung inflations. It is best to interpose breathing without any pause in compressions since cerebral perfusion drops to zero with any cessation of compression.

As soon as the patient arrives in the emergency room, a competent person should quickly pass an endotracheal tube, and intermittent positive ventilation with high concentrations of oxygen should be continued.

Although artificial ventilation by exhalation will deliver about 16% to 17% oxygen, supplemental oxygen is desirable by bag-valve-mask or bag-valve-tube administration as soon as possible. Bag-valve-mask devices should be employed only by persons well versed in their use. One should become adept at the use of the bag-valve-mask as soon as possible. Squeezing the bag and at the same time maintaining the head at proper extension, keeping the lower jaw elevated, and securing an optimum mask fit requires practice. The use of the endotracheal tube and oxygen-powered mechanical breathing devices as well as manually activated chest compressors should be a part of one's armamentarium but will not be discussed in this text on immediate care.

OTHER IMMEDIATE CONSIDERATIONS

Once a cardiac arrest is suspected or is diagnosed, the victim should be immediately placed in a supine position or with the head slightly downward. There is some disagreement about this advantage of lowering the head but, in general, it seems advisable during the first few minutes of resuscitation.

Certainly, if one has reasonable assurance that the heart is not entirely stopped, there is a restorative action of head lowering that produces an actual, significant, rapid, and demonstrable increase in the blood pressure to the brain. It is known, for example, that a period of 4 to 8 seconds of asystole will produce coma when a patient with Stokes-Adams syndrome is in the erect position. If the patient is recumbent at the time of the attack, however, 12 to 15 seconds are required before coma develops. Therefore, to stretch that delicate period between reversibility and irreversibility of cerebral cortical activity, it would seem that the head-down position does have some merit. In addition the Trendelenburg position tends to prevent aspiration of vomitus and gastric contents following pressure on the sternum and epigastrium; it also have the advantage of decreasing the likelihood of air emboli reaching the brain in rare cases where air emboli form.

As soon as the initial resuscitative efforts have been carried out, the patient should be placed in a supine position, since the impingement against the diaphragm by the viscera may significantly reduce vital capacity in some individuals and may increase the risk of further cerebral edema.

Another important measure that can be carried out almost at once is that of elevation of the patient's lower extremities. The beneficial rush of blood into the large veins depresses vagal tone by reflex action, and this allows the inhibited heart to escape the vagus restraint. Sudden augmentation of venous refilling of the heart may produce its desired effect simply by stretching the cardiac fibers. With elevation of the legs, venous return may be increased by making as much as 1,000 ml of additional blood available. This stretching effect of distending the right atrium or right ventricle may, in itself, provoke a heartbeat on the basis of Starling's law of contractility of the heart. In some instances and where there are adequate personnel available, additional venous blood may need to be returned to the heart by wrapping the extremities with elastic bandage.

Precordial percussion or thump

An often neglected but sometimes effective technique that can be immediately employed, even during the brief time spent in arriving at a diagnosis, is that of precordial thumping of the chest. This simply means that one strikes the left chest in the precordial area with a clenched fist with at least three quick heavy blows in succession. There is no question but that a sharp blow delivered with a clenched fist or with the ulnar border of the hand high upon the chest may activate the heart, producing several ventricular complexes and, in some instances, getting the heartbeat reestablished. Many persons advocate that precordial percussion should always be tried briefly before external cardiac massage is instituted. Certainly the speed and ease with which the precordium may be struck justifies the trial of such a procedure. Numerous proved cases of cardiac arrest have been restored to a regular rhythm simply by precordial concussion.

I have seen several of these instances. In two cases the electrocardiogram was recording the patient's cardiac complex when a straight line revealed sudden absence of activity. A good slap to the left anterior chest produced a subsequent cardiac contraction, and after several of these blows sustained cardiac activity returned. Patients whose hearts have suddenly stopped following a vagovagal reflex or as a result of Stokes-Adams disease are especially good candidates for precordial concussion. Obviously no great amount of time should be spent with precordial concussion since it will, in most instances, be ineffectual if the arrest has been present longer than just a few seconds.

Ventricular fibrillation

Ventricular fibrillation refers to an irregular, uncoordinated activity of the ventricles of the heart or to a quivering motion with almost complete absence of any cardiac output. Death will result from ventricular fibrillation in the untreated patient as quickly as it will from cardiac asystole.

Since ventricular fibrillation can seldom be diagnosed without either the aid of an electrocardiogram or direct visualization of the heart action, it is probable that ventricular fibrillation can only be a suspected diagnosis in cardiac arrests occurring outside of the hospital. It should again be emphasized that the need to defibrillate the heart does not, in itself, constitute a first priority in the scheme of one's efforts, although defibrillation is highly desirable at the earliest possible moment. Providing that adequate cardiac output is being maintained by closed-chest resuscitation and that adequate oxygenation is being provided by mouth-to-mouth or mouth-to-nose respiration, the patient can be maintained in a reasonably satisfactory state for some time. Most patients can be transported to a defibrillator, or vice versa, in the necessary time period.

I recall such a situation in the early 1950's when I was a resident at Bellevue Hospital in New York City. At that time we had one of the few cardiac defibrillators in the city. One morning we received a call from a hospital over 100 blocks away and on the opposite side of Manhattan. Ventricular fibrillation had occurred in a patient while he was on the operating table. Adequate resuscitative efforts were carried out by the hospital personnel during the time that it took us to arrive by ambulance through heavy traffic to the hospital. The patient was promptly defibrillated and the surgeon proceeded with the operation.

Defibrillation can be accomplished by electric countershock with either direct or alternating current. Generally speaking, the direct current countershock defibrillator is preferable. Using a direct external countershock, a setting of 400 watt-seconds is frequently used to defibrillate the adult heart and 100 watt-seconds for a child's heart. This recommended energy level may have to be raised in large, diseased hearts or under certain other conditions in which defibrillation is difficult.

It is important to remember that electrode paste must be applied generously to the skin or the the electrodes, which should be free of old, dried paste from previous defibrillation attempts. Saline-soaked gauze sponges are good conductors. One electrode is placed just below the right clavicle medially and a second electrode over the apex of the heart beneath the left breast. We prefer to apply our own countershock either by a foot or hand switch rather than delegate this to an assistant because of the danger of inadvertent shocking of the resuscitation personnel. The objective in defibrillation is to produce a synchronized depolarization of all heart muscle, to eliminate all uncoordinated ectopic foci of activity, and to converge all electric activity into one single contractile effort.

If the patient appears to be resistant to defibrillatory attempts, the intravenous or intracardiac injection of epinephrine may change the fibrillatory action of the heart to a coarser nature and increase the likelihood of defibrillation. Sodium bicarbonate injections may need to be repeated just prior to a defibrillation attempt. Between countershocks, of course, the patient should be well oxygenated and closed-chest compression should be continued. It is important to remember that almost all hearts can be defibrillated.

Occasionally the heart may be successfully defibrillated prior to either ventilatory assistance or external cardiac massage. This situation probably arises only in an area such as the coronary care unit where the electric activity of the heart is being constantly monitored. During President Eisenhower's last illness he required fourteen separate attempts at defibrillation. These were successful in several instances even without a loss of consciousness by the patient. "Blind defibrillation" in the unconscious, pulseless patient is becoming increasingly employed even though ventricular fibrillation has not been confirmed electrocardiographically, provided that artificial ventilation and chest compression efforts are not delayed.

Very seldom can one rely on the possibility of spontaneous defibrillation. It does occur, however. For example, ventricular fibrillation suddenly developed in a young lady during a cardiac catheterization procedure. Full monitoring observations were available and within a few seconds of adequate closed-chest compression the heart was seen to spontaneously defibrillate.

We will no doubt soon see the widespread introduction of portable external cardiac defibrillators as more satisfactory models become available.

All medical personnel should be knowledgeable in the use of the electric external cardiac defibrillator and, ideally, should have had practice in its use in the animal laboratory.

PHARMACOLOGIC AIDS IN CARDIAC RESUSCITATION

Although there are over thirty drugs that may have a part to play in helping to successfully resuscitate a heart, in the majority of cases one need only by concerned with a relatively few agents. One's best friend in such emergencies is probably epinephrine. For well over 60 years this drug has been employed in resuscitation, but its potentialities may be more nearly realized of late. Some physicians recommend an initial dose of epinephrine within the first 2 minutes of cardiopulmonary resuscitation. I am somewhat more inclined to wait a few extra minutes before the use of epinephrine since a considerable number of cardiac resuscitations can be achieved without the use of drugs. A cardiotonic drug may provide the additional needed contractile force to help maintain myocardial oxygenation. If epinephrine is not available then either calcium chloride or calcium gluconate can be used. Epinephrine acts by improving coronary perfusion pressure, by improving myocardial conduction through direct effect on the myocardium and on the conduction tissue, thereby producing more forceful contractions of the myocarium, and by lowering the defibrillation threshold. It increases the speed of atrioventricular conduction.

It is unlikely that pharmacologic assistance in cardiopulmonary resuscitation will be readily available for the case occurring outside of the hospital, at least not until the ambulance arrives. As emphasized elsewhere, immediate efforts should be geared to doing as much for the patient as possible prior to transporting him to the hospital. In other words, much can be done to stabilize the patient's condition. For example, an intravenous route can be established through which drugs can be administered. While epinephrine can be given directly into the heart, such an injection usually takes time away from the external cardiac compression that is being given. In addition, there may be some difficulty experienced in getting the drug into the heart chamber because of the size of the needle, site of the injection, or intrathoracic pathology.

In any event epinephrine probably should be given as soon as possible, particularly if there is no evidence of an immediate return of a spontaneous heartbeat. If the intravenous route is available, a dose of 0.5 ml of a 1:1,000 solution diluted to 10 ml or 5 ml of a 1:10,000 solution may be given. A similar dose can be given directly into the heart. It was formerly feared that the epinephrine would throw the heart into ventricular fibrillation, but we now know that regardless of the heart action epinephrine may have a beneficial effect. If the heart is in asystole the epinephrine may help initiate the heart action once it is circulated through the myocardium. If weak ventricular fibrillatory actions are present, epinephrine will encourage the strength of the contractions and will help promote successful defibrillation.

There is a sizable group of pressor drugs available to the clinician. All of the pressor drugs are derivatives of epinephrine, but they differ from it in their potency and predominant mode of action. In addition, their stability varies in the presence of aminoacidosis. Because of their differences in molecular structure, some act primarily as vasoconstrictors and some act principally upon the heart and may cause vasodilation. Of the two kinds of receptors at sympathetic nerve endings, the alpha receptors are concerned with excitatory efforts such as pupillary dilation, peripheral vasoconstriction, and mobilization of glucose from liver glycogen. The beta receptors at the nerve endings are chiefly concerned with inhibitory effects and thereby produce vasodilation of blood vessels that supply skeletal muscles, reduction of tone of the smooth muscle supplying the bronchial tree, and an increase in the rate of the heartbeat and cardiac output.

Because epinephrine stimulates some nerve endings while inhibiting others, it is regarded as both an alpha and a beta receptor. Levarterenol (norepinephrine) produces its effect chiefly by action on the alpha receptors. It increases the rate of contraction of the heart in the presence of heart block. In addition to causing vasoconstriction, pupillary dilation, and a rise in blood glucose level by liberation of glycogen from the liver, levarterenol also increases coronary flow and may produce slowing of the heart through reflex vagal inhibition as the blood pressure rises. Marked constriction of the vessels of the gut and reduction of bowel motility may occur with levarterenol infusion. Adrenergic blocking agents are able to block the alpha receptors but are not effective in blocking the beta receptors.

Among the pressor amines, other drugs are phenylephrine, methoxamine, and metaraminol. By acting mainly upon the alpha receptors, this group of drugs raises the systemic arterial blood pressure during vasoconstriction of peripheral vessels. The force of contraction of the heart is not appreciably altered, but coronary blood flow and cerebral blood flow are increased when hypotension is present.

Other pressor amines in addition to epinephrine that act mainly upon the heart and in the production of vasodilation are ephedrine, methamphetamine, and mephentermine.

In administering vasopressors during cardiac resuscitation and in the immediate postresuscitative period, care should be taken to avoid local tissue necrosis by using large catheters in large veins and by using dilute solutions. Obviously, one should use the smallest dose that will provide the desired effect. The action of pressor amines is less effective in the presence of uncorrected metabolic acidosis. Vasoconstrictors increase diastolic pressure during cardiac resuscitation and materially improve the chances for return of spontaneous circulation. The vasopressors, which act mainly on the alpha receptors, do raise diastolic pressure; their value seems to lie primarily in the improvement of the peripheral vascular tone.

There is complete absence of body perfusion during either cardiac asystole or ventricular fibrillation. This state is often followed by the marginal perfusional status of cardiopulmonary perfusion efforts, and both situations add up to a severe metabolic acidosis. The acidosis contributes to atony of the myocardium, to decreased peripheral vascular tone, and to interference with catecholamine (endogenous epinephrine and norepinephrine) production and action. When severe metabolic acidosis is present in association with attempts to resuscitate the fibrillating heart, success is unlikely since the arrhythmia rapidly recurs even after defibrillation.

While rapid correction of this acidosis occurs with establishment of adequate perfusion, sodium bicarbonate may be effectively used in the meantime—one ampule of 7.5% solution (44.6 mEq) may be given every 10 minutes during closed-chest resuscitative efforts or 500 ml of a 5% solution (297.5 mEq) given per hour.

Nearly all studies concerned with pH determination made during resuscitative attempts concur in finding rather marked metabolic acidosis as a result of oxygen deficit and accumulation of carbon dioxide and fixed acids. Under such conditions, catecholamines are interfered with. Once the pH is returned to normal, however, endogenous epinephrine and norepinephrine again act on the vascular tree.

The beneficial effects of maintaining a near-normal blood pH are multiple. For instance, the ventricular fibrillation threshold is considerably higher in an alkalotic heart than in an acidotic heart. The incidence of spontaneous difibrillation is also considerably higher in an alkalotic heart, as is the likelihood that the arrhythmia may extinguish itself.

As mentioned, cardiac arrest represents a *zero* perfusion state. During resuscitative efforts, this situation may improve only to the point that a low perfusion state exists. In any event, metabolic acidosis enters the picture along with its own inherent adverse features such as decreased arterial pressure, reduction in cardiac output, and a gradual rise in both central venous pressure and peripheral resistance. Cardiac slowing, sinus arrhythmias, sinus pauses, and sinus arrest (all suggestive of increased vagal activity) may be seen. Certainly the threshold for ventricular fibrillation is lowered.

Atropine sulfate may be effective in preventing arrest in profound sinus bradycardia secondary to myocardial infarction and under conditions of marked hypotension. By enhancing atrioventricular conduction and accelerating cardiac rate in sinus bradycardia, the acceleration of the heart rate may so improve cardiac output that the likelihood of ventricular fibrillation is reduced. If a severe bradyarrhythmia is encountered, a dose of 0.5 to 2.0 mg may be administered intravenously.

Lidocaine is proving to be a particularly effective agent from both a preventative and a therapeutic standpoint. Multifocal premature ventricular beats or episodes of ventricular tachycardia may be encountered in the patient during or shortly after a myocardial infarction episode. Rapid administration of 50 to 100 mg of lidocaine intravenously may effectively exert antiarrhythmic qualities and prevent cardiac asystole or ventricular fibrillation. Similarly, after cardiac rhythm has been established the heart may again revert to ventricular fibrillation. By depressing myocardial irritability, the ventricular fibrillation threshold may be raised sufficiently to protect the patient. After the intravenous bolus of lidocaine has been given, a continuous infusion of up to 3 mg/minute (500 mg in 500 ml of dextrose in water) is instituted.

A detailed presentation of the other aspects of the pharmacology of resuscitation is probably best left for a more definitive discussion. Because of its marked ability to increase myocardial contractility, enhance ventricular excitability, and prolong systole, calcium may be useful in certain patients not responding to epinephrine. Calcium can be injected intravenously as a dose of 5 ml of 10% calcium chloride or 10 ml of 10% calcium gluconate at 10-minute intervals. It should not be administered together with sodium bicarbonate because of the resulting precipitation of calcium carbonate.

IMMEDIATE POSTRESUSCITATIVE CARE

Although this book is not concerned with definitive care to any great extent but instead with the immediate measures that should be applied to the acutely ill or injured patient, some mention should be made of the postresuscitative care in patients experiencing cardiac asystole or ventricular fibrillation. The long-term results and recovery of the patient may hinge very directly upon what immediate postresuscitative care is given. In cases where there has been sufficient cerebral anoxia to prevent the immediate return of spontaneous respirations or consciousness, one should make every effort to obviate the neurologic sequelae that may develop. One method to reduce the oxygen needs of the brain as well as to reduce cerebral edema is the use of general body hypothermia. This should be started almost at once after resuscitation of the heart has been accomplished. Large doses of steroids have been effective in reducing the cerebral edema, as has the use of urea. Shortly after resuscitation there may be a period of hypercoagulability of the blood, which may lead to microembolization of the brain. Whenever possible, heparinization of the patient at an early point should be instituted. Adequate hydration and careful monitoring of the electrocardiogram is indicated. Antiarrhythmic drugs such as lidocaine or propranolol may be instituted by the cardiologist. Mechanically controlled ventilation through the endotracheal tube or via a tracheostomy tube may be required if the blood gases so indicate, if there has been much aspiration, or if there are signs of severe hypoxemia.

Because of antisludging properties and particularly because of their ability to aid in the prevention or reduction of cerebral edema, corticosteroids are usually indicated in the immediate postresuscitation period. Methylprednisolone (30 mg/kg every 6 hours) is recommended.

COMPLICATIONS AND PITFALLS IN CARDIOPULMONARY RESUSCITATION

Ill-advised or poorly applied resuscitation carries with it significant hazards of serious complications. Unless one is familiar with the hazards of resuscitation, many otherwise successful efforts may be lost. The consequent death of the patient may become the result of a sincere but nevertheless tragically fatal attempt to maintain life. The list of complications is a long one and includes injury to most of the anatomic structures within the chest and upper abdomen including the bony thorax. Overly enthusiastic pressure on the sternum may produce myocardial contusion, laceration of the heart, cardiac tamponade, and localized trauma to the heart such as injury to the coronary vessels.

Lacerations of the liver have been reported. In fact, one postmortem study of forty-six cardiac arrest patients on whom closed-chest resuscitation was applied showed an instance of 11% rupture of the liver. Because of a proportionally larger liver in childhood, the likelihood of rupture appears to be higher in the young patient. One should never compress the abdomen and chest simultaneously.

Trauma to the chest wall is unusually common. Multiple rib fractures, unfortunately, are seen frequently, particularly when closed-chest resuscitation is carried out on elderly patients with a relatively inflexible rib cage. In such instances the broken ends of the ribs present sharp edges that may lacerate the lung, pulmonary veins, or even the heart. Less frequent is a fracture of the sternum. Fractures of the scapula have been reported. The costochondral cartilages are also a common site of injury.

During closed-chest resuscitation, the act of bending and compressing bones such as the rib cage may lead to microfractures within the medulla of ribs and sternum with an increased marrow pressure. This permits entry of fat into the venous circulation. Even without fracturing the sternum or ribs, a significantly high instance of pulmonary marrow emboli may thus be produced. Just how much fat embolization influences ultimate survival is not yet known. Clinically significant fat embolization to the brain has been documented on numerous occasions. This may be an additional factor contributing to mental deterioration following cardiac resuscitation, particularly when cortical cells are already depressed following prolonged anoxia.

Pulmonary edema may be a complication of prolonged closed-chest cardiac compression. Part of this explanation may be that with closed-chest cardiac compression retrograde venous flow into the pulmonary veins occurs. Like trauma to the lungs, this no doubt is a contributing factor.

Another complication that can be largely prevented is that of a laceration or rupture of the stomach. Gastric dilation during artificial respiration is a frequent possibility, particularly when endotracheal intubation has not been employed. Tremendous dilation may occur. If one is conscious of the possibility, however, one can prevent the problem by simple pressure on the epigastrium from time to time to deflate the stomach. Without an endotracheal tube, the possibility of gastric dilation should always be suspected. Lacerations can also occur at the gastroesophageal junction. Trauma to other abdominal viscera is also reported with closed-chest resuscitation. Rupture of the transverse colon is one example. Ruptured spleens occasionally are reported, and even a transection of the inferior vena cava is a known complication.

Therefore, it behooves one to be clearly cognizant of the dangers of resuscitative efforts in that they may compound an ordinarily tragic situation into a failure. Training manikins are of help in giving one a certain degree of skill, but the novice should also attend as many "code blues" as possible in order to further observe proper techniques. The novice should remain with the patient since he may be allowed to apply closed-chest resuscitation to briefly relieve a member of the hospital staff.

One should be aware of the fact that vomiting may occur with a high degree of frequency in situations requiring oral resuscitation, particularly of asphyxiated patients. While vomiting is not present in all cardiac arrest situations, it does represent a potential complicating hazard. Use of suction equipment will be possible in many situations, but when it is not available the patient should be placed in such a position that the vomitus will not be aspirated. Mechanically tilting the patient and turning his head to the side will often prevent aspiration.

Many of the postresuscitative complications of cardiac arrest depend upon how quickly resuscitative efforts are employed and how effective they are. For example, the renal problems ensuing after cardiac arrest are much the same as with any shock-producing cardiovascular collapse. Any impairment of renal function caused by hypoxia with associated metabolic acidosis and hyperkalemia is a serious threat. The definitive care of the postresuscitative victim is outside the scope of this book, but certainly the problems can be minimized if the patient receives properly applied resuscitative efforts.

The most serious and dreaded complication of cardiac resuscitation results when cerebral anoxia produces serious neurologic sequelae. Depriving the brain of adequate oxygenation for even a matter of 3 to 4 minutes may have an adverse effect on the central nervous system. Anything over this period of time may result in irreversible damage. The amount of time that the brain will withstand complete ischemia without permanent damage has never been altogether established. Even if this were known, other factors such as age, oxygenation of the patient at the time of the arrest, and temperature of the patient and the environment all play a part. The brain apparently is somewhat more sensitive to metabolic derangements at some age periods than at others. The first sign of brain damage is, of course, unconsciousness. The respiratory center is knocked out, the pupils are dilated, the body is without reflexes, and electroencephalographic activity may be extremely slow or absent. Hopefully, however, most of these features can be reversed if oxygenated blood is quickly rushed to the most critical portion of the body, the brain.

What can one do on an immediate basis to reduce the likelihood of cerebral damage? Although the technique is somewhat controversial, I believe that the patient should be immediately tilted in a 10- to 15-degree Trendelenburg position (head down). Not only will this position improve venous return to the heart but there is some evidence that irreversible brain damage can be delayed a bit.

The crucial period of time can be compromised by several factors. Of first importance is the effectiveness of the individual in his ability to compress the heart manually. Ordinarily one should be able to maintain a systolic blood pressure of at least 60 to 70 mm Hg, produce an easily palpable pulse in the peripheral vessels, maintain normal skin color of the patient, and keep the pupils constricted. If such is not the case, the likelihood of neurologic damage is great.

If there is a serious question that severe brain damage may have occurred, the sooner one can apply effective measures the better. Therefore, even on the way to the hospital, large doses of steroids may be started and the patient's body temperature may be lowered with whatever means are available. Because of the adverse effect of metabolic acidosis produced by anaerobic metabolism in the absence of oxygen, sodium bicarbonare should be given as soon as possible. Lactic and carbonic acids, products of the anaerobic metabolisms, rapidly lower the pH of body tissues, and this action is thought by some to cause coagulation of the blood in the small vascular channels, such as within the brain.

The medical-legal aspects of cardiac arrest and resuscitation are discussed in Chapter 37, along with other medical-legal relationships to the delivery of immediate care.

Continuation of resuscitative efforts

If one compresses the heart for a prolonged period of time without success and if artificial ventilation is adequate, he should systematically review all the potential sources of error before deciding that further resuscitative efforts are of no avail. Prolonged heart massage for over 3 hours with complete recovery has been reported in several instances.

As a general rule cardiac resuscitative efforts should be maintained at least until the patient is brought to the hospital where electrocardiographic and even electroencephalographic tracings can be made.

In spite of precordial concussion, artificial ventilatory efforts, and closed-chest cardiac compression, very frequently a regular heart rhythm will not resume. Often directly related is the fact that ventricular fibrillation is present in a high percentage of arrests occurring outside of the hospital. Those cases associated with accidental electrocution, coronary occlusion, and occasionally drowning are particularly likely to be fibrillating. Ordinarily a heart that is fibrillating under such circumstances will not spontaneously defibrillate. Electric defibrillation will be indicated. The main point to remember is that life can be maintained and cerebral damage prevented simply by the *augmentation* of the cardiorespiratory system. This can be accomplished for an indefinite period if performed in optimal fashion. Certainly it can generally be maintained for a long enough period to allow the patient to be brought to a hospital or to allow more definitive care to be brought to the patient.

Open-chest cardiac compression and defibrillation, as mentioned elsewhere, should definitely be a part of every physician's armamentarium, whether he is a surgeon or not. There are times when closed-chest cardiac compression is less likely to be successful. Some of the situations that might be best managed by the open-chest approach include the following:

1. The patient with a pectus excavatum or marked pectus carinatum
2. Massive air embolism
3. Cardiac tamponade
4. The patient with a bilateral pneumothorax, or tension pneumothorax
5. Lack of availability of an external defibrillator in the presence of ventricular fibrillation
6. A failure to respond adequately to closed-chest compression (should the patient be in the operating room under a well-controlled situation, one should open the chest in 2 to 3 minutes)
7. In some instances of severe mitral stenosis (commissurotomy may be the emergency procedure of choice)
8. Pregnancy (third trimester)
9. Flail chest
10. Massive pulmonary embolism
11. Evidence of intrathoracic hemorrhage or severe trauma to the chest
12. Penetrating thoracic injuries
13. Ventricular herniation after cardiac surgery
14. When the heart's anatomic position is not in the midline
15. When one desires visual monitoring of the heart
16. With other causes of intracardiac obstructions, such as a left atrial myxoma
17. When the chest is already opened

Prognosis

How often are cardiopulmonary resuscitative efforts likely to be needed outside of the hospital? The full scope of the picture is yet to emerge but it is known that over 800,000 individuals in this country die each year of heart attacks. Over 50% of those patients dying of heart attacks die before reaching the hospital. In fact, over 50% of those dying of severe injuries die before reaching the hospital. There is good evidence that a substantial percentage of these patients could be saved if adequate resuscitative efforts were immediately available.

What can one expect of his resuscitative efforts? At the time of this writing, even resuscitative efforts under the most ideal conditions in the hospital are seldom producing successful results in more than 20% of the instances. There has been a permanent success rate in just over 16% of over 5,000 reported cases. Since resuscitative efforts outside the hospital are fraught with many additional problems, it seems unlikely that the success rate will soon approximate that within the hospital. It is likely, however, that these efforts should ultimately yield considerable dividends with improved ability to reach the victim quickly through more effective communications and through the proper training of large numbers of individuals capable of providing resuscitation.

The crux of successful resuscitative efforts revolves around the vital importance of the time factor. Certainly this principle is most important and needs to be reemphasized time and again. Beyond the need for active resuscitative measures, the need for consciousness of the urgency of this situation must play a part in any thoughts relative to cardiac arrest. If the percentage of permanent survivals is to be increased and if neurologic complications are to be reduced, then every possible source of delay in beginning immediate manual systole must be eliminated. In an early study of the first 1,200 recorded cases of cardiac arrest, it became apparent that 94% of the successfully and permanently resuscitated patients had cardiac massage within the first 4 minutes. In other words, cerebral circulation must be artificially augmented within this time period or else permanent irreversible changes will occur.

It is still too early to know what can be accomplished with cardiopulmonary resuscitation for the patient experiencing a sudden arrest from a myocardial infarction. Adequate numbers of cases are still not available. Permanent success with 15% to 20% of such cases has been reported in relatively small series. A group at the Royal Victoria Hospital in Belfast, Northern Ireland, has had remarkably high success rates with their mobile coronary care unit.

There may be a number of factors that may contribute to the failure to successfully resuscitate the heart. While much of the success rate may be dictated by the nature of the pathology, some degree of blame can probably be placed on the fact that there may have been an inexcusable delay in instituting proper resuscitation, the resuscitative measures were not adequate, or the individual applying resuscitation had inadequate knowledge. Obviously, proper means of compressing the heart will be completely negated if there has been a failure to establish adequate ventilation. Premature discontinuance of resuscitative efforts may be involved. Out of 300 fatal cases of cardiac arrest in one series, for example, almost one third were associated with totally inadequate attempts at resuscitation.

It seems most reasonable to assume that in the near future all medical personnel will be well versed in the techniques of cardiopulmonary resuscitation at an early stage. Practice sessions on resuscitation of the dog heart are essential. There are few better ways to acquaint one with the technique of cardiac resuscitation than by actual experience in the animal laboratory followed by observation of resuscitative efforts on the ward. Formal periods of instruction on cardiac arrest and resuscitation should be repeated each year. There is no reason to neglect training physicians in cardiopulmonary resuscitation, especially at a time when every effort is being made to provide lifesaving technique training to members of the nursing and allied health professions and members of rescue squads.

chapter 11

Immediate emergency management of cardiac arrhythmias and the myocardial infarction victim

Richard H. Martin

It is customary to organize a discussion of the treatment of cardiac arrhythmias by specific diagnostic categories. When considering the definitive therapy of each arrhythmia such an organization is appropriate, since a correct diagnosis should generally be established before treatment is begun. Unfortunately, under emergency circumstances, the equipment necessary to make a definitive diagnosis may not be available. On occasion it may be necessary to begin therapy without electrocardiographic confirmation of the specific type of arrhythmia, based upon careful consideration of the probable diagnoses that might be present, the risk of delaying therapy, and the potential hazard of immediate therapy.

The organization of this chapter therefore will be based upon the clinical presentation of the patient, before an electrocardiogram is available. The discussion will stress emergency measures that can be carried out with reasonable safety before reaching the hospital and will deal only with those steps of diagnosis and treatment that are appropriate in the home, the field, or the emergency room. The treatment of rhythm disorders requiring hospital or coronary care unit admission is beyond the scope of this discussion and is well covered in numerous other sources. Similarly, there will be no attempt here to cover details of electrocardiographic diagnosis of arrhythmias, which can be reviewed in standard textbooks of electrocardiography.

REGULAR TACHYARRHYTHMIAS

In the adult 100 beats per minute is the arbitrary upper limit for resting heart rate. An infant may have a normal sinus rhythm as fast as 200 per minute at 1 month of age, but the resting sinus rate should not exceed 140 per minute after 1 year of age. It is not unusual to find a heart rate of 200 per minute in a young adult during extremely strenuous exertion. Other causes of physiologic sinus tachycardia are fever, emotional stress, and severe pain. In general the sinus tachycardia accompanying these conditions in the adult does not exceed 150 per minute. A potentially more serious cause of sinus tachycardia is thyroid storm complicating thyrotoxicosis.

In a patient with a rapid regular pulse the diagnostic considerations are sinus tachycardia and three types of ectopic tachycardia: (1) supraventricular tachycardia (a categorical term that includes atrial tachycardia and atrioventricular junctional tachycardia), (2) atrial flutter, and (3) ventricular tachycardia. *Sinus tachycardia* requires no treatment except that which may be required for the underlying cause. In the presence of serious underlying heart disease, any rapid ectopic tachycardia can potentially lead to the serious complications of pulmonary edema or cardiovascular collapse.

Certain features are useful in attempting to establish a preliminary diagnosis. Ectopic supraventricular tachycardias usually produce a heart rate in excess of 150 per minute, in contrast to sinus tachycardia, which is rarely faster than 140. It is important to listen to the heart tones to establish the heart rate, since there may be a peripheral pulse deficit at very fast rates as a result of pulsus alternans in the patient with serious myocardial disease. The rate of sinus tachycardia generally varies by 5 to 15 beats per minute over a period of several minutes, in contrast to ectopic tachycardias, which are likely to be quite constant.

Carotid massage characteristically will slow sinus tachycardia slightly, but this may not be detectable without an electrocardiographic recording during the massage. In contrast, there will be no change in rate or abrupt return to normal sinus rhythm during carotid massage in the patient with supraventricular tachycardia. Atrial flutter may show a step-wise decrease in pulse rate because of increased atrioventricular block resulting from the augmented vagal tone induced by carotid massage. Ventricular tachycardia does not change during carotid massage. A hallmark (but not a sine qua non) of ventricular tachycardia is the presence of atrioventricular dissociation. This may be detected by the presence of jugular venous A waves dissociated from the first and second heart sounds and intermittent jugular cannon waves caused by right atrial contractions during ventricular systole against a closed tricuspid valve. The jugular veins on occasion may also establish a diagnosis of atrial flutter by revealing flutter waves (at a rate of 250 to 350 per minute).

The most important determinant of the potential need for treatment before an electrocardiogram can be obtained is the clinical setting in which tachycardia is observed. A healthy young woman with the sudden appearance of tachycardia of 170 per minute, moderate dyspnea, and lightheadedness is likely to have *paroxysmal atrial tachycardia.* There is often a history of previous episodes or possibly of an electrocardiographic diagnosis of Wolff-Parkinson-White syndrome. She generally does not require immediate treatment. Indeed, carotid massage should be deferred until an electrocardiogram is recorded in order to establish a diagnosis. After the diagnosis has been documented on one or more occasions, it is acceptable to treat recurrences in the home. Often the patient can be taught to terminate paroxysms by a Valsalva maneuver or gagging, both of which augment vagal tone. Carotid massage is generally somewhat more effective but is not without hazard, particularly in the elderly patient. It should not be maintained for more than 5 seconds and should never be applied bilaterally. If drug therapy is required, the patient should be monitored by electrocardiography in an emergency room or the physician's office. Normotensive young patients may convert when mild hypertension is induced by methoxamine, 10 to 20 mg intramuscularly or 5 to 15 mg intravenously. Edrophonium (Tensilon), 5 to 10 mg intravenously, is usually well tolerated and has effectively terminated supraventricular tachycardia in many patients since this use of the drug was introduced in 1969. If the tachycardia is well tolerated, a hypnotic drug may allow the paroxysm to terminate during sleep. If more urgent conversion is warranted, digitalis glycosides generally are the most effective drugs, particularly if manifestations of congestive failure are present. After administration of 0.5 mg of digoxin, carotid massage should be repeated, since the vagal effect of both measures will be additive. Propranolol, 1 to 2 mg intravenously, may also be effective. If the situation is critical or if rapid certain conversion to sinus rhythm is desirable for other reasons, synchronized precordial shock (cardioversion) under light sedation with diazepam or sodium pentothal will usually terminate supraventricular tachycardia immediately.

Atrial flutter is relatively uncommon and usually accompanies underlying mitral valve or congential heart disease. It occasionally complicates acute pulmonary embolism, which should be suspected in a previously healthy individual who suddenly develops atrial flutter or atrial fibrillation associated with acute dyspnea, with or without chest pain or hypotension. In contrast to atrial fibrillation, which is differentiated at the bedside by its irregular ventricular rate, the ventricular rate in atrial flutter often fails to slow after administration of digitalis. Misguided efforts to slow the pulse rate in atrial flutter with large doses of digitalis commonly result in digitalis intoxication. Because of this problem, it is often best to promptly terminate acute atrial flutter with synchronized precordial shock before administering digitalis, which can make cardioversion somewhat hazardous. Quinidine may also terminate atrial flutter. It should never be administered in an attempt to convert atrial flutter until after adequate digitalization has been accomplished, because of the risk of reducing atrioventricular block, leading to a 1:1 ventricular response to each flutter wave at a rate in excess of 200. Quinidine should not be given in doses exceeding 0.4 gm every 6 hours because of the risk of cardiac or respiratory arrest with high doses of this drug. High-dose quinidine therapy has been replaced by cardioversion, which is much safer and much more likely to terminate the arrhythmia.

Tachycardia detected in a patient with crushing substernal pain, diaphoresis, and a sensation of impending doom (the classic symptoms of acute myocardial infarction) may represent sinus tachycardia, supraventricular tachycardia, atrial flutter, or ventricular tachycardia. *Ventricular tachycardia* is a particularly life-threatening problem in this setting. It usually produces a heart rate between 100 and 180 per minute. It is more likely to cause hypotension or loss of consciousness than are the supraventricular arrhythmias. If ventricular tachycardia is a significant consideration in a patient with severe cardiovascular distress, an attempt should be made to terminate the rhythm without delay.

Occasionally a sharp blow delivered with the fist to the precordium will terminate a paroxysm of ventricular tachycardia; this is particularly true if the blow is delivered within a few seconds of the onset of ventricular tachycardia induced by a premature ventricular beat occurring in the vulnerable period of the cardiac cycle. If such a blow does not promptly break the arrhythmia, lidocaine should be administered in a dose of 100 mg intravenously. If the rhythm is actually sinus or supraventricular tachycardia, lidocaine will be ineffective but the dose will have done no appreciable harm. If a precordial blow or lidocaine administration terminates the arrhythmia, a continuous drip of lidocaine, 1 to 4 mg per minute, should be maintained during transport of the patient to a hospital or coronary care unit. After electrocardiographic confirmation of the diagnosis, if lidocaine has not been effective, precordial shock should be administered as soon as possible, since ventricular fibrillation may supervene as a result of several factors that include further reduction in coronary blood flow to already ischemic areas of the myocardium.

IRREGULAR TACHYARRHYTHMIAS

A rapid irregular rhythm may result from premature atrial (or junctional) contractions, premature ventricular contractions, atrial fibrillation, or multifocal atrial tachycardia. Multiple premature beats generally produce a patterned irregularity, while atrial fibrillation and multifocal atrial tachycardia cause the rhythm to be totally irregular. Premature beats occur commonly in normal individuals and usually require no treatment. Acute *atrial fibrillation*, likewise, is usually fairly well tolerated, allowing time for transport to a hospital for definitive diagnosis and treatment. When atrial fibrillation results in a very rapid ventricular response in a patient with a serious underlying heart disease, emergency treatment may be indicated prior to admission to the hospital. In the presence of mitral stenosis, the sudden onset of atrial fibrillation with a fast ventricular response may quickly lead to pulmonary edema.

Efforts should be directed toward slowing the ventricular rate rather than immediate conversion. This can usually be accomplished with digitalis glycosides. Care should be taken to avoid overdosage since such patients have often already been receiving digitalis. Digoxin given intravenously in 0.25- or 0.125-mg increments every 2 to 4 hours will usually be effective. Rarely, propranolol may be necessary, in combination with digitalis, to secure adequate slowing. Caution is required with propranolol, however, for its myocardial depressant effects may aggravate congestive heart failure. It is contraindicated if there is a history of bronchial asthma. Conversion of acute atrial fibrillation is most safely and surely accomplished by cardioversion, which should be carried out unless the prognosis for prolonged sinus rhythm is very poor or unless conversion occurs spontaneously, after digitalization, or after administration of quinidine, 0.2 to 0.4 gm every 6 hours (given primarily to minimize the likelihood of reversion to atrial fibrillation after cardioversion).

Multifocal atrial tachycardia is impossible to differentiate from atrial fibrillation without an electrocardiogram. It is usually encountered in severe, life-threatening illnesses such as septic (or less commonly hemorrhagic) shock or acute respiratory failure. There is no effective means of controlling this arrhythmia or slowing the heart rate in this condition; pushing digitalis in attempting to do so is a certain way to produce digitalis intoxication.

Premature beats in the setting of a suspected acute myocardial infarction frequently warn of impending, more serious arrhythmias. The peripheral pulse may feel as though there are dropped beats and thus may suggest intermittent second-degree heart block. Auscultation of the heart while palpating the carotid pulse should resolve this problem. It is impossible to differentiate between atrial and ventricular premature beats without an electrocardiogram (even with one this is often difficult). There are so many exceptions to the "rule" that premature ventricular contractions have a fully compensatory pause that this feature is useless in making decisions regarding therapy. It is reasonable to act on the assumption that all premature beats early in the course of an acute mycardial infarction are premature ventricular contractions. Thus premature beats in this setting should be treated promptly with intravenous lidocaine (50- to 100-mg bolus followed by a drip of 1 to 4 mg per minute during transport to the hospital and coronary care unit), particularly if the frequency of premature beats exceeds 6 per minute. As in the case of sustained tachycardia during an acute myocardial infarction, it would appear to be far safer to administer lidocaine unnecessarily (and ineffectively) for atrial arrhythmias than to allow a ventricular arrhythmia to progress to ventricular fibrillation because a relatively innocuous drug has been withheld.

BRADYARRHYTHMIAS

Although the accepted lower limit of normal sinus rhythm in adults is 60 beats per minute, it is not unusual to see physiologic *sinus bradycardia* with a rate of 40 or 50 beats in healthy adults of all age groups. Sinus bradycardia may be seen in patients under treatment with propranolol for prevention of tachyarrhythmias, reserpine for hypertension, and on occasion a variety of other drugs. Any condition associated with increased vagal tone—for example, nausea and vomiting—may produce sinus bradycardia, as may myxedema, hypothermia resulting from prolonged cold exposure, obstructive jaundice, and cerebrovascular accidents associated with increased intracranial pressure.

A particularly common syndrome in which profound sinus bradycardia is a frequent finding is *vasodepressor (vasovagal) syncope,* the common fainting spell. Such fainting may occur at any age but is most characteristically seen in young healthy individuals subjected to a sudden emotional stress such as threatened or imagined bodily injury. The patient has generally been noted to have collapsed to the floor, usually without warning. He may appear to be near death, with profound hypotension, marked pallor, and diaphoresis. The pupils may be dilated. Respiration may be shallow or deep and sighing. There may be alarming bradycardia (rates of 20 to 30 beats are not uncommon). Heart tones may be distant, suggesting severe cardiac disease. Clonic movements may occur, localized to the face and upper body or occasionally generalized.

The ultimate mechanisms underlying vasodepressor syncope have fascinated investigators for many years and remain the subject of some uncertainty. It is evident that there is profound autonomic activity during the faint; this factor is responsible for the bradycardia (vagal effect). The hypotension results from pooling of blood in capacitance vessels of the body, so that venous return cannot keep up with the demand for increased cardiac output that would ordinarily accompany the drop in peripheral resistance characteristic of this syndrome. These physiologic mechanisms provide the rationale for therapy, which consists of placing the victim supine with the head and trunk lower than the legs (to augment venous return) and giving reassurance verbally and by maintaining a calm environment about the patient. The syndrome will usually clear quickly without further therapy; occasionally intravenous atropine, 0.5 to 1.0 mg, may be necessary to reverse the marked bradycardia, and rarely vasopressor agents may be needed if hypotension is prolonged.

Some patients may develop a syndrome similar to vasodepressor syncope during acute myocardial infarction. The age of the patient and the presence of severe chest pain (usually but not invariably present) help to differentiate this life-threatening problem from the benign simple vasodepressor faint. Diaphragmatic wall myocardial infarction is particularly likely to produce this *bradycardia-hypotension syndrome,* which, like vasodepressor syncope, is usually associated with diaphoresis and other signs of autonomic hyperactivity. Bradycardia in this setting is particularly dangerous, since it predisposes to the development of ectopic beats, which may lead to ventricular tachycardia or fibrillation. In addition the bradycardia, coupled with the limited stroke volume of an acutely damaged left ventricle, impairs cardiac output and intensifies the hypotension, which initially results from inadequate peripheral resistance and venous pooling. Hypotension may then beget further reduction in mycardial perfusion and further myocardial ischemia or necrosis, or both, and may lead to a vicious circle and death. Morphine, given appropriately to relieve chest pain and allay anxiety in the patient before transport to the hospital, causes dilation of arterioles and veins that can intensify this process. Therapy consists of elevating the lower extremities to increase venous return to the heart, administration of vasopressors if necessary to maintain a blood pressure of 90 to 100 systolic (in a previously normotensive subject, higher in the hypertensive patient), and the immediate intravenous injection of atropine, 0.5 to 1.0 mg. Atropine should be injected slowly (over 1 to 2 minutes) in this circumstance because on rare occasions rapid injection of the drug may cause a sudden release of acetylcholine from cardiac vagal nerve endings and produce a paradoxic vagal effect with complete asystole or heart block.

Marked bradycardia or asystole may also result from *heart block* or less commonly from *sinoatrial arrest.* These two conditions generally occur in patients over the age of 50 years, as a result of degeneration of the specialized fibers of the cardiac conduction system and sinus node, or coronary heart disease. Such patients most commonly seek help because of an episode of syncope or near-syncope. There is usually no associated chest pain. The pulse pressure is usually wide because of the large stroke volume accompanying the slow idioventricular rhythm that generally becomes established after several seconds of asystole. Hypotension is unusual once an escape rhythm appears. Ausculation may reveal atrial sounds dissociated from S_1 and S_2, and occasional cannon waves may be seen in the jugular veins. Asystole may recur at any time in such patients, who should be observed continously until such time as effective therapy with a transvenous pacemaker has been established.

In this electronic age, physicians often feel helpless without an oscilloscopic electrocardiographic monitor under such circumstances. They forget that each patient has been endowed with a very effective built-in heartbeat detector: the peripheral pulse. A finger on the pulse continuously will detect recurrent asystole before sufficient time has elapsed for the patient to lose consciousness. A sharp blow to the precordium during this interval will do little to further a budding doctor-patient relationship but will usually mechanically stimulate the myocardium sufficiently to trigger ventricular depolarization and obviate the need for cardiac massage, a most difficult procedure during transport to a hospital. In the absence of a specific electrocardiographic diagnosis in such a patient, it is reasonable to administer atropine, which may increase the heart rate and reduce the risk of recurrent asystole if the mechanism has been marked sinus bradycardia, sinus arrest, or heart block in the atrioventricular junctional region. Atropine will have no effect in the statistically more likely event that the block in such a patient occurs below the atrioventricular node, in the bundle of His, or its more distal ramifications. Isoproterenol increases the irritability of myocardial cells with pacemaker potential in the sinus node, atrium, atrioventricular junction, and ventricle; in addition, its effect on the atrioventricular node may reduce block at that level. Thus this drug may be effective regardless of the cause of the asystole. If atropine has not resulted in a heart rate of at least 60 per minute within 5 minutes, an intravenous drip of isoproterenol should be begun (1 to 2 mg in 500 ml at an infusion rate of 0.01 to 0.03 µg/kg/minute). Even if this does not increase the heart rate, it may reduce the chances of prolonged asystole or make the myocardium more responsive to the occasional precordial blow required for episodic asystole. The patient should be transported to a hospital with facilities for artificial pacemaker implantation without delay. Therapy of heart block with sodium lactate infusion, corticosteroids, or potassium solutions has no place in the emergency treatment of the patient with asystole.

An increasingly common cause of asystole and bradycardia is sudden failure of an implanted cardiac pacemaker. Pacemaker failure generally results from cessation of effective pacing, and the patient should be dealt with in a manner outlined above. Less commonly an implanted pacemaker may accelerate to a dangerously high rate, also leading to near-syncope. In this circumstance antiarrhythmic drugs will not be effective, and the pacemaker must be inactivated and replaced by another unit as soon as possible.

PROPHYLACTIC ANTIARRHYTHMIC DRUGS IN ACUTE MYOCARDIAL INFARCTION

The major impact of the coronary care unit in reducing the mortality of acute myocardial infarction has resulted not from the original goal of prompt resuscitation of cardiac arrest but instead from *prevention* of cardiac arrest. This has been accomplished by identifying warning arrhythmias and initiating antiarrhythmic therapy before the appearance of ventricular tachycardia, ventricular fibrillation, or asystole. It has been established that the risk of serious arrhythmias resembles a logarithmic function of time from onset of infarction, with the highest risk immediately after the onset of the chest pain and a diminishing risk thereafter. Thus it appears reasonable to extend the principles of coronary care to the suspected victim of myocardial infarction before he reaches the coronary care unit and thus into the earliest moments after infarction, when the risk of cardiac arrest is highest. Mobile coronary care units have achieved notable results with this approach. However, it seems unlikely that mobile coronary care will be available to the majority of patients sustaining acute myocardial infarction in the foreseeable future. The question thus arises whether the principles of prevention of life-threatening arrhythmias cannot be applied in the absence of the sophisticated electronics of the mobile coronary care unit.

The preceding discussions of ventricular tachycardia, premature ventricular contractions, and the bradycardia-hypotension syndrome in acute myocardial infarction have been in large part based upon the as yet largely untested assumption that such prophylaxis is indeed applicable. Recently it has been suggested that this approach be extended to include all patients with suspected myocardial infarction, even in the absence of a detectable arrhythmia. It has been proposed that lidocaine be given to all such patients (50 mg intravenously, 100 to 200 mg intramuscularly) provided that the heart rate is above 60. If the initial rate is below 60, lidocaine carries the risk of suppression of "backup" idioventricular pacemaker foci, which might be needed if sinus arrest or complete heart block were to ensue. Thus in such patients a small dose of atropine (0.3 mg intravenously) has been recommended in place of lidocaine, on the assumption that bradyarrhythmias are the most likely threat to the patient. It should be kept in mind that there are as yet no data to support the use of these approaches, which are, however, based upon reasonably sound assumptions and are being adopted quite widely at the time of this writing.

chapter 12

Immediate management of airway emergencies

Few emergencies create such panic in the victim or in the observer as those having to do with sudden airway obstruction. There are few considerations of an emergency nature that will require a more thorough understanding of the anatomy and physiology involved than those associated with the respiratory emergency. Cardiopulmonary resuscitation has been considered in some detail in Chapter 10. A number of the principles considered in that chapter will be applicable here also. Furthermore, Chapter 13, Near-Drowning, includes special aspects of artificial ventilation.

Airway emergencies include a wide gamut of etiologic factors. Aspirated foreign bodies are responsible for an inordinately large percentage of accidental deaths in the young child. In the adult, there is a condition termed the "cafe coronary." This refers to the clinical observation suggesting an apparent sudden heart attack when in actuality it represents the inadvertent swallowing of too large a bolus of food with resultant airway obstruction and often death.

How long does it take for complete airway obstruction to cause death? Asphyxia for a period of between 5 and 10 minutes is all that is required. The hypoxia as well as hypercapnia (accumulation of carbon dioxide) obviously represents an emergency of almost the same time proportions as sudden cessation of cardiac output. Under conditions of asphyxia the heart may continue to beat for several minutes but all available oxygen stores are rapidly depleted. Cardiac output rapidly becomes ineffective and ventricular fibrillation may be initiated.

It may seem that airway obstruction would be readily recognized. Such, however, is not always the case. In the unconscious patient whose head and neck muscles are relaxed and whose neck in a partially flexed position, the tongue may be relaxed so as to press against the posterior pharyngeal wall. Not all victims become cyanotic. In some there may actually be a vasodilation set off by the hypoxemia that is present. An appraisal of the color of the nail beds, conjuctiva, or mucous membranes may be misleading, particularly in dark-skinned individuals. In some patients there may be no airway obstruction, but respiratory movements of the chest or abdomen cannot be detected. Under such a profound state of hypoventilation as may be found in patients somnolent from hypercapnia or suffering the effects of massive drug overdose, one may need to hold a wisp of cotton in front of the patient's mouth or nose to detect any air current.

There are various degrees of partial airway obstruction. Depending on the degree of obstruction, intrathoracic pressure fluctuations are increased along with the efforts of breathing. Gradually the respiratory center becomes less sensitive to the usual stimulant from a buildup of carbon dioxide.

Marked activity of the accessory muscles of respiration in the neck and supraclavicular and intercostal areas should alert one to the presence of severe or even complete airway obstruction. If the airway obstruction is complete one will hear no air flow; if it is incomplete various degrees of noise intensity may be provoked, depending upon the degree of obstruction. Snoring is probably the best known example of partial airway obstruction and is simply produced by hypopharyngeal obstruction by the tongue. The wheezing effect of the asthmatic patient caused by partial bronchial obstruction is well known. Laryngospasm produces a characteristic crowing sound. Foreign matter obstructing the airway may occasionally produce a gurgling noise.

Dr. Peter Safar has repeatedly stressed the principles necessary for the recognition and management of airway obstruction. He recommends that a sequence of activities be followed until one is satisfied that an open airway exists:

1. The unconscious patient should be properly *positioned*. He should be supine with the head tilted back. The unconscious patient should not be placed in the prone position for a number of reasons. Not only is the face inaccessible for mouth-to-mouth respiration, but such a position may further promote mechanical obstruction.

2. Perhaps the most effective step one can take in promoting an open airway in the unconscious patient is to simply *tilt the head backward* by placing one hand under the patient's neck and the other at the patient's forehead. This maneuver stretches the tissues between the larynx and the mandible and lifts the base of the tongue from the posterior pharyngeal wall. In some instances elevation of the patient's shoulders may further facilitate the tilting of the patient's head. The patient's mouth will usually open when the head is tilted back and this may, indeed, be advantageous, particularly when there is partial or complete nasal obstruction.

3. Mouth-to-mouth or mouth-to-nose respiration should be applied by exhaling into the patient's air passages. The *positive airway pressure* may help overcome obstruction by increasing the pressure gradient for air flow and by dilating the air passages.

4. In approximately one out of five patients the preceding steps will still not result in an open airway, and an additional maneuver should be performed, namely the *forward displacement* of the mandible. This can be done simply by lifting the mandible with one's hands at the ascending rami or placing one's thumb in the mouth and pulling the mandible forward. If the mouth does open with the backward tilting of the head, then one should separate the patient's lips and teeth in the event that an expiratory nasal obstruction is present.

5. The airway may still not be open. *A foreign body may be in the back of the pharynx* and can be quickly removed by turning the patient's head to the side, forcing the mouth to open, and wiping the pharynx and mouth clean with the fingers or, if available, by the use of suction. Obviously one must not risk further spinal cord damage by twisting the cervical spine in cases of possible fracture of that area.

The most recent advice disseminated to the lay public by the American Heart Association for the immediate handling of something stuck in the throat of an infant or small child is to pick the infant up and turn him upside down over one's arm. The infant should then be slapped or hit between the shoulder blades. Frequently this will dislodge the foreign body. In the adult, however, one may harm the individual by a hard slap on the back because it may cause the victim to take a deep gasping breath and instead of coughing out the food or foreign body, he may well suck it further down into the airway.

6. *Artificial oral airways* may be necessary to hold the base of the tongue forward and maintain the lips and teeth in an open position. The nasopharyngeal tube, if available, may be particularly valuable in the patient with trismus (spasm of the jaw muscles preventing easy opening of the mouth). The familiar S shaped oropharyngeal airway may be used, as may the simple comma shaped airway, often referred to as the Guedel airway. If a nasopharyngeal tube is not available, the mouth may be forced open by sliding the index finger backward between the cheek and the teeth and then wedging the tip of the index finger behind the last molars. If the jaws are not clenched, the oropharyngeal tube may be inserted by forcing the mouth open with the thumb and index finger crossed, inserting the tube over the tongue, and twisting it into position. The Brook airway is an oral airway that prevents any throat obstruction by the tongue by hyperextending the victim's head. Unlike the oropharyngeal airway, it is not likely to stimulate vomiting and cause aspiration of the gastric contents in the partially comatose patient. Occasionally an oral airway may even reach beyond the pharynx and obstruct the air passage by impacting the epiglottis.

Each individual can serve as an effective pulmonary resuscitation unit. The air we breathe contains over 20% oxygen and 0.04% carbon dioxide. Our exhaled air contains 16% oxygen and 4% carbon dioxide. Instinctively, one will breathe more deeply when applying mouth-to-mouth resuscitation, thereby enhancing the quantity and quality of his expired air. The victim will subsequently receive twice his normal tidal volume of air containing as much as 18% oxygen and 2% carbon dioxide. Generally speaking, after about 15 seconds or five deep inflations, the victim's lungs will contain near-normal amounts of oxygen and carbon dioxide.

7. *Tracheal intubation* may be required. When it is imperative that the tracheobronchial tree be rapidly suctioned, when gastric contents have been aspirated, and when the preceding steps have not been sufficient to maintain adequate oxygenation, a rapid insertion of the endotracheal tube is indicated. Obviously the endotracheal tube may not be available in many emergency situations, but it should be a part of the equipment on every ambulance. The endotracheal tube will not be tolerated easily by the conscious or partially conscious patient. Most medical students will not have had opportunity to learn the technique of rapid passage of the endotracheal tube at an early period in their medical school curriculum but certainly by the end of the junior year this should be a part of their armamentarium.

Of immediate urgency in the event that endotracheal intubation is impossible may be the need to perform a rapid cricothyrotomy. This technique simply denotes puncture of the cricothyroid membrane. Puncture of this membrane may be accomplished with relative ease by using a knife blade or a large-bore needle. Acute obstructive laryngeal edema from an allergic reaction to penicillin, hemorrhage into neck tissue planes, or an engorgement of particulate matter such as food in the larynx all provide indications for immediately establishing an airway via the cricothyroid membrane puncture. If an inability to inflate or deflate the lungs is noted upon mouth-to-mouth respiration, obstructions of this nature can be suspected.

Entry through this relatively avascular membrane is easily made because of its superficial position and adjacent cartilagenous landmarks. The cricothyroid space is quite large and can accept fairly large tubes. Posterior perforation may occur, but protection is offered by the heavy posterior projection of the cricoid cartilage. In order to perform a cricothyroid membrance puncture, one should stabilize the larynx between the left thumb and the middle finger. The skin is incised by scissors or knife over the cricothyroid space. The scissors or knife is then guided down the index finger to puncture the membrane. One of the major advantages of the cricothyroidotomy is that it is a quick, easy technique with no major blood vessels in the area, and there is very little tissue between the skin and the trachea. As soon as the knife blade enters the trachea, the resistance gives away and the incision can be enlarged to at least 1.5 cm. A tracheostomy tube can be put in place if one is available.

If one notices that the suprasternal notch is drawn upward when the patient takes a breath, one may suspect that the foreign body has lodged above the level of the cricothyroid membrane puncture site and that the emergency procedure may be lifesaving.

Tracheostomy is often described as an emergency procedure and is frequently used as such. Actually, it is poorly suited as an emergency technique and for all practical purposes should not be strongly considered at this point. Tracheostomy should be performed under ideal situations, most frequently in the operating room with the patient well oxygenated via an endotracheal tube, if possible. The tracheostomy is best reserved for individuals who will need to have assisted ventilation over a prolonged period of time. Theoretically, the tracheostomy might be reserved for upper airway obstruction if the cricothyroid membrane puncture is not effective. Usually the tracheostomy is indicated for patients who for one reason or another cannot bring up their secretions. These are usually patients with neurologic trauma or injuries, severe inanition, or chronic lung disease and bronchitis. Patients who have had severe trauma may often require a tracheostomy. Particularly do we employ a tracheostomy in patients with a flail chest. Patients with conditions such as a fractured larynx or an acutely obstructing carcinoma of the larynx may require an emergency tracheostomy, but in each instance a cricothyroid membrane puncture will be more rapidly accomplished.

Because of the belief that an emergency tracheostomy is generally outside the scope of this book, its detailed description of the technique will not be included.

Occasionally a bronchoscopy may be necessary as an emergency procedure for lower airway obstruction, aspiration, and atelectasis, but this will be reserved for the individual skilled in its use.

Once the airway is patent, artificial ventilation may be satisfactorily accomplished. This can best be accomplished by intermittent inflation of the lungs with positive pressure applied to the airway. Mouth-to-mouth, mouth-to-nose, mouth-to-tube, or a bag-mask ventilation apparatus may be used. In most instances the most available technique will be either the mouth-to-mouth or mouth-to-nose ventilation approach.

During mouth-to-mouth respiration, the nose should be compressed with one hand; the other hand should be used to apply pressure over the patient's upper abdomen and epigastrium to prevent distension of the stomach by air. The mouth of the patient may be covered by several thin layers of gauze, a handkerchief, or even a thin paper towel. Prior to expiration, the operator should take a deep inspiration and then immediately apply his widely opened mouth over the mouth of the patient and made a forcible exhalation. The uninitiated will be surprised at the degree of inflation produced by this method. The patient's chest will be observed to expand as the air is blown into his mouth, and when the operator raises his mouth from that of the patient, a rush of air will be heard coming from the patient's lungs. This latter aspect can be improved be forcible pressure on the patient's chest. As in all other methods of artificial respiration, the tongue must be brought forward, since it may occlude the oral pharynx. Again it should be pointed out that one may have confidence in one's ability to perform mouth-to-mouth respiration when it is recalled that 16 mm Hg pressure is the level of oxygen pressure developed by most of the positive-negative pulmonary resuscitators. Men can exhale with a force of 50 mm Hg, and this figure may even reach 100 mm Hg. A rate of at least twelve times a minute is suggested. One should exhale twice one's normal resting tidal volume (about 1,000 ml). Inadequate oxygenation is often the result of exhalations that are too slow.

Caution should be observed in the use of mouth-to-mouth respiration with infants, since a pressure may be exerted by the operator that will be sufficient to rupture some of the alveoli. As in all types of artificial respiration, there is the problem of keeping the airway patent. This can be aided by pulling the tongue forward or, most ideally, by insertion of the endotracheal tube or catheter. If one uses excessively high inflation pressures during artificial ventilation, some of the air will be forced into the stomach by means of an open esophagus. Don Michael,* concerned about the inflation of the stomach that occurs in the course of routine mouth-to-mouth respiration, has developed an airway that can be easily introduced into the esophagus and can be manipulated so that a balloon obliterates this orifice.

Artificial respiration may be best applied by the mouth-to-nose technique in several instances. For example, the individual applying artificial respiration may be unable to completely seal his mouth around the patient's mouth. If transient rigidity, trismus, or convulsions are present, mouth-to-nose respiration should be used. A patient with a broken jaw may have his teeth wired. Even so, blowing between the teeth may be successful.

The mouth-to-tube device ensures that adequate volume of sufficient gas composition is delivered to the patient. Unlike other forms of artificial respiration, the mouth-to-tube method does not depend upon the operator's observation and judgment to determine whether ventilation of the patient is adequate. The mouth-mask or mouth-to-tube methods have advantages over the simple mouth-to-mouth procedure in that both hands of the operator are available to maintain patency of the upper airway. The operator is able to sense any increase in pulmonary resistance by the amount of exertion it takes to deflate his own lungs.

The mouth-to-tube method of respiration has several points in its favor besides that of prevention of hypocapnia in the operator. These include the prevention of cross-contamination between the operator and the patient if a disposable filter is placed in the breathing tube. The method can be continued for long periods of time, and no special position of the patient is required by the operator. The equipment is of minimal expense, and adequate ventilation is ensured in spite of abnormalities in airway resistance and in lung compliance.

Most ambulances carry the self-refilling bag-valve-mask units for artificial ventilation using the above-mentioned means of keeping the airway open. The mask is applied to the

---

*Brunswick Manufacturing Co., Inc., 90 Myrtie Street, North Quincy, Mass. 02171.

face with one hand and the bag is squeezed rhythmically with the other hand. The nonrebreathing valve should permit inhalation of oxygen from the bag during spontaneous and artificial respiration.

Generally speaking, automatic resuscitators have very little place in emergency artificial respiration and particularly in conjunction with cardiac resuscitation. External cardiac compression triggers the termination of the inflation phase prematurely, and flow rates and pressures are usually inadequate.

CARBON MONOXIDE POISONING

Carbon monoxide, an odorless and colorless gas, is responsible for death under a variety of circumstances. In some large city hospital emergency rooms it is the second most common cause of poisoning death, next to alcohol.

The treatment of carbon monoxide poisoning is obviously of a most urgent nature. Even though permanent brain damage may have occurred before treatment is begun, one cannot, of course, be immediately aware of this fact. The first thing one does is to remove the victim from the environment contaminated with carbon monoxide. Artificial ventilation must be started at once, with mouth-to-mouth respiration being a satisfactory approach. It is with carbon monoxide poisoning that oxygen under high pressure is important, more so than with patients who have nearly drowned or who have been exposed to electric shock. Pure oxygen under 2.5 atmospheres of pressure will reduce blood carboxyhemoglobin by 50% in approximately 40 minutes. With room air the same reduction would take 250 minutes. The high oxygen pressure chambers are ideal for carbon monoxide poisoning, but unfortunately they are not easily available to most patients around the country.

Morphine sulfate is not indicated with carbon monoxide poisoning. Respiratory stimulants are of little value. Whole blood transfusions have been advocated by some but are of questionable value. Methylene blue is no longer used. If there has been a question of considerable cerebral anoxia, it may prove helpful to put the patient in a hypothermic state as soon as the hospital is reached.

The question of giving carbon dioxide is often raised. The British Medical Council recently voiced an affirmative vote in favor of the 5% mixture of carbon dioxide. Those advocating a carbon dioxide mixture do so with the belief that a high level of carbon dioxide increases the ventilation, helps carboxyhemoglobin dissociation, and may serve to raise the oxygen pressure. On the other hand, the respiratory center may have already experienced excessive carbon dioxide exposure, and by giving carbon dioxide one depresses the amount of oxygen that can be delivered. In summary, the question of the use of carbon dioxide in carbon monoxide poisoning is not entirely clear at this moment.

Newspapers carry accounts of carbon monoxide poisoning almost daily. Carbon monoxide may result from any fire in a closed space. Faulty exhaust pipes and wornout mufflers or manifolds often lead to carbon monoxide leakage into the closed automobile. An automobile engine that is idling will double its rate of carbon monoxide exhaust. Children have been fatally poisoned in closed cars while waiting for parents in grocery stores or on other errands. The heater takes in exhaust fumes from the car in front, and the carbon monoxide level within the car may build up rapidly. Birds building nests during the spring and summer often plug flues, which in turn may produce carbon monoxide poisoning to the members of the household in the fall. A flue plugged with soot may do the same thing. It is dangerous for one to move his barbecue grill into a closed garage in case of inclement weather. The use of the grill may provide an excellent opportunity for the accumulation of carbon monoxide within the closed, unvented garage. Guards in tunnels and workers in kilns are subjected to high levels of carbon monoxide inhalation. Drivers on crowded roadways are often required to creep along bumper to bumper for a considerable distance. The carbon monoxide drawn into the car from the car in front may be enough to produce a dangerous level of carbon monoxide poisoning in the driver. This may be responsible for faulty judgment on the part of the driver. Unfortunately, carbon monoxide gas has no odor, but its presence should be suspected whenever an unconscious patient is found in a garage or inside a closed building.

The *subjective complaints* experienced by the patient include headache, vertigo, irritability, frequent yawning, ringing in the ears, a feeling of tightness at the forehead, weakness, dimmed vision, aching limbs, a throbbing heart, a feeling of lethargy, vomiting, collapse, and unconsciousness.

The patient may not present the pathognomonic cherry red color at the onset but may be somewhat dusky in color. Muscular twitching, a rapid pulse, hyperreflexia, warm skin, dilated pupils, and Cheyne-Stokes respirations may be evident. Coma and unconsciousness may be evident when the patient is first seen.

The hypoxia and poisoning of tissues by carbon monoxide results from the special affinity of hemoglobin for carbon monoxide. This affinity is 200 to 300 times greater than that which hemoglobin shows for oxygen. Carbon monoxide and hemoglobin combine to form carboxyhemoglobin. Respiratory enzymes have a greater affinity for carbon monoxide than oxygen. There is evidence that carbon monoxide acts directly on cerebral tissue and causes brain damage, particularly in the area of the globus pallidus.

chapter 13

Near-drowning

Before considering the immediate measures necessary to resuscitate a submersion or near-drowning victim, one should be reminded of several considerations. For one thing, it is no longer considered desirable to spend precious early seconds during the resuscitation period in trying to remove water from the patient's lungs. If the drowning has occurred in fresh water, this hypotonic solution will be rapidly absorbed through the lungs. Although the water is less rapidly absorbed in instances of saltwater near-drowning and drowning in chlorinated water pools, simply establishing an airway and allowing postural drainage will allow any trapped water in the lungs to escape. There is strong evidence in some instances that very little water at all enters the lung because of early occurrence of marked larynogospasm.

To a large extent, resuscitation of the nearly drowned patient is simply an extension of the principles of cardiopulmonary resuscitation with the interjection of several specialized components.

PRIORITIES

With these preliminary considerations in mind, what are the immediate priorities that must be met in the resuscitation of the near-drowning victim? Immediate efforts to establish ventilation receive top priority. This may even be instituted before the victim is removed from the water. After removal, the mouth and pharynx should be cleared quickly and mouth-to-mouth ventilation begun. One can use somewhat greater exhalation pressure than ordinarily used because of the beneficial effect of positive pressure breathing on any intrapulmonary shunts and pulmonary edema present. If means are available, the oronasopharynx should be suctioned, an oral airway inserted, and ventilation maintained by means of an Ambu bag. Sometimes the victim will already show efforts at breathing. Coughing may be present. In such instances, an improvement of the airway and assisted ventilation are indicated. Postural positioning of the patient will permit drainage of what little water there is in the lungs.

Obviously, ventilatory support will be of no benefit unless adequate circulatory efforts are taking place. Using the same criteria for establishing the presence or absence of an adequate cardiac output as mentioned elsewhere in the book, one must quickly make a decision whether or not closed-chest cardiac compression is needed. If there is any doubt, manual compression of the chest as detailed in Chapter 10 is begun, along with the maintenance of artificial ventilation.

For many years it has been customary in most communities to call the fire department whenever a near-drowning has occurred, with the idea that the fire department was most likely to have a pulmonary resuscitator available. It may be difficult to realize that mouth-to-mouth ventilation along with closed-chest cardiac compression of the immersion victim are measures that have been generally employed around the country for less than a decade.

VENTRICULAR FIBRILLATION

During transportation to the hospital, 100% oxygen administration via positive pressure breathing is desirable. Obviously, closed-chest resuscitation should be continued if there is an ineffective or absent cardiac output. If the ambulance is equipped with an electrocardiogram (hopefully, all ambulances should have portable electrocardiograms and defibrillators), then the patient should be defibrillated as soon as possible. Originally it was believed that perhaps half of the people who drowned in fresh water experienced ventricular fibrillation. The ventricular fibrillation was thought to be a potassium fibrillation. In dogs the increase in potassium was attributed to anoxemia and to hemolysis with subsequent release of intracellular potassium. This increased incidence of ventricular fibrillation in fresh water drowning has not been adequately documented in clinical cases, however. In any event there are undoubtedly many cases of cardiovascular collapse in which a ventricular fibrillatory rhythm may be established during cardiopulmonary resuscitation.

METABOLIC ACIDOSIS

In addition to the prompt establishment of an adequate airway and, if indicated, cardiac resuscitation via closed-chest massage, other immediate efforts are likely to be most valuable. It now appears that there is an almost inevitable metabolic acidosis associated with these patients and that the sooner the metabolic acidosis is corrected by adequate ventilation and administration of sodium bicarbonate, the sooner adequate perfusion will occur. For this reason an adult should have at least 1 ampule of sodium bicarbonate administered intravenously. Each ampule consists of 44.6 mEq of bicarbonate and comes in a 50-ml ampule of water. If the patient is unconscious or nearly so, 2 ampules may be given in rapid succession. With small children, intravenously administered sodium bicarbonate may be given in a dosage of 1 mEq/kg of body weight. Often the administration of sodium bicarbonate will result in rather immediate dramatic clinical improvement of the patient.

Frequent oronasal suctioning should be instituted as soon as a suctioning device arrives. In addition a cuffed endotracheal tube insertion is advantageous at an early stage for several reasons. Since a large percentage of near-drowning victims vomit during resuscitative procedures, it is desirable to aspirate the gastric contents via a nasogastric tube in order to prevent aspiration of vomitus into lungs that are already severely compromised.

EMERGENCY ROOM CARE

Immediately upon arrival at the emergency room, the effectiveness of ventilatory efforts must be rechecked, electric activity of the myocardium monitored, and closed-chest resuscitation continued as long as necessary, following much the same procedure routine as outlined in Chapter 10, which will not be duplicated at this point. Because a marked metabolic acidosis and hypoxemia may not be clinically apparent, blood samples should be immediately drawn for arterial oxygen and carbon dioxide tensions along with acid-base studies consisting of blood pH and base excess. Blood pH levels below 6.96 have been reported in near-drowning victims who subsequently recovered along with base deficits of -26 mEq/liter. Almost empirically one can administer 1 ampule of sodium bicarbonate to an adult or a graduated dose in a smaller individual.

It is at this point that a mechanical ventilator will most likely have its first usage. Mechanical ventilators at the scene of the drowning or on the way to the hospital are sometimes ineffective because of the unfamiliarity of the rescuer with the equipment.

CONTINUING OBSERVATION

After the patient has arrived in the emergency room and spontaneous respirations and adequate heart action have resumed, much of the immediate action is over. However, further definitive care is almost always necessary since many near-drowning victims may take a turn for the worse several hours after initially successful resuscitative efforts. For one thing, corticosteroids should be administered in large doses if there is any suspicion of prolonged cerebral anoxia and in an effort to reduce subsequent cerebral edema. A dosage schedule as suggested in Chapter 10 may be used. Steroids may also reduce the inflammatory reaction subsequent to aspiration and the resulting aspiration pneumonitis.

The emergency room physicians will obtain chest films, serial electrocardiographic observations, and repeat blood gases. The blood gases will be monitored carefully in order to determine the need for additional buffer solutions such as sodium bicarbonate.

Antifoaming agents such as 20% to 30% ethyl alcohol as an aerosol may be helpful in treating the patient's pulmonary edema, and there is some rationale for use of isoproterenol to reduce bronchospasm. This may be administered either by aerosol inhalation or by the intravenous route. Antibiotics such as ampicillin are usually given as a prophylactic measure. As mentioned earlier, some hemodilution or hemolysis may occur. In most instances in which these factors have been documented, they have been relatively minimal. An intravenous route is maintained. Ideally, lactated Ringer's solution is given at the rate of 10 ml/kg of body weight for the first hour.

In summary, much can be done for the near-drowning victim. Studies of Dr. J. H. Modell at the University of Florida in Gainesville and Dr. Hasan and associates at Mount Sinai in Miami Beach have placed resuscitation of the near-drowning victim on a more rational plane by their careful clinical observation of large numbers of these patients. It is important to remember that the intensity of the cardiopulmonary resuscitative efforts should be maintained throughout, just as they are when any other etiologic factor is involved. The danger of irreversible brain damage always looms as a potential threat, and its likelihood must certainly not be accentuated by any inadequacies on the part of the rescuer.

part three

Mechanical trauma requiring immediate care

chapter 14

Immediate management of injuries to the extremities

Marshall B. Conrad

The application of an emergency splint should not be a complicated or difficult maneuver. Any ambulance that purports to provide emergency service should be equipped so that emergency splints can be applied with facility. However, other materials that are usually readily available can be very adequately utilized. These include triangular bandages or folded towels or sheets to be used for slings and swaths, cardboard or magazines to make excellent short splints, a pillow or blanket wrapped around an injured extremity, or the simple expedient of securing an injured lower extremity to the uninjured leg with adequate padding between them.

It is important to remember that fractures of the spine and pelvis are difficult to detect; the only indication may be the complaint of pain in the affected area. If the victim is unconscious or cannot communicate, the possibility of such an injury must be kept in mind and the victim must be handled accordingly.

FRACTURES OF THE SHOULDER

Fractures about the shoulder involving the scapula, clavicle, or upper humerus should be suspected if the victim complains of pain or tenderness or both in the area of the shoulder. The involved extremity will be protected by the victim, and the shoulder on the involved side may sag. These injuries can be adequately splinted by means of a sling and swath using two triangular bandages. One is applied as a sling and the second used to immobilize the upper arm to the chest wall. Unless other injuries preclude it, these victims are usually more comfortable if transported in a semi-sitting position. Fractures of the upper arm between the shoulder and elbow can be splinted in a similar manner. Fractures about the elbow may be splinted by sling and swath when the elbow can be bent without resistance or increased pain. If the elbow cannot be flexed, then the victim is best transported by a stretcher with the extremity splinted at the victim's side, with adequate padding between the arm and the body.

FRACTURES OF THE ARM

Fractures of the upper extremity below the elbow should be splinted using adequately padded boards extending from the elbow to the fingertips. The extremity is then placed in a sling. Padded boards are recommended since these are widely available and can be

81

considered to be disposable. Inflatable plastic splints are excellent but require special training in their use. Also, they are more expensive than boards and sometimes are hard to retrieve after use. Injuries of the hand must be managed in a similar manner, with a dressing over wounds and immobilization on an adequately padded splint. The hand should be supported on soft padding with the fingers and thumb comfortably flexed.

FRACTURES OF THE LEG

Emergency splinting of fractures involving the lower extremities is a little more complicated but the same principles apply. This can be quickly accomplished by adequately trained personnel, provided the necessary equipment is at hand. For fractures at or above the knee the half-ring traction splint is best. This requires that equipment be available and the attendants be trained in its use. Padded board splints are certainly acceptable, provided that the outer board extends from the axilla on the affected side to below the sole of the foot. The inner board extends from the groin to below the foot. Both boards must be well padded. The application of either of these splints requires a two-man team whereby one man supports and applies gentle traction to the extremity while the second man applies the splint. Plastic inflatable splints are only suitable for fractures below the knee. Other means of splinting injuries below the knee serve equally well, such as a pillow reinforced by boards on the outside. Well-padded boards extending from midthigh to below the foot can be used and are easily obtained. Any open wounds should be covered with a clean or sterile dressing, of course, prior to applying the splint. It will frequently be necessary to realign the extremity if gross deformity is present before the leg can be splinted. This can easily be done by cautiously applying gentle traction. Fractures about the hip are best managed by applying a half-ring traction splint but are equally well handled by supporting the injured extremity on a pillow with the hip and knee flexed slightly and the extremity stabilized by gently strapping it to the stretcher or to the uninjured leg. Fractures of the pelvis usually require no special splinting but the patient should be transported with care on a firm surface. Frequently the patient will be less uncomfortable if the legs are strapped together with adequate padding between them.

DISLOCATIONS

Dislocations of major joints may present special problems. The term *dislocation* may be defined as the complete and persistent displacement of the articular surfaces of a joint. Except for certain major joints, these injuries can be splinted in the same manner as a fracture. Dislocations of the shoulder and the hip, however, usually result in gross deformity such that splinting is difficult. Force in attempting to realign these injuries should never be used, and the involved extremity should be supported in the least painful position.

Most dislocations of joints of the lower extremity can be easily splinted provided voluminous padding is used. As mentioned before, however, a dislocated hip presents a special problem. Dislocations of this joint usually occur as a result of a powerful force applied in the long axis of the femur with the thigh adducted. This results in a posterior dislocation with or without a fracture of the acetabulum and causes a characteristic deformity. The hip is flexed and adducted and cannot be brought down into normal alignment until the dislocation is reduced. Anterior dislocations occur more rarely, and in this injury the deformity of course is in the opposite direction and results in the affected thigh being flexed slightly and externally rotated. A patient with such an injury must therefore be transported with the limb supported and immobilized in the position of deformity. This can best be accomplished by supporting the extremity on multiple pillows or blankets and gently strapping it to the stretcher.

DIAGNOSIS

The following are *symptoms and physical signs* that indicate that a fracture probably occurred:
1. Complaint of pain in the area of injury, provided the victim is conscious and can talk
2. Tenderness elicited by gentle pressure at the site of injury
3. Deformity of the extremity
4. False or unnatural motion at the fracture site
5. Swelling and discoloration

If any of these findings is present, the patient should be handled as if a fracture were present. The possibility of nerve or vascular injury must always be kept in mind and should be noted at the time of the initial examination at the scene. Such information is most useful in evaluating the patient's condition and in planning definitive treatment. It will be most helpful to the treating physician to know whether or not there was evidence of vascular or nerve injury at the scene of the accident or whether competent observation indicated that these structures were intact and that by the time the victim has arrived at the medical facility evidence of vascular or nerve injury has appeared.

As a general rule a fracture, even an open fracture, is not a life-threatening injury. The proper immediate care of fractures is important, however, because of their frequency. Proper emergency splinting will also do much to prevent or control shock. It follows, then, that after the life-threatening conditions have been dealt with, fractures should be splinted before transportation is attempted. Assuming that a quick but thorough survey indicates that no life-threatening conditions are present, then the victim should be checked for soft tissue wounds and for fractures.

The term *fracture* means a break in the continuity of a bone. This results, except in special cases, from the application of considerable force either directly or indirectly. It is important to note the general area of injury and whether the fracture is open or closed. Closed fractures are those in which the skin over the fracture site is intact. These may be displaced or undisplaced and may or may not be comminuted. Open fractures are those in which the skin is open so that there is communication between the fracture site and the exterior. These are more serious injuries but, from the standpoint of immediate care, demand only the application of a clean (preferably sterile) dressing before a splint is applied. Other injuries may include abrasions, contusions, sprains, lacerations, and dislocations. It may be difficult even under ideal circumstances to tell whether or not there is a fracture associated with these other injuries. It is good practice, therefore, to handle such an injury as if there is a fracture, that is, an appropriate splint should be applied in addition to a dressing, if indicated. Major bleeding can usually be controlled with a properly applied pressure dressing. A tourniquet is practically never indicated unless a traumatic amputation has occurred or unless a limb is so badly damaged that it cannot be salvaged.

chapter 15

Initial care of the critically burned patient

Boyd E. Terry

The seriously burned patient deserves and requires maximum compassion from the physician. Unpleasant features of burns often call forth a defeatist attitude from those observing the burn. This attitude may explain why many burned patients receive minimal initial care often poorly suited to their needs. Transportation of the burned patient without initial care frequently ends with disaster.

Frequently the question is asked: is there a method such as immediate immersion in cold water that will prevent a superficial burn from becoming a full-thickness burn? The answer is no, unless the physician is present and can douse the patient in cold water at the moment of the burn, when it may theoretically have some importance. In terms of initial physician care this is a helpful maneuver for the alleviation of pain in superficial burns. The critically burned individual, on the other hand, rarely complains of pain and is usually quite calm; therefore, it is important not to treat one's own emotions by giving narcotics for anticipated pain. Deep burns actually destroy the nerve endings and pain is absent.

Another puzzling observation is that the severely burned patient may frequently be ambulatory. One wonders how this could be possible in the patient with impending "burn shock." Such reasoning leads to the underestimation of the severity of burns. If the patient is given adequate initial fluid therapy, burn shock is rare because it is prevented without appearing in a diagnosable state. Burn shock does not occur rapidly as does hemorrhagic shock but appears over a period of hours in the untreated patient.

AIRWAY

Of primary importance in initial care of the severely burned patient is the need to assure an airway. One might think that a severely burned patient will have burns into the bronchi of the respiratory tract, but this is rarely true except in burns incurred in a closed-room steam explosion. Reflex mechanisms ordinarily close the glottis to heat stimuli, thus protecting the lower respiratory tract; however, the pharynx, nasopharynx, and mouth may be burned. The damage to the lower respiratory tract from smoke inhalation ordinarily manifests itself several hours after the burn is initially seen. The hazard of upper respiratory tract obstruction is most easily circumvented by insertion of a nasotracheal or orotracheal tube. The patient burned in the head and neck area will generally have serious burns over the usual tracheostomy site. Tracheostomy is best avoided as an initial measure because it compounds the possibility of later pneumonia and sepsis from the extended burn wound.

Edema is of greatest concern in initial management, particularly in the infant and child. The subsidance of edema after 48 to 72 hours allows for the nasotracheal tube to be removed. Certainly if one is in the position to dictate transport of the patient who has been burned in the head and neck area, he must do this only with the assurance of adequate airway placement and care as the patient is transported. On rare occasion it is necessary to perform escharotomy of the circumferentially burned upper torso to allow expansion of the chest wall (as explained under Associated Injury).

A major problem confronting the severely burned individual is acute gastric dilation, which may cause airway problems by aspiration of vomited gastric contents. Nasogastric intubation is important as a preliminary step to nasotracheal or orotracheal intubation to prevent aspiration. Well-intended large doses of narcotics (seldom needed in the severely burned patient) may be the factor that compounds an already severe airway problem.

EVALUATION

History and physical and general evaluation are singularly important in the initial care of the burned patient and are most frequently overlooked. The patient has obvious physical findings but frequently there are associated injuries and conditions that will have much to do with the outcome of the burn. These must be determined early. Initially the burned patient will be lucid and able to converse, whereas several hours later he may not be so because of delirium that frequently occurs in larger burns. The dictum that "burn patients die not of their burn but of the complications of the burn" serves to emphasize the importance of determination of pertinent history and physical findings. It is evident that the evaluation of the cardiorespiratory and renal systems by history will be valuable in the initial management. This will allow for the anticipation of significant problems likely to be made worse by the burn.

Age, size of burn, amount of full-thickness burn, and general health are of greatest value as predictors of ultimate patient survival. Patients under age 3 and over 50 years have higher mortality. The "rule of nines," though a rough approximation, will help estimate size of burn (head 9%, each upper extremity 9%, each lower extremity 18%, and 18% for anterior and posterior trunk respectively). Full-thickness burn is defined initially by absence of response to pinprick and ultimately by requirement of skin graft.

FLUID REQUIREMENTS

Early initiation of resuscitative fluids to the burned patient is a preventive measure against burn shock. It is equally important to prevent another complication of the severely burned patient: acute renal failure. Traumatic acute tubular necrosis is common in the burned patient. Hemolysis of red cells in damaged capillaries causes deposition of pigments in the renal tubules at a time when urinary flow in the tubules is low. Maintenance of adequate tubular urine flow will prevent irreversible damage should tubular necrosis occur. Particularly in the patient with an electric burn (in whom there is circulating myoglobin pigment in addition to heme pigment), it is important to ensure adequate tubular urine flow.

The essential fluid requirement can be satisfied with a balanced electrolyte solution such as Ringer's lactate. The administration of blood is contraindicated as a resuscitative agent unless there is blood loss from another injury. Intravenous solution will be necessary for all burns over 20% and for many pediatric burns, which are smaller in area. Burns around the head and neck preclude early oral intake of fluid even though the burned surface area is small; they indicate the need for intravenous fluids. The route of intravenous fluid administration is important. Many times extremities cannot be used for intravenous fluid because of the burn, and particularly in the severely burned patient it may be necessary to give fluid through the subclavian vein by percutaneous puncture. Such entry through a cleansed area of the burn with subsequent changes of the catheter on a frequent basis is much safer than cutting down through burn tissue or the use of lower extremities, which precludes the monitoring of central venous pressure.

Urinary output must be monitored on an hourly basis in the severely burned patient; placement of a Foley catheter becomes necessary as an initial event. This monitoring provides information as to the volume of urine produced and frequently indicates the presence of heme pigment. The use of intravenous mannitol may then be warranted to provide immediate tubular diuresis should there be a lag in the production of adequate urinary flow.

How much and what kind of fluid can be decided in all burn patients by providing lactated Ringer's solution initially in such amounts as to produce urinary output in the range of 50 ml/hour in the adult and approximately 1 ml/kg/hour in the infant and child.

ASSOCIATED INJURY

The presence of other injuries in the burned patient is frequently obscured and must be assiduously sought by careful examination, particularly extremity ischemia and eye injury. The former is caused by edema with circumferential burns leading to distal ischemia, primarily in the extremities. Escharotomy is rarely necessary but is limb-saving when there is vascular compromise. Escharotomy is performed by incising the skin to the level of the subcutaneous fat in a longitudinal direction on either side of the extremity.

Eye injuries are uncommon because of the very adequate protection the eyelids afford. In the occasional burn of the eyelids the primary requirement, initially, is immediate coverage of the cornea by tarsorrhaphy (suturing together of the upper and lower eyelids). Edematous lids swollen shut are good protection and rarely hide corneal damage. However, early examination is essential!

IMMEDIATE ACTION TO TREAT INFECTION

The burned patient becomes a risk from airborne and contact sources of contamination from the immediate environment and must be protected from infection. Tetanus toxid, or tetanus immune globulin (human) in those who have not been immunized, is a specific requirement for burned patients. Removal of clothing, rapid cleansing of the burn wound with Betadine "scrub" solution, and removal of any loose dead tissue will minimize contamination of the burn wound. The patient should be managed with clean if not sterile technique. Once cleansed, the burn wound should be covered with sterile dressings or at least by a sterile sheet, with provision for conservation of body heat with blankets. Elevation of the ambient temperature to 30° to 32° C with external heaters will prevent shivering and add to patient comfort. Caloric and vapor losses through the burned skin are very large and require particular attention in the infant and child.

Antibiotics are best withheld for the treatment of specific infection rather than being used prophylactically. Cultures of the burn wound should be obtained upon initial inspection.

chapter 16

Emergencies caused by environmental temperature extremes

Although the various terms for heat emergencies are occasionally misused, it is important to differentiate at least three types of clinical situations resulting from exposures to excessive heat: heat exhaustion, heat pyrexia, and heat cramps. Emergency care can be lifesaving, providing the proper therapy is instituted.

HEAT CRAMPS

Heat cramps are characterized by severe muscle pains and cramps, particularly in the lower extremities and sometimes in the abdomen. They are, of course, more of a problem in a hot environment and in individuals who do a lot of sweating. Since heat cramps may progress to heat exhaustion, the systemic picture may include faintness, dizziness, and a marked weakness.

The immediate measure needed is the replacement of sodium chloride. In fact, drinking large quantities of water may increase the severity of the cramps. Enteric-coated sodium chloride tablets mixed with water will usually be sufficient. If the patient is brought to the hospital or is in the emergency room, an infusion of isotonic sodium chloride will be ideal.

HEAT EXHAUSTION

Heat exhaustion can be recognized by the clinical feature of general peripheral collapse, which is usually of a mild to moderate degree. The patient may complain at the onset of generalized weakness and lassitude and may even faint. Helpful in identifying heat exhaustion is the pale, clammy skin presented by the patient. The temperature of the skin may be either normal or decreased. In addition to profuse sweating, nausea and vomiting may be seen. There is a fast, weak pulse and usually a decreased blood pressure. The pupils may be dilated.

The immediate care of a heat exhaustion victim dictates moving him into a cooler environment, if at all possible. Clothing is loosened and fluids are encouraged, particularly water with sodium chloride added.

If syncope has occurred, the patient should be placed in the supine position with the feet elevated. An intravenous infusion of isotonic saline solution will hasten the patient's return to a more normal state. Coffee may serve as a beneficial stimulant, and aromatic spirits of ammonia may be helpful.

A patient suffering from heat exhaustion will, by the nature of his peripheral vasomotor collapse, have a definite pallor. This is in marked contrast to the reddish blush presented by the patient suffering from heat pyrexia or heat stroke.

Placing cold applications on the patient's body, especially around the forehead, will be beneficial, as will the reduction in body temperature aided by an electric fan blowing over the patient.

Since heat exhaustion is characterized by the pooling of large quantities of blood in the skin, the reduced amounts of circulating blood can be partially corrected by elevating the legs well over the body and, if necessary, applying elastic bandages so as to increase blood return to the right side of the heart.

HEAT PYREXIA (HEAT STROKE OR SUNSTROKE)

In contrast to heat exhaustion, heat stroke, more effectively termed *heat pyrexia,* is an emergency of greater magnitude. Heat exhaustion occurs more commonly in females, heat stroke is seen most often in males. Like heat exhaustion, heat pyrexia indicates poor acclimatization to excessive heat usually associated with high humidities. The individual is unable to adjust to the heat by the body's temperature-regulating mechanisms. Accordingly, sweating ceases, causing a further rise in body temperature. Unlike the normal or slightly subnormal temperatures of heat exhaustion, patients with heat stroke may be found with temperature elevations well over 106° F. Such temperatures cannot be tolerated by the body's vital organs, especially the brain, and death may result. As mentioned earlier, these patients have a reddish flush to the skin. Cardiac output is increased, as reflected in the elevated blood pressure and a strong, bounding pulse.

At the onset the patient may experience dizziness, headache, and marked dryness of the mouth. Unconsciousness may quickly ensue.

Immediate measures demand as rapid a fall in body temperatures as possible. If emergency treatment is delayed until the reddish flush of the skin turns to a grayish color, the prognosis becomes increasingly worse. All possible measures should be utilized to reduce the body temperature. These may include placing the patient in a tub of ice cold water or continued washings with rubbing alcohol. Wrapping the patient in cold, wet sheets with an electric fan blowing on the patient is an effective measure.

Frequent recordings of the temperature are indicated, since it may again rise after an initial fall if continued efforts to cool the patient are not maintained. Unlike the heat exhaustion patient, the patient with heat stroke is best placed in a head-up or partially reclining position. Immediate efforts to reduce body temperature should not cease until the temperature has been reduced below 102° F.

One should be cautious not to administer large amounts of intravenous fluids too rapidly. Cardiac congestive failure is frequently associated with heat pyrexia.

All patients with heat pyrexia should be hospitalized. If immediate care of the patient has been deficient or slow in arriving, permanent brain damage or disabling neurologic deficits may persist.

FROSTBITE

A relatively simple approach is required in the immediate treatment of a portion of the body subjected to freezing temperatures for a sufficiently prolonged period to produce severe vasospasm and the even cessation of circulation. If the extremities, for example, have progressed from an initial tingling and painful condition to that of numbness and total anesthesia, the sequelae of the frostbite may require prolonged definitive care. In order to reduce the time of the cold exposure, efforts should be made at once to rewarm the affected area. Moderately rapid rewarming is to be desired over earlier concepts supporting very gradual rewarming. Placing the frozen extremities in a water bath heated to the vicinity of 110° F will provide rapid rewarming. Attempts should not be made to improve circulation and to rewarm by massaging the affected part since this may increase the tissue damage.

Any constricting garment or dressings should be removed. Blisters should not be opened and only gentle manipulation should be attempted. If pain is severe an analgesic may be administered. Smoking should be denied the victim. The victim should not be allowed to ambulate or bear weight on the affected area.

One should avoid obvious contamination. Although various modalities of definitive therapy may be employed at a later hour, the individual administering immediate care should specifically note whether or not tetanus toxoid or tetanus antitoxin has been administered. Tetanus prophylaxis is essential. Prophylactic antibiotic therapy may be begun as a part of the initial definitive therapy. In any event the patient should be admitted to the hospital if definitive therapy is required.

chapter 17

Decompression sickness and air embolism

Jefferson C. Davis

Until very recently, pressure-related emergencies were the sole province of a limited group of physicians working in support of commercial or military deep-sea diving, tunneling, bridge building, or high-altitude or space operations. Developments within the past few years have made it mandatory that all physicians, regardless of specialty, become familiar with the life- and function-threatening consequences of sport as well as commercial exposures to these environments.

The ready availability of excellent quality self-contained underwater breathing apparatus (scuba) has made diving one of the world's fastest growing individual sports. Scuba diving has been considered to be limited to seacoast and resort areas, but a weekend visit to almost any body of water in the United States will quickly show that notion to be erroneous. Scuba divers can be found in every city; besides diving in local lakes, a common practice is for a group or club to charter an aircraft, fly to a popular diving area, dive, and then fly home. In either event, any physician could be faced with the clinical manifestations of decompression sickness or air embolism at any time. Definitive therapy is quite specific and requires expeditious immediate management and coordinated emergency transfer to the nearest recompression chamber.

Similar clinical manifestations with comparable diagnostic features, emergency management, and definitive therapy required can result from exposure to high altitudes in nonpressurized aircraft or sudden loss of cabin pressurization in a pressurized aircraft flying at a high altitude.

The numbers of people exposed to both environments with their attendant risks have reached a significant level, but we are presently only on the threshold of vast expansion in both areas.

TERMINOLOGY

The following terminology includes most of the effects of changes in barometric pressure:

    I. Mechanical effects (Boyle's law)
        A. Barotitis ("ear squeeze," "ear block")
        B. Barosinusitis ("sinus squeeze," "sinus block")
        C. Barodontalgia ("tooth squeeze," "tooth block")

       D. Trapped gastrointestinal gas expansion (ascent to altitude)

       E. Pulmonary problems

         1. "Lung squeeze" (breath-hold diving)

         2. Pneumothorax

         3. Pneumomediastinum

         4. Air embolism

    II. Decompression sickness (Henry's law)

       A. Bends

       B. Chokes

       C. Neurologic decompression sickness

       D. Vasomotor collapse (shock)

       E. Skin manifestations

       F. Aseptic bone necrosis

This chapter will consider only those disorders requiring emergency use of the recompression chamber: air embolism and the first four listed manifestations of decompression sickness.

AIR EMBOLISM
Etiology

    Cerebral air embolism is the result of breath-holding ascent from depth by a scuba or surface-supplied diver. It has also occurred rarely in breath-holding during rapid decompression of a pressurized aircraft cabin. Expansion of the volume of gas trapped in the lungs by a closed glottis as barometric pressure decreases accounts for distension. If the tensile strength of the lung is exceeded, air is introduced directly into pulmonary veins through lung rupture.

Clinical manifestations

    The most significant factor in the diagnosis of cerebral air embolism is the sudden onset of neurologic symptoms during or immediately following decompression from a dive with scuba or surface supply of air or other gas mixture. The neurologic pattern may be most confusing in that many small bubbles may occlude arterial supply to diverse areas of the brain. Commonly, the first manifestation is seizure activity, either focal or generalized. The patient may be suddenly rendered unconscious, show visual field defects or blindness, or have any imaginable combination of other sensory or motor deficits. Shock and death may occur if the volume of bubbles is great and if recompression facilities are not immediately available.

Treatment

    The overriding factor in management of the cerebral air embolism patient must be to get him to a recompression chamber as rapidly as possible. During transportation the patient must be kept in a Trendelenburg position, preferably also tilted 15 degrees to his left side. If oxygen is available, it should be administered by mask to achieve as near as possible to 100% inspired concentration. An intravenous infusion of low molecular weight dextran should be started. It is reemphasized, however, that there should never be a delay in transportation to a recompression chamber to institute any other therapy. The *one* determining factor in the outcome of the case will be the time delay between onset of symptoms and recompression therapy. Every minute lost decreases the chances for complete recovery or at best prolongs cerebral ischemia and cellular hypoxia with resulting tissue edema and leads to a difficult course of therapy. A recent case illustrates this problem.

A 19-year-old male was being given "free ascent" training at a lake. In this portion of scuba training, the student and his instructor descended normally to 30-foot depth. The student removed his mouthpiece and with the instructor ascended to the surface, exhaling all the way. All was normal until immediately after surfacing, when the student became rigid and lost consciousness. He was rescued by the instructor, and on the shore he remained comatose with clonic jerking of the entire left side. A helicopter was dispatched and flew the patient at low altitude, to avoid bubble expansion, to the nearest recompression chamber, 80 miles distant. Recompression therapy was begun 2 hours after onset. At the chamber, examination revealed response only to noxious stimuli, plantar Babinski reflex on the right, and extensor reflex on the left. Corneal reflexes were absent, pupils equal and reactive. The left lower extremity was rigidly extended. He was treated in the recompression chamber according to U.S. Navy Treatment Table VIA for air embolism. This table includes 30 minutes at an air pressure equivalent to 165 feet of sea water (6 atmospheres absolute [ATA]) to achieve maximum bubble volume reduction. This was followed by prolonged intermittent oxygen-air breathing at 60-foot and 30-foot equivalents in the chamber to provide not only slow decompression but also hyperbaric oxygenation to hypoxic tissues.

During the treatment he recovered orientation, and rigidity of the left lower extremity disappeared. However, despite repeated and prolonged therapy, vision did not return for 12 hours, apparently because of the 2-hour delay in reaching the chamber. Besides hyperbaric oxygen, dexamethasone and intravenous mannitol were used to combat cerebral edema. The patient was fully recovered at 24 hours following the incident.

This case is important in suggesting another etiologic mechanism for cerebral air embolism during decompression. Despite the fact that the patient did exhale during ascent, air was apparently introduced into the pulmonary veins. It is considered most likely that localized air trapping in blebs or bullae accounted for lung rupture into vessels.

Prevention

With a satisfactory air supply, divers simply breathe normally during ascent from depth. If an equipment malfunction or depletion of air supply at depth makes this impossible, the diver must exhale continuously during ascent to vent the increasing volume of air in his lungs. Any evidence of chronic pulmonary disease should disqualify a candidate for scuba instruction. On rapid decompression in an aircraft, normal respiration is all that is required.

DECOMPRESSION SICKNESS
Etiology

Despite the fact that decompression sickness resulting from too rapid ascent from compressed air environments has been known since the development of the caisson in the mid-1880's, many features of basic etiology are still unclear. Synonyms for this disorder include "caisson disease" and "compressed air illness." Inasmuch as cases presented to the physician who does not specialize in diving medicine will generally be sport scuba divers, this section will concentrate upon this population and thus consider the breathing medium to be compressed air.

In order to balance the linear increase in water pressure (0.445 psi/foot of sea water) as the scuba diver descends, the breathing regulator is designed to provide air pressure equal to water pressure at any depth. As the alveolar air pressure increases at depth, the partial pressures of inspired gases increase. For example, at 99 feet of sea water (or 4 ATA), the absolute barometric pressure is 3,040 mm Hg. Approximately 79% of this pressure is nitrogen (2,400 mm Hg, compared to 600 mm Hg inspired nitrogen partial pressure [pN_2] at sea level breathing air). This results in an alveolar nitrogen pressure of approximately 2,360 mm Hg. This alveolar pressure is rapidly reflected in arterial blood and presented to all tissues. A highly complex set of variables including differences in tissue perfusion and solubility factors results in a family of tissue nitrogen uptake curves throughout the body. Tissue nitrogen saturations achieved in diving then are a function of depth and time.

The U. S. Navy and other decompression schedules are based on calculations and testing of ascent methods to avoid exceeding safe rates of decompression after diving. The tissues can tolerate a certain degree of supersaturation, but if barometric pressure is lowered beyond a critical level of nitrogen supersaturation that can be held in the tissues, it comes out of solution as bubbles. The result is a series of events caused by bubble embolization of various tissues, agglutination of platelets caused by the intravascular bubble foreign bodies, tissue ischemia, and hypoxia resulting in edema. Venous bubbles are swept through the pulmonary artery to produce pulmonary embolism, and possibly bubbling occurs de novo in tissues. The resulting symptoms and signs make up the family of disorders known as decompression sickness.

Clinical manifestations

Bends. Mild to severe deep, dull pain usually located in or around joints may occur immediately after surfacing from a dive or may begin up to several hours later. Any area may be involved but most commonly pain is in the knees, ankles, shoulders, or elbows. Usually no objective findings are present, although occasional patients have shown some edema around affected joints. There may or may not be tenderness in the involved areas. In some cases, local pressure as with a blood pressure cuff gives temporary relief if applied directly over the joint. While bends itself is not life-threatening, it indicates that bubbles have formed. Some patients progress to more serious manifestations if left untreated. Bends is by far the most common type of decompression sickness.

Chokes. Chokes is a much more serious form of decompression sickness characterized by burning substernal pain, dyspnea, and a nonproductive cough. The exact pathophysiology is not clear, but animal studies have shown great volumes of bubbles or foam in the pulmonary artery, right ventricle, and atrium following unsafe decompression. It is considered likely that chokes actually represents massive bubble pulmonary embolism. Patients with this rare form of decompression sickness may go rapidly into profound shock or may develop neurologic forms of decompression sickness.

Neurologic decompression sickness. In both diving and altitude-induced decompression sickness, some patients proceed through a pattern of bends, chokes (with or without vasomotor instability), or neurologic manifestations. Others develop one form only as an isolated event without any of the other forms. When this is neurologic decompression sickness, the event may be very confusing in that any level of the brain or spinal cord may be embolized. The diver is more likely to develop spinal cord lesions with the onset (soon after decompression) of severe, girdling, abdominal pain either with or without sensory and motor impairment of lower extremities, with loss of bowel and bladder control according to the level and extent of embolization. In altitude decompression sickness, neurologic involvement is more likely to result from single or multiple arterial emboli to the brain. Because many bubbles of varying sizes may result in involvement of diverse brain areas, the neurologic examination can be very confusing and could erroneously indicate hysteria. There may be scintillating scotomata, visual field defects, blindness, aphasia, vertigo, patchy sensory or motor losses, loss of consciousness, and focal or generalized seizures. With neurologic manifestations, a shock picture may supervene so that vital signs must be carefully monitored.

Vasomotor decompression sickness. A very small percentage of persons develops severe shock with hemoconcentration. The precise mechanism is still not clear, but it is considered most likely that bubble embolization, ischemia, hypoxia, and bubble-induced changes in blood elements result in loss of fluid from the intravascular to the extravascular spaces. Shock may also occur secondary to the massive pulmonary embolism of chokes described previously. While adequate fluid replacement is important, experience has shown that decompression sickness patients often respond poorly until recompression therapy is instituted.

Treatment

Of paramount importance is a high index of suspicion. Unfortunately, sport scuba divers will often be unable to give precise times and depths of their diving, so that the physician must take the history of diving and then proceed to manage the patient according to his clinical picture.

It is important to do a complete physical examination if at all possible; but again, as with cerebral air embolism, in the serious cases transportation to a recompression facility is the overriding consideration. It must be remembered that the patient who presents with a chief complaint of simple bends pain or a seemingly minor neurologic manifestation may have a more serious neurologic deficit demonstrable on complete examination.

As first aid and during transportation to a recompression chamber, the use of 100% oxygen by mask is indicated. The major purpose of oxygen administration is to wash out nitrogen, so anything less than 100% oxygen will not be as effective. An anesthesia mask or aviator's breathing mask is suggested to achieve this goal. Because of the known platelet agglutination secondary to bubble embolization, it has been suggested that low molecular weight dextran be used as an adjunct to recompression therapy, and it may be started before transportation.

It is important that each physician and each emergency room be aware of the nearest civilian or military hyperbaric or recompression chamber and how to contact it immediately in an emergency. Time is of the essence in treatment of decompression sickness as it is in air embolism.

Transportation to the chamber must be made by the most expeditious means available. During transportation oxygen administration and intravenous fluids should be continued and the patient placed in the Trendelenburg position. If the recompression chamber is not within short reach of surface transportation, movement by air ambulance must be considered. In both decompression sickness and air embolism, it is crucial that the patient not be exposed to significant altitude, since bubbles will enlarge as a result of a decrease in barometric pressure. It is preferable to move the patient in an aircraft with a pressurization system capable of maintaining sealevel equivalent pressure, although unpressurized helicopter movement at low altitude has been successful.

It is beyond the scope of this chapter to discuss details of definitive treatment in recompression chambers. The basic mechanisms of action are to reduce bubble volume throughout the blood and other tissues, restore normal perfusion, eliminate excess nitrogen, and provide hyperbaric oxygenation of hypoxic tissues. All adjunctive measures are continued or may be instituted in the chamber.

chapter 18

Injuries caused by lightning

The number of deaths from lightning shock in the United States each year has been estimated at around 300. This number is only one fourth of all persons struck by lightning. Most injuries from lightning do not result from the mainstream of the bolt but are caused by current flowing through the victim from direct contact with the charged ground. Many of the injuries from lightning result from the fires it causes. Approximately 75% of all reported farm fire losses originate from lightning, and more than 80% of all livestock losses from accidents are a result of lightning.

Often as many as a dozen individuals will be knocked to the ground by a bolt of lightning. In such a situation the rescuer should avoid the general axiom that one centers his first aid efforts on the living rather than the apparent dead. If an individual shows signs of life, the chances are good that he will survive. On the other hand, many of those individuals who are apparent fatalities can be revived if cardiopulmonary resuscitative efforts as outlined in Chapter 10 are followed.

Dr. Taussig has pointed out in a study on "death" from lightning that metabolic activity as well as heart action and respiration stops almost instantly when a person is struck by lightning. The heart may start again in sinus rhythm. The onset of degenerative changes is apparently delayed by the sudden cessation of metabolic activity to the extent that successful resuscitation may be achieved in the victim who has apparently been "dead" for longer than 4 minutes. Therefore, vigorous efforts at resuscitation following lightning shock are often most rewarding.

An amazing variety of clinical findings may be present immediately following lightning shock even though the patient appears to be only stunned by the lightning. The patient may be unable to move his extremities. Deafness or blindness may be present. Fortunately, many of the complications are only transient but, obviously, the victim should be transported to the nearest medical center where definitive care can be administered.

While some individuals may be only momentarily stunned following a lightning shock, others will require cardiopulmonary resuscitation. Artificial respiration, as described elsewhere in the book, as well as closed-chest cardiac massage, should be begun immediately. Cardiopulmonary resuscitation may be necessary during transportation to the hospital, and respiratory depression may be such that artificial maintenance of respiration will need to be continued for several days. In addition, cardiac defibrillation may be required in a certain percentage of patients. Originally it was believed that most patients fibrillate following a lightning shock; however, there is now additional evidence that a majority represent simple asystole.

One should assume that multiple skeletal injuries may have occured from the tremendous repulsive force. The skull and extremities should be checked by the rescuer for the possibility of fractures. Temporary paraplegia may be caused either by the effect of lightning on the central nervous system or by spinal cord injury.

The rescuer should be prepared for the victim to complain of deafness, blindness, and other neurologic deficits. Fortunately most of these are temporary. A postlightning shock psychosis is reported.

A word concerning prevention is always in order. To the golfer in an electric storm goes the advice to get rid of his clubs, get away from trees or golf carts, and lie down on the ground in the area of greatest depression. A thick woods is a relatively safe spot.

During an electric storm an automobile with a metal top is one of the safest spots. Certainly one should avoid being in a swimming pool, near a single tree, near horses or cattle, or on the top of a hill or mountain; one should always avoid either being the tallest object or being near the tallest object in a given vicinity. One should *never* raise an umbrella over his head in an electric storm.

chapter 19

Initial care of the hand injury

John P. Adams

There is a great tendency in initial care of hands to do too much, too early. When in doubt, one is better off doing too little. Incised wounds that are not severely contaminated should be cleaned. Suturing can usually be done immediately after irrigation and cleansing. The soft tissue is best supported in a firm compression dressing or a splint with the wrist and hand placed in the position of function—that in which the wrist is in neutral position, the fingers flexed at least 45 degrees at each joint, and the thumb held in abduction and opposition.

Patients who have initial wound suturing in the emergency room must be seen promptly by the physician who will give aftercare because even with minor injuries, fingers tend to stiffen, and permanent disability may ensue. In circumstances where major injuries are present and initial care is not immediately available, the best treatment is to thoroughly irrigate the wound. If the wound is of suitable type it should be sutured (if infection is imminent, the wound should be left open), covered with a compression dressing, placed in a supportive position with the wrist and hand as near to the functional position as possible, and the patient transferred to a facility where difinitive care can be carried out. Certain types of *wounds contaminated by foreign material* such as tear gas, paint, grease, turpentine, or paint solvents require thorough cleansing of the wound as early as possible in whatever facility is available; in these circumstances, the wound should remain open and no definitive further care should be carried out at that time.

Wounds that involve *open fractures, tendon lacerations,* or *nerve lacerations* more severe than a digital nerve laceration or wounds in which *avulsion of the skin* is part of the primary injury require hospitalization and definitive care in the operating theater. As a general rule no definitive surgery to any deeper structures should be carried out in the emergency facilities unless there are unusual circumstances. *Minor lacerations* may be sutured in the emergency room; however, major wounds should be admitted to the hospital for adequate care. In many instances definitive care must be deferred for several hours for reasons such as a full stomach, injuries, inability to secure skilled surgical personnel, or unavailability of operating room space. In such instances, thorough irrigation of open wounds by copious amounts of saline should be carried out; if saline is not available, tapwater should be applied to the wound for initial debridement and then sterile dressing reapplied. Once the wound is covered with a sterile dressing the emergency nature of the injury has been altered to one of semielection, and definitive surgery, if indicated, may be carried out several hours later without increasing the complication rate.

A great deal of time and effort in reconstructive hand surgery are devoted to the care of hands with disabilities that could have been prevented or substantially reduced if initial care had been adequate. Compared with disabilities of other parts of the body, hand injuries occupy a substantial position. The upper extremity is the most frequently injured part of the body.

INITIAL EXAMINATION

Care of the hand within the first few hours after injury often determines the degree of the patient's future physical impairment. The injured hand should be considered a surgical emergency, particularly if the wound is open, and should receive prompt treatment. Treatment of any injury, but particularly an organ system as complex as the hand, wrist, and upper extremity, requires an accurate diagnosis at the onset. Such a diagnosis can only be made by an examination embracing the basic components of this organ system:

1. The integumentary system
2. The intactness of the nerve supply
3. The motor function as reflected in joint motion
4. The skeletal system
5. The ligamentous system

The *initial examination* should be conducted as follows. After inspection to ascertain the general nature of the wound, the degree of gross contamination, and whether the wound was produced by an avulsing or crushing type injury, the wound should be covered with a well-applied, clean, preferably sterile compression dressing. If hemorrhage is a problem, it can normally be controlled by a sterile compression dressing and elevation. Other than superficial inspection of the wound, no examination should be carried out through the wound itself. After the dressing has been applied, a detailed examination can be carried out, always distal to the site of injury. This means, then, a careful assessment of sensation in the autonomous zone of the ulnar nerve in the pulp space of the little finger, of the median nerve in the pulp space of the index finger, and of the radial nerve in the small area in the dorsal skin overlying the web space between the thumb and index metacarpals. Motion is determined by having the patient move individual joints. In spite of severe injury, if the digit is properly supported the patient will be able to perform specific functions, and this can be ascertained and recorded. The detailed examination of possible fractures, joint subluxations, or dislocations should be accomplished by adequate roentgenologic examination; usually this should include x-rays taken in at least three planes: anteroposterior, lateral, and oblique. For specific suspected injuries, a single digit may be outlined in more detail. The vascular status of the extremity can be assessed by the blanching characteristics of the nailbed and the general color and temperature of the part.

IMPORTANCE OF FULL HISTORY

Initial care will obviously include a careful history of the accident. It is more important to know whether the wound was caused by a sharp object, such as a knife, in which crushing of tissues is not apt to occur, or whether laceration was caused by a fall on a broken bottle or some blunt object. It is also important to determine whether there was heat applied to the wound through friction or any other external cause.

Information should be obtained as to wound contamination by possible noxious agents, such as tear gas or chemicals like turpentine, paint, or grease. If at all possible, the position of the hand at the time of injury should be ascertained, because only then can one accurately determine the levels of tendon laceration, such as in the palm and finger. For example, if the laceration occurs with the fingers in full extension, then the skin and tendon lacerations will correspond to the same level. If the hand is in flexion, however, such as in grasping a knife, then the tendon laceration will always be distal to the skin laceration when the fingers are placed again in their anatomic position. Injuries caused by human or animal bites are in special category and will be considered later.

BURNS

Hand burns usually fall into one of three categories: thermal, chemical, or electric. Of the three, the electric burn carries the poorest prognosis. Initial care in the emergency room of any burn to the hand is normally application of a sterile dressing, which should be supported with a splint, and hospital admission if the burn is obviously greater than first degree. Definitive care of deep second- or third-degree burns should not be carried out in an emergency room setting. Initial inspection of most thermal burns will easily distinguish between first degree (redness), second degree (blistering), and third degree (full-thickness skin loss with possible loss of deeper structures). One exception is the burn produced by hot liquid; in this case skin injury may be minimal while injury to deeper structures may be severe. Electric burns also tend to show more deep tissue injury than is apparent from superficial inspection.

BITES

Human and animal bites are a common type of acute hand injury and must be considered separately. Human bites are rarely, if ever, made by a rabid individual; therefore, the primary concern is assessment of skin and deeper tissue damage. Wounds in the area of a joint must be suspected of having penetrated the joint. The local treatment is debridement and thorough irrigation. Local cauterizing agents should not be used. Lavage with antibacterial agents such as 1% neomycin solution may be indicated if the wound is seen within 1 hour. After cleansing, the wound should always be left open and closed secondarily. Systemic antibiotics may be indicated.

An injury similar to a human bite is the penetration of the hand or finger by materials used in orthodontia. The wires and other appliances may penetrate deeply and may produce a closed-space infection.

Pets are the most common source of animal bites, and the general management is as for human bites. The possibility of rabies is high in cases of bites by animals such as bats, and use of rabies antisera may be essential. Snake bites should be incised and should have a venous tourniquet applied if seen immediately. Appropriate antivenom should be given locally and systemically.

PSYCHOLOGIC EFFECT

The psychologic effect of hand injuries is great. This is not surprising when one realizes that much of the information placed in our brains gets there because of activities of the hand. Therefore, any hand injury is a threat to the livelihood of either the working man or the professional. The psychologic reaction is much greater than that of injury to any other part of the body with the possible exception of the genitalia. It is of utmost importance that the initial examining physician be judicious in any statement he may make to a patient as to either prognosis or the exact nature of the injury. In most cases the emergency room physician should explain only in general terms what has happened; the specific prognosis should be given by the surgeon who will provide definitive care. First impressions are often the most lasting ones, and an inaccurate statement made by a physician at the time of initial treatment may jeopardize the entire future treatment and rehabilitation program.

In outline form are listed the steps toward providing initial care of the hand:

1. The hand injury should be recognized as a bona fide emergency and not relegated to care at the convenience of emergency room personnel.

2. An accurate history of mechanism of injury, possible contaminants, and condition of the hand at the time of injury should be ascertained.

3. After superficial inspection, the wound should be covered with a clean, preferably sterile dressing.

4. The examination for definitive injury should be carried out distal to the wound.

5. Adequate x-ray examination, rather than physical examination, should be utilized to ascertain bone and joint injury.

6. After an accurate estimate of disability has been made, definitive care of an injury to deeper structures should not be done in the emergency room but only after the patient's admission to the hospital.

7. In general, tendon lacerations in the palm and fingers are best treated by delayed repair; repair of tendons in these areas may be carried out primarily only under ideal circumstances in which highly trained individuals are available to evaluate and treat the patient.

8. In wounds where there is no question as to whether they will heal by primary intent and where there are lacerations of flexor tendons at the wrist level or above, primary repair may be carried out; this same principle applies to extensor tendon injury.

9. Injuries of mixed nerves (motor and sensory) should be treated by initial wound closure and delayed nerve repair in 4 or 6 weeks.

10. When the patient is recovering from soft tissue repair and awaiting further repair of deeper structures, he must be followed closely, and joint mobility must be maintained. He should be placed in the hands of the surgeon who will give the followup care early after the injury.

11. The prognosis in severe hand injuries is often guarded as to restoration of normal or nearly normal function, even with treatment by the most skilled surgeons. Therefore, the initial physician must be extremely careful in offering any opinion to the patient on the final outcome.

12. No emergency room physician can be criticized for his initial care of a hand wound providing his diagnosis is accurate, his findings are recorded, and his attention is directed toward the wound itself.

13. Bites, human and animal, are a special type of injury; these wounds must be thoroughly cleansed and not closed.

14. All hand wounds, because of potential contamination, must be considered to be a possible source of tetanus and gas gangrene. In animal bites rabies is an additional cause for concern. Antitetanus measures must be instituted in all injuries. Prophylactic use of

gas gangrene antitoxin has not proved to be effective. The use of antirabies serum will depend on the state of health of the wounding animal. Snake bites should be treated with appropriate antitoxin.

chapter 20

Early management of abdominal trauma

Despite antibiotics, despite blood replacement and blood substitutes, and despite other refinements in treatment, the morbidity and mortality from major abdominal trauma is still excessively high. The crux of the problem—the hope for increased survival rates—rests on the early management of patients with abdominal trauma. Early management is basically a matter of prompt diagnosis in order to institute immediate and effective treatment.

Delays in diagnosis are attributable to several factors. Patients arrive in the emergency room with multiple injuries, injuries of more *apparent* urgency than whatever trauma has been provoked within the abdomen. A shock-like state may mask the signs of intraabdominal trauma to the extent that the clinical picture may be considerably altered. The patient with alcoholic intoxication is difficult to diagnose accurately at an early stage. Some drug addiction problems present a similar picture, and the unconscious patient can give no history and his abdominal examination may be difficult to interpret. The onset of peritonitis from sharp or blunt perforation may be insidious and may escape early detection. If the patient arrives in the emergency room within a few minutes after receiving the trauma, there may be no intraabdominal signs to indicate perforation of a hollow viscus.

The pathology may include a multitude of possibilities and combinations of injuries. With any blunt or penetrating injury of the abdomen, one should keep in mind the possibility of a lacerated liver, a ruptured spleen, trauma to the pancreas, torn mesentery, diaphragmatic rupture, urinary bladder rupture, laceration of the vena cava or aorta, retroperitoneal hematoma or renal injury, ruptured duodenum or jejunum, gastric or colonic perforation, or injury to the gallbladder, portal vein, or abdominal portion of the esophagus.

The general priorities previously emphasized apply equally to the patient with suspected abdominal trauma. Patients with abdominal injury often have associated fractures of extremities, head injuries, and thoracic injuries. A proper assessment of the overall importance of these injuries must be made.

As always, the need for adequate ventilation is obvious. Nasogastric suction should be started. A cutdown for an intravenous infusion using a large-bore needle is accomplished. In some instances a subclavian catheter should be inserted to obtain central venous pressure monitoring. Regardless of the complaints of the patient, analgesics or narcotics should not be administered until a diagnosis is made. At the time of venipuncture, blood should be obtained for typing and cross-matching as well as for measuring serum electrolytes and serum amylase.

The history of the injury may provide important clues. The location and nature of any blunt trauma should be noted. Initial complaint of radiation of pain to the left supraclavicular fossa may be noted after a splenic tear, for example.

In observing the patient, the respiratory excursions are noted. With intraabdominal hemorrhage or peritoneal contamination, splinting of the abdominal muscles is observed and respiratory activity is generally of a thoracic nature. If abdominal contents are exposed, prompt covering with the most sterile dressing available is indicated.

Undue apprehension and thirst should lead one to suspect abdominal hemorrhage. These are often complained of before a significant fall in blood pressure is noted. Palpation of the abdomen for areas of maximal discomfort, muscle guarding, or rebound tenderness should be carefully done. If the patient is in shock the findings may be partially obscured. Evidence of rebound tenderness indicative of peritonitis will usually take a matter of several hours to develop.

Percussion will be significant if the usual area of liver dullness is absent as a result of the accumulation of free air in the peritoneal cavity over and above the liver. On auscultation the absence of bowel sounds is significant, particularly if one has listened carefully for a period of 2 to 3 minutes in each quadrant.

Despite suggestive findings on inspection, palpation, percussion, and auscultation, early diagnosis of an intraabdominal catastrophe may be delayed unless one exhausts one's armamentarium while the patient is still in the emergency room.

ABDOMINAL PARACENTESIS

Of greatest help is the abdominal paracentesis to determine the presence and nature of any free intraabdominal fluid. Different techniques are described for the abdominal paracentesis, including the four-quadrant tap. We prefer the single midline abdominal paracentesis. A small subcutaneous wheal is made with procaine hydrochloride (Novocain) or lidocaine (Xylocaine). After a scapel has incised the skin for several millimeters, a No. 14 needle is inserted into the anterior abdominal wall through which an intracath or appropriate polyethylene catheter is inserted. As the needle is slowly advanced, so also is the catheter within the needle. At the moment the needle advances beyond the posterior rectus sheath and the peritoneum into the intraabdominal cavity, the catheter will advance freely beyond the needle. At this point the needle is withdrawn and the catheter is inserted to the desired depth and to some degree in the desired direction. Of particular aid is proper positioning of the patient in order to aspirate a representative quantity of intraabdominal fluid content. The knee-chest position has proved to be of particular value for small quantities of fluid that will gravitate in such a manner that aspiration is possible. If aspiration fails to reveal any blood or fluid, then the catheter should still be maintained in place and observed at several-minute intervals, since one often obtains a positive tap simply by capillary action of the fluid within the polyethylene catheter. By insertion of the catheter with proper positioning of the patient, a positive tap will almost always be obtained if there is any free abdominal fluid. One can diagnose a ruptured spleen or intraabdominal hemorrhage within a few minutes of the patient's arrival in the emergency room and thereby facilitate prompt removal to the operating room. High amylase readings in the aspirated fluid may indicate trauma to the pancreas. Aspirated fluid with high leukocyte counts points to early peritonitis; occasionally, bile may be aspirated. We have never aspirated urine but such a possibility may occur. A urinary catheter is generally inserted at the time of the patient's admission, however, to rule out a urinary tract injury.

The same tubing used for the paracentesis may also be used for a peritoneal dialysis. This test has become increasingly popular as an adjunct in determining intraabdominal complications.

Fluid removed from the abdomen can be checked for peritoneal ammonia. Levels above 3 mg/ml suggest a perforated bowel or urinary extravasation.

DIATRIZOATE TEST FOR INTESTINAL PERFORATION

In the case of perforation of the stomach, small intestine, or occasionally the colon, we have found the urine precipitation test for diatrizoate salts after the ingestion of Gastrografin to be a valuable diagnostic aid. Gastrografin is not normally absorbed to any appreciable amount within the gastrointestinal tract. If, however, it escapes into the peritoneal cavity, it is rapidly absorbed and subsequently excreted by the kidneys. Its early detection in the urine can be made by adding *concentrated* hydrochloric acid a drop at a time to a testtube specimen of the patient's urine. If a white, chalky precipitate is seen, the diagnosis of a perforation of the colon can be made, providing the patient has not been taking penicillin. Penicillin salts will precipitate in a similar fashion. The latter problem can be circumvented, however, by first checking a control sample of the patient's urine for a precipitate. In this case, the specific gravity of the patient's urine can be measured at 15-minute intervals to note whether or not diatrizoate is present, as indicated by the gradual rise in urine specific gravity. In several instances we have seen the specific gravity rise rapidly within 30 minutes to 1.050. The diatrizoate salts can be administered via the nasogastric tube. With adults 50 to 60 ml is an appropriate dose. In babies the hypertonicity of the Gastrografin may contraindicate its usage.

As mentioned, it is important to avoid a false-positive test by first doing a control or by utilizing specific gravity determinations. A false-negative reaction will be obtained if dilute instead of concentrated hydrochloric acid is used.

X-RAY DIAGNOSIS

What about the use of abdominal x-rays? While the abdominal x-ray may provide useful information, the urgency of the information is lessened by the above-mentioned examination and test. In the case of a foreign body such as a bullet, the path of the bullet and the nature of the injuries may be more nearly ascertained or suspected by the location of the bullet or foreign body. A rupture of the diaphragm may be suspected early from the chest film. In many instances the patient is not able to stand in an upright position for an accurate determination of free air beneath the diaphragm because of the semishock state. For an accurate determination of the intraabdominal air, the patient should be in an upright position for at least 3 to 5 minutes. The lateral decubitus can be obtained in lieu of the upright film and, while its accuracy is somewhat less, its value is still a real one.

Controversy continues over the early management of stab wounds of the abdomen. The advocates of mandatory laparotomy point to the risk of undiagnosed perforation of a hollow viscus or laceration of the liver, spleen, or a major vascular component. Those urging selective management with a conservative approach in a sizable number of cases stress the reliability of current diagnostic observations.

DUODENAL INJURY

A stab wound with questionable peritoneal penetration can be investigated through an incision, longitudinally placed by preference, about 3 cm to the side of the stab wound and carried down to the peritoneum by muscle-splitting action. This is not best performed in the emergency room, of course, but should be done in the operating room where the exploration, if positive for intraabdominal penetration, can be further extended into a laparotomy. Avoiding a laparotomy is particularly advantageous in the alcoholic patient or in an individual with upper respiratory or active pulmonary disease. The patient may have just eaten and the possibilities of vomitus aspiration increase the risk.

Renal and major venous injuries in penetrating abdominal trauma can be anticipated preoperatively by use of a venogram.

Although pancreatic injury should be suspected in any trauma to the upper abdomen, particularly as in an automobile accident, the preoperative diagnosis is difficult to make. A rise in serum amylase determinations is, however, usually noted within a few hours of injury.

Diagnostic peritoneal lavage may be performed with 1,000 ml of Ringer's lactate solution in an adult or 300 to 500 ml in children. The connected infusion bottle is then lowered to floor level, creating a siphon to return the peritoneal fluid. As little as 75 ml of free blood in the peritoneal cavity colors the perfusate salmon pink, an indication for laparotomy. In addition to amylase determinations, microscopic examination for fecal material or bacteria should be done.

In summary, the immediate care of the patient with abdominal trauma must, in addition to emphasizing the possibilities of other injuries elsewhere in the body, center on the urgency of an early diagnosis. With the present diagnostic armamentarium of adjuncts in addition to a careful evaluation of the circumstances of the injury and the physical findings, prompt diagnosis should usually be established.

chapter 21

Early management of chest trauma

Thoracic injuries present with certain differences not found in other anatomic areas. Particularly do we refer to the normal presence of a negative intrathoracic pressure. When this pressure relationship is disturbed, the cardiopulmonary dynamics are altered. Therefore, the immediate goal in the management of the patient with a thoracic injury is concerned with a restoration of cardiopulmonary function as nearly to the normal state as possible. This even supersedes the control of hemorrhage. Ventilation takes precedence.

Of first priority is a necessity to inflate the lung. If ventilation does not occur properly, there exists an immediate need to locate the cause for an unexpanded lung or portion of lung. As emphasized before, the patient should be completely disrobed in order to adequately view the chest wall for any evidence of paradoxic motion, open wounds of the chest, signs of rib fractures, or stab wounds.

CARDIAC TAMPONADE

Once one is assured that ventilation is occurring, the next procedure of immediate priority relates to the possibility of the pericardial tamponade. Since rapid filling of the pericardial sac with blood markedly compresses the vena cava and the chambers of the heart, the venous return to the heart is seriously impaired. Adequate diastole or filling of the ventricular components of the heart is prevented, thereby limiting the amount of cardiac output with a resultant fall in coronary artery filling and decreased blood pressure. Because of the nature of steering wheel injuries and many other examples of blunt trauma to the chest, a cardiac tamponade effect can occur, involving a laceration or puncture wound of the heart or intrapericardial portion of the aorta.

One can suspect acute hemopericardium of sufficient nature to cause a cardiac tamponade by clinically observing distended neck veins along with a low peripheral arterial pressure and a high systemic venous pressure.

Immediate decompression of the pericardial sac is indicated and can be done through a needle aspiration of the left parasternal fifth or sixth interspace. This effort at decompression will often enable the patient to be transported to the hospital where a thoracotomy, pericardiotomy, and correction of the underlying pathology can take place.

108

PNEUMOTHORAX

If lung ventilation is impossible on one side of the chest, a tension pneumothorax may be present. In such a situation there is a rapid buildup of intrapleural tension causing a collapse of the lung on the involved side with displacement of the mediastinal structures to the opposite side. In displacing the mediastinal structures, the heart and great vessels including the large veins are compromised and cardiac filling is disturbed. This progressive buildup of pressure must be relieved by venting the intrapleural air to the outside. A large-bore needle may be the only means available, and if the needle is not available, even a stab wound may be lifesaving. While a large-bore tube ideally should be inserted or attached to an undersealed drain, the above approaches may be mandatory on an immediate basis.

The problem of the open pneumothorax may seem more obvious. The same mechanisms are involved with an open pneumothorax except that there is a swinging of the mediastinal structures toward the injured side. A marked swinging from one side to the other may occur during the respiratory cycle. By applying a dressing sufficiently large to cover the sucking wound, one can stabilize the situation long enough to get the patient to the emergency room or to eventually get an adequate thoracotomy tube inserted.

MASSIVE BLOOD LOSS

Massive blood loss within the chest may occasionally pose an insurmountable problem. In many instances the bleeding is from low-pressure vessels. If the blood volume interferes markedly with lung volume, a repeated thoracocentesis may stabilize the patient. When possible the insertion of a thoracotomy tube is indicated. In spite of severe exsanguination, many patients with stab wounds of the heart or injury to the great vessels can be salvaged.

FLAIL CHEST

The markedly reduced ventilation occurring as the result of paradoxic motion with a flail chest can be improved by a number of rather simple techniques. Simply inserting a cuffed endotracheal tube and inflating the lungs under positive pressure ventilation may stabilize the flail chest. Simply turning the patient onto the injured side or maintaining pressure against the involved side may prevent some degree of paradoxic motion. Efforts to further stabilize the chest can be taken in the emergency room by mechanical means and a tracheostomy can be performed there.

RUPTURE OF DIAPHRAGM

Although it is relatively uncommon, there may be sufficient trauma of either a penetrating or blunt nature to rupture the diaphragm. This complication calls for early surgery and its diagnosis is usually confirmed by roentgenograms. Of an immediate nature is the need to give intermittent positive pressure respiration if the patient is in marked cardiorespiratory distress from compression of pulmonary tissue by the abdominal viscera that have been drawn up into the thoracic cavity.

EMERGENCY TRACHEOSTOMY

Even under optimum conditions, a tracheostomy may be a difficult technical procedure. There are few times when an emergency tracheostomy should be performed on an immediate basis, because an endotracheal tube can establish an effective airway in a much more rapid fashion. The cricothyroid membrane puncture as described in Chapter 10 is much more rapid if an endotracheal tube is not available and if an airway obstruction is present. The matter of a tracheostomy can be resolved later in the hospital. Because endotracheal tubes generally are not left in place over long periods of time, a tracheostomy will usually be performed in such trauma conditions as a flail chest. The immediate means of pulmonary ventilation by mouth-to-mouth respiration and mouth-to-tube or mask and bag ventilation have been reviewed in Chapters 10 and 12 and will not again be discussed in detail here.

RECOGNIZING A CHEST INJURY

In many instances the presence of chest trauma will be obvious, but in instances of multiple injuries including unconsciousness from a head injury, the intrathoracic injuries may not be so apparent. Of particular importance is the observation that the patient is experiencing dyspnea, is complaining of chest pain, has hemoptysis, or is coughing. A rapid respiratory rate, mucous membrane or nail beds indicative of inadequate oxygenation, or the presence of blood-tinged sputum should certainly alert one to the fact that all is not well within the chest. Other very significant clinical observations include a chest wall that is moving in a paradoxic fashion, the obvious presence of a sucking wound of the chest, distended neck veins in the presence of shock, deviation of the trachea in the suprasternal notch, absent or distant breath sounds or heart tones, stridor or a crowing type of respiration, and marked restlessness. Most of these findings, if allowed to persist by failure to correct the underlying pathophysiology, will rapidly lead to respiratory failure and shock.

The frequently emphasized point throughout this book again is pertinent here and needs to be repeated: to adequately examine and diagnose the problem, one must disrobe the patient and observe the chest wall, palpate, and auscultate. Unless one does so, the presence of paradoxic motion, an open wound, or crepitus will be overlooked. (Crepitus in this case refers to the presence of air within the superficial layers of the chest wall.)

With inadequate ventilation and perfusion, the patient may rapidly become confused and agitated. The resulting depressed state of consciousness leads one to believe that a head injury is present. The patient's cerebration may be rapidly restored if adequate respiration once again takes place.

PHYSIOLOGIC CONSIDERATIONS

Although one is exposed to a great deal of instruction concerned with the physiology of respiration, a brief review of pulmonary function is in order since the proper working understanding of the pathophysiology of urgent life-threatening thoracic injuries is the crux of an understanding of proper therapy.

If one considers the respiratory process as one in which there is an adequate exchange of gases between the patient and his environment, one can break down pulmonary function into the phase or process of ventilation and that of gas exchange.

Ventilation simply refers to the ability or technique of getting oxygen into the lungs. Once it is there, the mechanism by which oxygen gets into the circulating blood volume and carbon dioxide exits from circulation is referred to as gas exchange. Adequate gas exchange or the diffusion of oxygen and carbon dioxide across the alveolocapillary membrane is, of course, dependent upon the adequate circulation of blood through the lungs themselves.

Where can things go wrong? The answer is that interference with the mechanism of either the ventilatory or the gas exchange phase can lead to serious disruption.

To begin with, the arrival of oxygen in the lungs can be interfered with in a number of ways. If the lung volume is reduced by a pneumothorax, the air within the pleural cavity collapses the lung on the involved side and often interferes with the expansion on the opposite side. Blood in the thoracic cavity (hemothorax) likewise reduces lung volume and thereby diminishes ventilation. If the integrity of the diaphragm has been interfered with as in a traumatic rupture, the abdominal viscera may herniate into the thoracic cavity to the extent that lung volume will be markedly reduced.

With ventilation there is an important time relation as the lung volume has to be expanded and collapsed over a time period. The term *tidal volume* refers to the volume of air that enters or leaves the respiratory tract with each breath. This aspect of ventilation may be interfered with if there is an obstruction of the airway by vomitus, blood, or foreign objects. When a massive crushing injury to the chest has occurred, producing a stoving-in effect or a fracture of multiple ribs, the chest expansion will occur in a paradoxic fashion in that one will observe an inspiration expansion of the uninvolved side of the chest and a collapse of the flail portion. With expiration the involved side shows expansion. The ventilation in the normal side may be expired not only into the trachea but to the abnormal side as well. A somewhat similar effect is produced with an open pneumothorax or a so-called sucking wound. In such an injury where there is an open wound to the chest, air is sucked through the wound into the thoracic cavity on inspiration, thus collapsing the lung on the side of the injury and moving the mediastinum to the opposite side. This decreases ventilation on the uninvolved side and also decreases cardiac output. Pulmonary ventilation is dependent upon other factors such as central nervous system control of respiratory rates and depths, normal functioning of the respiratory muscles used in respiration, and an effective elasticity of the lungs. This last factor is called lung compliance. None of these last factors will be considered to be of major importance in the immediate care of lung or thoracic injuries.

In addition to adequate pulmonary ventilation, effective and adequate pulmonary gas exchange must be present, otherwise respiratory failure and shock quickly occur. The relationship of ventilation and gas exchange is fundamental. If ventilation perfusion inadequacies are of significant magnitude, obvious signs of hypoxemia or hypoventilation are present. Examples of chest trauma that may produce a marked derangement of the ventilation perfusion rate are hemothorax, pneumothorax, and bronchial obstruction. *Immediate* care of the patient suffering thoracic trauma is followed as soon as possible by the more definitive measures available in the emergency room and operating suite of the hospital. As with other seriously injured patients, an intravenous route should be rapidly established to replace any blood loss and to combat hypovolemia. Measures as outlined in Chapter 4 are employed. Occasionally a patient will benefit by being moved directly to the operating room, where more effective resuscitative measures can be effected. For example, a patient with a penetrating wound of the heart can be taken first to the operating room and further observation, probably pericardial paracentesis, and ideal monitoring can be accomplished.

Again, it should be emphasized that the *immediate* measures employed for patients with serious chest trauma are of the utmost importance and, if properly employed, will be extremely rewarding. Generally speaking these measures are relatively simple. Some of these measures have been outlined in this chapter. One should refer also to Chapters 4, 10, and 12 because of an obvious overlap.

chapter 22

Injuries resulting from animal contact and their initial care

William V. Miller

SNAKE BITES

Throughout recorded history, men have feared the serpent. Objectively, the appearance of snakes is hardly more terrible than that of some other creatures of the earth, but religion, superstition, and old wives' tales make the snake an object of horror. This fact is important in a consideration of treatment of snake bite, since treatment of bites by poisonous reptiles is entirely different than treatment of the nonpoisonous variety. The emotional effect upon the patient of snake bite must be as well assessed as the character of the wound if overtreatment is to be avoided.

To be sure, poisonous snake bite does constitute a problem in America today. Various estimates place the number of poisonous bites at 180 to 300 per year, yet the death rate is very low, only ten to twenty deaths per year.

Poisonous snakes are found in all the states with the exception of Maine and Alaska. The number of snakes—and bites—is highest in the South, especially in Florida, and the Southwest.

As is well known, the pit viper (Crotalidae) injects venom through paired fangs located near the front of the mouth. This family includes the rattlesnake, the copperhead, and the cottonmouth water moccasin. The coral snake is the fourth poisonous snake in the United States. A member of the family Elapidae, its poison is not injected through fangs in a quick strike; rather, it is released from glands located at the rear of the mouth as a response to tenacious chewing movements.

While coral snake bites comprise only 5% to 10% of the total number of annually reported snake bites, the venom is the most toxic of all. Surprisingly, the bite of the western (Sanoran) coral snake has produced no fatalities, but a number of deaths from the eastern coral snake are recorded.

The bite of the coral snake manifests two important differences when compared to that of the pit viper: the mild local reaction and a delay between the time of the bite and onset of symptoms.

Essentials of treatment

Prevent spread of venom. Application of a tourniquet proximal to the location of the bite will limit the spread of venom through the subcutaneous lymphatics. It should therefore be applied tight enough to occlude only these vessels. As the edematous area expands, the tourniquet should be applied to the wrist or ankle. The tourniquet will obviously be difficult to utilize in treating bites of the trunk, head, or neck.

Application of ice was formerly thought to be useful in preventing the spread of venom. This regional hypothermia now appears to be of questionable benefit, and it may produce further tissue damage.

Since movement increases circulation and lymphatic drainage, it is to be avoided if possible. If the patient must move some distance under his own power for decisive treatment, a compromise must be effected between a slow pace to prevent spread of the toxin and a more rapid pace to hasten treatment.

Neutralize or remove toxin. It is at this juncture that the major controversy in treatment of snake bite has arisen. Should an attempt be made to remove the toxin, or should the wound be left closed and treated only with antivenin? If antivenin is more than 4 to 6 hours away or if there is no antivenin available, then the familiar X shaped incisions, ¼ inch long and ¼ inch deep, should be made. Mechanical suction should then be applied. Oral suction should be used only as a last resort. However, if the antiserum is close at hand, it is probably best to take steps to prevent the spread of the venom and to support the patient pending its administration.

Controversy has developed from contradictory experimental data concerning toxin removal. Some workers find that the amount of venom extracted from a wound is often sufficient in amount to kill an experimental animal; however, others report the inability to duplicate this finding. They believe that incision and suction present little advantage over no treatment at all. Furthermore, careless incision increases the amount of dead tissue that is susceptible to gas gangrene. We feel that careful incision and suction does no harm and may be beneficial.

The route of administration of antivenin has also been the subject of considerable discussion. While it has been customary to inject the serum subcutaneously around the bite, intravenous use of the serum may produce prompt cessation of edema, necrosis, and systemic manifestations of venenation. In any event, it is important that the patient be checked for hypersensitivity to horse serum before administration. Desenitization may be an aid, although it has been of questionable effectiveness.

Support the patient. Polyvalent Crotalidae antivenin (Wyeth) is generally available, but antivenin to coral snakes and other poisonous snakes must be obtained from special sources. Most large city zoos stock special antisera and a central file of antivenin is kept at the New York Zoological Park, The Bronx, New York.

Snakebite victims are frequently given copious quantities of alcohol, presumably as "psychotherapy." No treatment could be worse, since one of the inherent dangers is that of respiratory depression caused by curare-like effect of the venom. Alcohol serves only to aggravate the situation.

Proper support should include tetanus prophylaxis, vasopressors in the presence of shock or histamine release, sedatives to lessen anxiety and movement, and possibly antibotics and gas gangrene antisera as prophylactic measures. Cortisone is frequently used to reduce morbidity and mortality in cases of snake bite, as well as to reduce the severity of serum sickness in overdosage of antivenin. Disturbances in red blood cell count and electrolyte balance may resemble those found with third-degree burn, and the patient should be carefully monitored with these factors in mind.

Pathogenicity

Age and size of the victim are important to the outcome of bites by poisonous snakes, as are degree of penetration, size of the snake, and amount of venom injected. It should be remembered that snake bite is not synonymous with envenomation, since the snake may recently have exhausted the supply of venom in a previous strike.

Although the nature of the toxins found in snake venom remains an area of study, it appears that they fall into three general classes: *proteases,* which may produce necrosis at the site as well as remote visceral hemorrhage; *phosphotidases,* which are responsible for hemolysis through their action upon lecithin and which indirectly produce hypotension through histamine release; and *neurotoxins,* which may produce a curare-like effect as they interfere with neuronal conduction or act directly upon the central nervous system to produce death through bulbar paralysis. The coral snake produces a venom that is chiefly neurotoxic. Venom of the water moccasion produces intravascular coagulation. Copperhead venom has a curare-like effect, while the toxin of the rattlesnake venom includes the effect of each of the other venoms. Practically speaking, the toxins of the pit vipers are grouped together since they are treated similarly; however, bites produced by the Elapidae present a different problem.

Antiserum for the combined polyvalent pit viper toxins is prepared in horses and is available in a dry, powdered form that is rehydrated before use. The coral snake is a more serious problem, however, since the only antiserum available at the present time is that prepared in humans. While it is theoretically possible to immunize everyone, it is, of course, highly impractical except in high-exposure groups.

INSECT BITES AND STINGS

Of all of man's "natural enemies," insects probably cause him the most discomfort. Insects are vectors of hundreds of diseases. Their uncomfortable bites and stings are dangerous and represent a constant and a considerable menace to health.

General approach

Treatment of the bites of ants, mosquitoes, gnats, flies, chiggers, and other biting insects, as well as those that sting, is essentially prophylactic and symptomatic. The host of available insect repellents which are primarily hydrocarbon in nature, work with varying degrees of effectiveness, in some cases affording real protection against many species. In the case of other insects, control of their population with insecticides is more effective.

The usual insect bite represents a minor acute inflammation of the skin and it may be treated with calamine lotion, either pure or combined with a local anesthetic. The acid of bee stings may be effectively neutralized by application of a paste of baking soda. In applying symptomatic treatment, it should be borne in mind, of course, that insect-related disease is a distinct possibility in almost all regions of the United States.

Allergic reactions

The major danger to the patient bitten or stung by insects is that of allergic reaction. While overwhelming envenomation can occur, it is very rare; intravenous stings are so rare as to be almost academic in consideration. In the years between 1950 and 1959, however, 50% of deaths from all animal venoms was caused by bees, wasps, hornets, and yellow jackets (order Hymenoptera). Death occurred mainly in adults and usually within 1 to 2 hours of the sting.

The individual is usually aware of his sensitivity through experience with increasingly severe reactions upon repeated exposure, but the patient may occasionally fail to exhibit such a history. The reaction is a characteristically anaphylactic one. Epinephrine, antihistaminics, and corticosteroids are drugs of choice in treatment. Since movement of the patient in order to obtain medical aid is usually precluded by the short time between exposure and onset of severe symptoms, it is urged that the hypersensitive person make every effort to avoid exposure and that he always carry an antihistaminic as well as a sublingual sympathomimetic drug on his person. It is also recommended that he have readily available, both in his home and in his automobile, a syringe containing aqueous epinephrine, 1:1,000 and that he be instructed in its administration.

SPIDER BITES

The black widow ranges over almost the entire continental United States. It is easily recognized by its glossy black appearance, combined with an hourglass-shaped red area on the ventral aspect. Its fondness for outdoor toilets and other cool, damp outbuildings accounts for the high frequency of bites on the buttocks, genitocrural regions, and the extremities.

The black widow bite is manifested by immediate pain, local redness, and swelling. The systemic toxic effects are usually evidenced within 1 hour. Pain and muscle cramps begin in the region of the bite and spread until most of the major muscle groups are involved. The cramp-like pain and the abdominal rigidity at times suggest an acute surgical abdomen; however, an important feature in diagnostic distinction lies in the fact that the patient with this bite is quite restless and is seen to toss about. Although death rarely results, respiratory depression caused by intercostal spasm may be a problem. The venom is neurotoxic and may cause ascending paralysis as well as damage to peripheral nerve endings.

Tubocurarine has been used to lessen muscle rigidity, as have intravenous infusions of 10 ml of 10% calcium gluconate solution. Sedatives, hot baths, and intravenous procaine have all been used as a part of treatment, but most effective is the specific black widow antiserum prepared in horses. When properly administered, it is so effective that mortality is less than 5%.

Within the past decade, a second spider native to the southern and central United States has been shown to be responsible for bites followed by soft-tissue and muscle necrosis with long-delayed healing. The brown recluse *(Loxosceles reclusa)* prefers warm, dry places such as closets, garages, and clothing stored therein. Both male and female appear to secrete a potent venom that is poisonous to mammals, producing a characteristic necrotic lesion at the site of the bite.

A painful stinging sensation is usually felt immediately, but occasionally it is several hours before the victim is aware that he has been bitten. A small blister arises, and a large area around the site of venenation becomes edematous and congested, with indurated margins. The local pain is often quite intense, and the patient is frequently restless and febrile. During the following days, the affected soft tissue becomes necrotic and gradually sloughs, exposing underlying muscle or bone. These lesions may be small or quite large, ulcers up to 4 inches in diameter having been reported. Although the effects are generally local, there have been cases of systemic reaction accompanied by erythema, proteinuria, fever, and hematuria.

Treatment of the bite is a considerable problem since the action of the toxin is not understood. It has been suggested that it is similar to L-norepinephrine, with a powerful vasospastic action and resulting ischemic necrosis. Fresh bites do seem to be improved by administration of epinephrine antagonists. Few bites are seen at this stage, however. First-aid treatment is now confined to antisepsis and supportive therapy. Local infusion of antihistamines and corticosteroids has been used. The ulcer heals by granulation, leaving a large scar, and surgical debridement may be required. Prevention of the spider bite by eradication of the spider is the first line of defense. In addition, recognition of the spider and its habitat should reduce the chance of being bitten.

DOMESTIC AND WILD ANIMAL BITES AND SCRATCHES

Just as insect bites and stings represent injuries that are potential portals of entry for organisms of serious infectious disease, so are the bites and scratches of various higher animals. Cat-scratch fever, a viral disease, is well known. Cats have occasionally been implicated in the etiology of *Pasteurella* infections, as well. Dogs and a number of other animals harbor within their mouths various infectious agents including tetanus bacilli. The rabies problem is discussed in Chapter 36.

First-aid measures are essentially the same as for a similar wound of different etiology. Hemostasis, debridement, antisepsis, and closure should be accompanied by an ascertainment of the level of tetanus immunity. Antibiotic prophylaxis is not generally recommended.

STINGRAYS AND JELLYFISH

Cutaneous injuries resulting from contact with stingrays and jellyfish are common in coastal waters. In both, the toxin appears to be heat labile and best treated with debridement of the wound and prompt, copious warm water irrigation. The serrated spines of the integumentary sheath of the stingray may be especially difficult to remove and cause extensive tissue damage.

chapter 23

Athletic emergencies*

Fred A. Wappel

In order to properly understand athletic injuries, the trainer and the physician should know precisely how the injury was sustained, so that they will be able to visualize the areas receiving the greatest stress, the direction from which the stress came, and the damage that occurred to the joints and other areas of the body. Bilateral comparison in examination is helpful in detecting irregularity, bone displacement, swelling, and other symptoms that aid in diagnosing the injury.

Immediate examination on the field of play by the trainer has proved to be beneficial to the physician who sees the athlete. Marked pain, swelling, and stiffness are not always immediately present; thus the athlete may not be apprehensive during examination. A goal of immediate care on the field is to lessen swelling and decrease pain. It is important to calm the athlete and to offer reassurance.

INTERNAL INJURIES
Concussion

With a mild concussion, generally the athlete is incoherent and dazed, and occasionally he sees spots before him. There may be loss of memory and headache. There may be a period of unconsciousness during which the athlete should not be touched or moved. Return of consciousness may not bring coherency. Amnesia may be present. The neck as well as the head may be injured. Neurologic tests of pinching and pinpricking should be administered before the athlete is moved. Direct questioning should be avoided because of fear, emotion, and shock. Observation should be made of any pupillary dilation.

If these tests are negative, the athlete should be hospitalized for observation, particularly if he was unconscious for a lengthy period. The athlete who was never unconscious but who was incoherent or dazed, with a temporary loss of memory, should never be left alone. He must be accompanied by a friend, coach, or trainer and must be placed immediately in the hands of his family or roommate. He must *not* be left alone

---

*Athletic injuries are seldom discussed in the medical curriculum. In fact, few physicians feel confident to manage their immediate diagnosis and treatment unless they have had special exposure and experience to this specialized group of injuries. For one thing, these are injuries occurring in eager, young, and active individuals in the best physical condition. An improper decision may result in serious or permanent damage. Mr. Fred Wappel, a veteran intercollegiate trainer, presents a brief summary of immediate measures needed in the care of some frequently encountered athletic injuries.

because he may have a relapse, suffer amnesia, and wander off alone, not knowing who he is or where he lives.

On occasion the athlete may become violent. To anticipate this problem, the physician or trainer should kneel and straddle the athlete at the waistline and reassure him when he regains consciousness.

Finally, the athlete may "swallow his tongue." In this case, the jaws lock and the athlete will suffocate if prompt treatment is not initiated. An oral screw is used to pry open the jaws and the tongue should be placed in its normal position, using the tongue-seizing forceps. Usually, however, simply positioning the head as outlined in Chapter 12 will open the airway satisfactorily. Artificial respiration should be administered if necessary.

In the event an oral screw is not available, tongue depressors may be used by staggering them one on top of the other and taping them together. The bottom blade is placed between the jaws and they are wedged in as rapidly as possible until one of the fingers can remove the tongue from the airway. Needless to say this procedure must be accomplished within 4 minutes.

Ruptured spleen

The athlete who receives a blow to the left upper abdominal quadrant may suffer a ruptured spleen. The symptoms and signs of a ruptured spleen may be pain in the left upper abdominal quadrant and shoulder, weakness, rapid pulse, paleness, apprehension, thirst, and sweating.

Pain may be present in the left shoulder (supraclavicular fossa) because of an irritation of the diaphragm. The phrenic nerve innervates the diaphragm, and the pain in the shoulder is referred pain. An athlete who has any of these symptoms should be seen by a physician immediately or placed in the hospital for observation and examination.

Ribs in the left upper quadrant should be examined carefully before a hasty generalization is made.

Kidney injuries

With any trauma to the posterior lower aspect of the rib cage, a kidney injury should be suspected and proper examination should be made before the athlete returns to the contest. Generally there is pain in the back over the area of the kidney. A urine sample should be taken immediately to determine whether there is any hematuria. If blood is present, the urine sample should be retained and the athlete should be seen by a doctor immediately.

Needless to say, this athlete should not compete in athletics if marked kidney damage is present. An athlete who has only one kidney should never be permitted to participate in contact sports.

Bladder

Bladder injuries are rare in athletics. One reason is that the athlete generally keeps his bladder empty because of nervous tension.

Hematuria has been discovered after running. This is usually of no consequence. Examination should be made by the physician, however, as a precautionary measure.

Rib cage injuries

Injuries to the rib cage fall into two categories: injury to the ribs and injury to the costal cartilages.

The rib cage injury usually involves symptoms of pain, point tenderness, bony irregularity, inability to breathe deeply, and inability to lie down without discomfort.

Palpation will determine whether there is any bone irregularity. Usually injury to the costal cartilage produces a detectable separation. By no means should the athlete be picked up by the belt to restore respiration. The ribs may be fractured and the lung punctured.

The ribs should be taped until x-rays determine the extent of the injury. The athlete should exhale as the tape is applied. The hair should be shaved and tincture of benzoin applied to the skin, which is highly susceptible to tape rash.

The 6-inch elastic bandage is adequate to wrap around the rib cage for comfort and to eliminate the rash from tape, which may be then applied over the elastic bandage. Ice should be applied immediately and continued for a minimum of 12 hours.

Hyperventilation

Hyperventilation is defined as a greater respiratory rate and/or depth than is necessary for physiologic needs of the body. Hyperventilation is brought about by fright and apprehension following injury. Direct questions such as: "Do you have any feeling in your arms and legs?" will alarm the athlete further and should be avoided until the condition has been relieved. The athlete has a conscious feeling of needing more air, begins rapid breathing, and exhales too much carbon dioxide.

A paper bag is held in place over the mouth and nose to permit rebreathing of the expelled air, which is increasingly rich in carbon dioxide. The athlete is instructed to breathe slowly, which is not easily accomplished in this condition.

The bag should remain in place until respiration returns to normal. The athlete may lose consciousness, but he regains it in a short period of time. On occasion, heavy breathing begins again, and the same procedure is once more followed.

HEAD, NECK, AND BACK INJURIES
Sunstroke or heat stroke

These matters are treated in Chapter 16.

Nosebleed

Nosebleed is discussed in Chapter 35.

Cervical spine injury

When an athlete is lying motionless on the field, whether conscious or unconscious, he should not be moved until a doctor is summoned. Anything should be suspected at this point. The athlete should be observed to determine that he remains motionless and to rule out spinal injury. If he regains consciousness and moves his body, more precise examination may begin. The symptoms of cervical vertebral involvement are pain, stiffness in the neck, limited range of motion, muscle spasm, referred pain in the arms, and general lack of peripheral sensitivity. A physician should be summoned immediately. The athlete should not be moved, and no equipment should be removed, particularly the helmet, until there is voluntary head movement. The subject is discussed in further detail in Chapter 26.

An athlete who is exposed to a neck injury should not be permitted to return to a contest, particularly in a contact sport, until he has been properly x-rayed and cleared for competition. An x-ray study is made of all cervical vertebral injuries, no matter how minor they may seem. This is a hard and fast rule, and it must not be ignored.

Many athletes do not report neck injuries immediately. They feel the matter to be of no significance and after an athletic event may sit slouched over in front of the locker with marked pain, stiffness, and limited range of motion and in a partial state of shock. This athlete should be handled in the same way as the athlete on the field who is suspected of having a cervical vertebral injury.

SHOULDER INJURIES
Acromioclavicular separation

Acromioclavicular separation occurs as a result of falling directly on the shoulder or from a blow directly on the shoulder as in tackling. The athlete should be made comfortable and the arm must be placed in a sling with the elbow supported until the diagnosis is made by the physician. Normally, the complete or severe separation is easiest to detect. Elevation of the clavicle is distinctly prominent. The moderate separation will show partial elevation, and the mild separation will show slight elevation. Bilateral comparison of x-rays is important. Some athletes demonstrate normal elevation of both joints.

If the separation is severe, surgery may be performed; however, we find this procedure to be debatable. If the separation is mild, the arm should be placed in a sling and ice should be applied to the shoulder for a minimum of 6 hours. The sling should be worn until pain disappears. If the separation is moderate, the shoulder must be taped. Tincture of benzoin should be applied to the skin. A piece of ½-inch felt should be placed over the lateral aspect of the clavicle or on the point of elevation.

Application of 1½- or 2-inch adhesive tape or 3-inch elastic tape should begin on the posterior aspect of the shoulder. It will cover the felt and pass below the elbow and back up to the anterior aspect of the shoulder, where it overlaps. Mild tension should be applied to the tape, particularly when it is pulled up to the anterior aspect of the shoulder. A piece of sponge rubber should be placed under the elbow to cushion it. This procedure reduces the separation, enables the ligaments to heal, and reduces the strain placed on the shoulder girdle.

The taping procedure should be repeated three times, overlapping out to the tip of the shoulder. The tape should remain in place for a period of 14 to 21 days, and further x-ray study should determine the amount of reduction from the taping. The arm should be placed in a sling and ice should be applied for a minimum of 24 hours.

Dislocation

Shoulder dislocation in athletics generally occurs when the arm is in abduction and external rotation. The joint capsule will usually tear anteriorly and inferiorly. On rare occasions, most frequently in wrestling, the posterior aspect of the joint capsule will tear.

The dislocation of the shoulder is easily recognized by noting a hollow pit at the superior portion of the deltoid muscle. The condition is generally accompanied by fixation of the arm. The athlete is apprehensive at moving the arm from its fixed position. There is immediate muscle spasm, and reduction without administration of relaxants is not easily accomplished unless one is particularly skilled in this manipulation. When manipulation is being attempted without analgesics, one must be cautious not to apply a force so great that more extensive tearing will result. It is important, however, that reduction be accomplished immediately if at all possible, to minimize muscle spasm.

When the athlete is moved, the arm should be placed in a comfortable position and stress should be taken off the shoulder joint. This may be accomplished by placing towels, a pillow, or a similar bulky object under the elbow and upper arm so that the shoulder joint will be as relaxed as possible under the circumstances. The arm should then be placed in a sling, or a sling may be improvised by taping posteriorly from the shoulder girdle, under the elbow, and back to the shoulder girdle.

An x-ray study should be made immediately to eliminate the possibility of fracture. An effective method of reduction by the physician consists of placing the athlete on the affected side with the arm hanging off the end of the table, while resting his head on another table. A 10-pound plate with a tape extension is applied to the athlete's wrist and a reduction is accomplished by the hanging weight. Ice should be applied to the area immediately after reduction to minimize hemorrhage.

After reduction, the athlete should be placed in a Velpeau splint for at least 4 weeks, permitting the joint capsule to scar down and lessening the possibility of recurrence.

ELBOW INJURIES
Dislocation

Elbow dislocations generally occur at a time when the arm is extended with the hand stabilized on the ground or floor, so that the elbow is forced into hyperextension. Symptoms are displacement of the elbow joint, pain, fixation, swelling, and greatly diminished range of motion. A physician should be summoned immediately, or if the athlete is to be taken to the hospital, the elbow should be cradled in a pillow for comfort and held against his body. An x-ray study should be made to determine whether a fracture is present.

After reduction, the elbow should be wrapped with an elastic bandage from the hand up to the axilla. The elbow should be elevated, and it should be encased in ice for a minimum of 24 hours.

Hyperextended elbow

When the arm is extended with the hand fixed on the ground or floor, the elbow may be forced into hyperextension in such a manner that it does not dislocate but the ligaments, muscles, and joint capsule are stretched and distended. Symptoms include swelling of the medial condyle, limited range of motion, pain, and tenderness.

The elbow should be examined for swelling and to determine passive range of motion for flexion, extension, supination, and pronation. Palpation is helpful in determining any bony irregularity or chips.

The elbow should be elevated, wrapped with an elastic bandage, and encased in ice for 1 hour. It should then be wrapped with an elastic roller bandage and cushioned by foam rubber. The wrap should extend from the hand to the axilla. The arm should be placed in a sling, and the athlete should be referred for examination and x-ray study. Even when initial swelling and other symptoms are absent, the elbow should be iced and wrapped since it will usually swell and become symptomatic several hours later.

HAND AND WRIST INJURIES
Navicular fractures

The carpal navicular is more subject to injury than are any of the other carpal bones. It may be fractured in a fall, which forces the wrist into hyperextension, or by other violent action to the wrist. Pain, particularly in the snuff box area, limited range of motion, and swelling characterize the injury. Range of motion tests should be accomplished to determine the amount of immobility. Immediately after injury, pain, swelling, and limited range of motion are frequently absent; but these symptoms may begin several hours later.

Ice should be placed on the wrist immediately and should be maintained until x-ray study and examination are instituted. If the wrist is painful, a longitudinally halved type-carton or wooden splint padded with cotton or any soft material should be placed under the wrist; an elastic bandage should be used over this splint. An x-ray study should follow.

Many physicians cast this injury at once because a fracture is not always detected immediately. If a fracture is not detected upon a recheck x-ray after a week or 10 days, the cast is removed and the athlete may resume activity. Otherwise, the cast will be retained and the athlete will be removed from participation in athletics until the fracture unites. Healing is slow because of the poor blood supply, and in many instances this fracture does not unite.

Fracture of metacarpals

The reader is referred to Chapter 18 for a discussion of hand injuries.

Forearm injuries

Fracture of the radius or ulna is identified with displacement of bone, bone irregularity, swelling, pain, limited pronation and supination, and inability to grip with the hand. Any bony irregularity or displacement should be noted before active motion is accomplished. Pressing the radius and ulna together with the hand will elicit sharp pain if either bone is fractured, although pain may also be present with a contusion. After determining that pronation and supination can be accomplished, the athlete should be asked to grip the hand of the examiner firmly so that muscular strength may be evaluated. An x-ray study should follow.

When there is a question of fracture, the forearm should be wrapped with a 3-inch elastic bandage from the hand to the elbow and the arm should be placed in a sling. If a fracture is present, the forearm should be wrapped with an elastic bandage and placed in a pillow, blanket, or any available splinting material until a physician can give further treatment.

INJURIES TO THE CREST OF ILEUM AND THE GROIN
Groin

Although groin injuries have never presented a serious problem in athletics, muscle strains are frequently detected in this area. Symptoms include pain with hip flexion, abduction, hyperextension, and rotation. There is a limited range of motion, and the characteristic walk will favor the involved hip. Treatment of groin strain consists of ice for a minimum of 12 hours and rest. Moist heat will help restore muscle function in a few days. When the athlete is able to walk normally without pain, a spica wrap is applied to the upper thigh and lower abdominal area with 2- to 4-inch elastic roller bandage. This spica wrap supports the hip muscles and aids hip flexion, enabling participation in athletics even though there is slight pain. The injury is rarely disabling.

Crest of the ileum contusion

The crest of the ileum is subjected to trauma when the athlete fails to properly wear hip pads designed to protect this area. Pads are frequently worn too low, exposing the crest to trauma. Occasionally, a shoulder or helmet hits this point with terrific force and the injury cannot be avoided. Symptoms include marked pain and limited range of motion, particularly trunk rotation. There is swelling, and coughing or sneezing cause acute pain. Swelling will be noted upon visual examination. Fortunately, fracture of the crest of the ileum is rare and treatment for contusion is the same as that prescribed for other contusions.

KNEE INJURIES

Although the knee is considered to be a hinge joint, it is not a true hinge. In flexion, it has the ability to go into a medial or lateral rotation. The knee does not have a true joint capsule for stabilization as other joints do; therefore, it is particularly subject to a variety of injuries. The cartilages that lie on the condyles of the tibia are injured if forced rotation takes place. The collateral ligaments are injured if the stabilized knee is hit from a medial or lateral plane. The cruciate ligaments are injured if the body is hit from either the front or the back while the leg is in complete extension and the foot is stabilized. Multiple damage (to the medial collateral ligament, to the medial cartilage, and to the anterior cruciate ligament) occurs when the cleats of a football player are stabilized in the ground during forced medial rotation. This injury is classified as the "external triad" and has been occurring frequently in athletics during recent years.

When examining a knee injury, it is important to know how the injury occurred. The knowledge of this fact enables one to understand the structural derangement that takes place and the exact anatomic location of injury. Palpation is an excellent means of determining any irregularity around the joint, and point tenderness is an important indicator of ligamentous tissue damage or derangement. (Point tenderness over the joint margin, medially or laterally, may indicate either cartilage or meniscus damage.)

Medial collateral ligament involvement

The ligament may be torn or severed when the athlete is subjected to a forceful blow from the side while the foot is stabilized. The medial collateral ligament is longer than the lateral collateral ligament and has a deep branch that attaches at one point on the outer rim of the medial cartilage border. Generally, when the medial ligament is stretched, torn, or severed, the medial cartilage is also torn. There is inability to bear weight and point tenderness over the ligamentous area. Swelling is highly variable with time and with the degree of injury. There is pain, and the joint may be unstable.

A visual examination should be accomplished, before the individual is moved, in order to determine any displacement of bone. The athlete should be calmed and the leg should be completely extended before an abduction test is then applied. One hand is placed on the lateral aspect of the knee and the other hand is placed medially on the ankle. Pressure is exerted on the knee joint to determine whether there is any relaxation of the medial ligament. Then the knee is placed in partial flexion and the same procedure is repeated. Bilateral comparison with the opposite knee will make possible determination of the amount of relaxation of the ligament if there is any question of tearing.

If the medial ligament is stretched or slightly torn (which may only involve a few fibers), ice and pressure should be applied for a minimum of 1 hour, and I recommend application of ice during the entire evening. The knee will not become stiff and sore for several hours after activity. Foam rubber should be placed under 4- or 6-inch elastic roller bandage. Crutches are generally unnecessary with this type of sprain.

If the medial ligament is partially torn and relaxation is present, the athlete cannot bear weight well. In this case the knee should be wrapped with an elastic bandage before the athlete is carried from the playing area. Ice and pressure should be applied immediately. The ice should be placed in large plastic bags encasing the knee to control hemorrhage and swelling. Ice should remain for at least 24 hours. The extent of relaxation and gapping of the joint should be determined by x-ray during forced abduction. Avoidance of weight bearing and bed rest with elevation are important during the first 24 hours. When the medial ligament is completely severed, orthopedic consultation will naturally be requested.

Lateral collateral ligament involvement

The ligament is torn or severed when the knee is subjected to a forceful blow from the medial side while the foot is stabilized. The symptoms are generally the same as those encountered in medial involvement except that the athlete generally bears weight well with this type of tear or sprain. The lateral ligament is much shorter than the medial one and neither pain nor immobility is marked.

The examination procedure is reversed from that of the medial ligament, with one hand placed on the medial aspect of the knee and the other hand placed laterally on the ankle. Procedures to determine the extent of injury and the nature of treatment are the same as those for the medial collateral ligament.

Anterior and posterior cruciate ligament involvement

The anterior cruciate ligament is generally torn or severed by forced hyperextension at the knee. The posterior cruciate ligament is torn or severed if the tibia is forced backward while the knee is in complete extension. Both ligaments have been known to rupture when the athlete is struck below the partially flexed knee while the cleats of the football shoe are locked in the ground, thereby forcing medial rotation of the knee. Concomitant tearing at the medial collateral ligament and the medial cartilage may also occur. The extended knee generally lacks stability. Pain may be present, although little swelling is detected until several hours after injury.

During examination, the knee is flexed at 90 degrees and the drawer sign is used in the following manner to determine the extent of tearing or possible severing. The hands are placed below the knee with a firm grip around the leg; the leg is pulled forward and pushed backward. The distance that the leg glides forward and backward will determine the severity of injury. Slight displacement anteriorly or posteriorly indicates only mild damage; however, if the ligament is completely ruptured, the knee glides forward or backward with no resistance.

In mild and moderate tearing of ligaments, the knee should be immediately encased in ice to limit hemorrhage and swelling. The ice should be continued for a minimum of 24 hours and in some cases up to 48 hours. The leg should be wrapped from the foot to well above the knee with an elastic bandage, and it should be elevated. The physician may wrap the knee heavily with cotton wadding and place it in half or full cylindrical cast. Crutches will be issued. If the cruciate ligament is ruptured, surgical intervention will be decided upon by the physician handling the case.

Medial and lateral semilunar cartilage involvement

The medial cartilage is injured more frequently than the lateral cartilage. Its injury is caused primarily by the forced medial rotation of the knee from partial flexion while the cleats of the shoe are locked in the ground, thus tearing the cartilage. The cleated shoe is the largest cause of all cartilage injuries. The cartilage is also torn if the knee is hit from either the medial or the lateral side while partially flexed and while the shoe is stabilized. Forced medial or lateral rotation tears the cartilage. The primary symptom of any torn cartilage is locking of the joint in partial flexion. When walking, the knee may collapse or give way. The knee may also present a clicking sensation when walking or squatting. Pain and point tenderness are present at the joint margin, although these may be delayed symptoms. If an athlete says he "cuts up field and feels the knee give way," this is a positive indication of a cartilage tear. Walking is possible; but comfort depends on the degree of tearing. Fluid is not always immediately present, but if the cartilage is torn, fluid will increase or decrease, depending on the activity of the athlete.

If the medial ligament is sprained or ruptured, generally the medial cartilage will be torn. When the abduction test is applied, the cartilage will "pluck." The presence of the McMurray sign (the knee presents a "click" when going into extension) is a good indication of posterior tears of the cartilage. The athlete is placed on a table with the knee flexed at 90 degrees. The heel is grasped and rotated in external rotation and the knee extended by circling the leg. A "click" or pain from this action will indicate tearing.

The immediate treatment of a torn cartilage consists of ice, pressure, and immobility with crutches. Ice and immobilization should be continued for at least 24 hours. Crutches may be indicated for a longer period of time. A pressure bandage with foam rubber should be worn at all times to support the knee and control synovial fluid increase. Treatment is generally conservative until point tenderness and pain subside; however, if the knee cannot be unlocked with manipulation or traction, surgery is, of course, advised. Traction has been used to unlock the cartilage, and, with conservative treatment, the athlete has been able to complete a season with the knee taped without ill effects. It must be remembered that pain and the knee "giving way" should not be tolerated when the athlete is participating in an event.

During his convalescence, the athlete must maintain quadriceps tone by such methods as isometric contraction and progressive resistive exercise.

ANKLE INJURIES
Sprain

A sprain is fibrous tearing of ligaments, either partially or completely. The identifying features of a sprained ankle will differ markedly, depending upon the severity of the sprain. The manner in which the athlete walks will give an indication of the severity of his sprain. The symptoms are inability to bear weight, swelling resulting from internal bleeding (hemorrhage may or may not appear immediately; swelling, in many instances, does not begin for 5 or 6 hours), pain, and point tenderness over ligamentous tissue. Bony irregularity is an indication of fracture. Derangement of the ankle joint is an indication of severe ankle injury, which is not often seen in athletics but which is not beyond possibility.

On the field, the athlete should be calmed before any examination begins. An attempt should be made to determine how the injury occurred. Only after careful observation of the position of the ankle and foot should the shoelaces be cut, and the shoe should be removed with care. Pressing the tibia and fibula together helps to determine the possibility of a fracture, which is indicated by marked pain with this action. Palpation of the ligaments surrounding the joint reveals tenderness, swelling, or bony irregularity. If possible, determination of range of motion will enable evaluation of the degree of injury. If range of motion if limited, the athlete should be carried off the field and more complete examination should follow.

If range of motion is good and pain is not severe, bearing weight on the ankle will determine whether there is any limitation while standing. In the absence of pain and if the attending physician consents, the athlete may return to the game. It must be emphasized, however, that the injury may not present any immediate symptoms. If, with continued activity, the athlete begins favoring the ankle, he should be removed from the game immediately for treatment.

Treatment should be initiated with elevation, ice, and pressure. Ice should be packed entirely around the ankle and lower limb. Heavy ice-filled plastic bags have proved to be the most effective means for controlling hemorrhage. A regular icebag does not offer adequate hypothermia, and hemorrhage will not be controlled to any marked degree. Ice, pressure, and elevation should be continued for a minimum of 24 hours and in some cases as long as 48 hours or until a physician examines the injury.

Ice should be applied when the athlete returns home and should be continued throughout the night.

The use of foam rubber under the elastic pressure bandage, when swelling is present, is a general practice at the University of Missouri. The bandaging is removed when the athlete goes to bed and is reapplied when he awakens. He continues this procedure until swelling subsides.

The elastic wrap is applied with mild pressure, beginning at the toes, enclosing the ankle, and ending below the calf. If the toes swell, the wrap is too tight and should be reapplied. Elevation of the foot will reduce the temporary swelling.

chapter 24

Immediate handling of acute blood loss

Earl J. Wipfler, Jr.

Early one January morning several years ago, I was walking to the hospital from my home. A blanket of freshly fallen snow was on the ground. As I walked across the campus I noticed on the snow a trail of blood that led all the way to the hospital entrance. In the emergency room I found that a student had accidentally lacerated his wrist. Bleeding occurred through a small tear in the radial artery. Obviously, such massive blood loss was completely unnecessary. Had the injured student or one of his friends simply placed his thumb over the bleeding point of the radial artery, almost no blood loss would have occurred. Most copious blood loss at the time of accidents is caused by the inadequate application of pressure over the bleeding point.

A second and more massive bleeding episode comes to mind when I recall a case of a 15-year-old school boy who was practicing the "fast draw." Unfortunately he pulled the trigger on the gun much too soon and the bullet exploded into the right upper thigh, tearing the femoral artery and vein for a considerable length. He was alone with his mother in their home in the country and his mother was unable to drive a car. Almost at that instant, however, a neighbor drove into the yard. Driving as fast as possible, they arrived at the University of Missouri Medical Center (approximately 5 miles away) and were immediately seen in the emergency room where the victim was gradually losing consciousness and was without any palpable pulse or blood pressure. Immediate direct firm pressure was placed on the bleeding area in lieu of only partially occluding pressure that had been applied. Ringer's lactate solution and dextran were immediately started and the patient was rushed to the operating room where adequate control of the bleeding was accomplished, a prosthetic graft was placed between the two torn ends of the femoral artery, and the femoral vein was reconstituted.

Bleeding from a laceration of a peripheral vessel is usually not a great control problem. On the other hand, the problems presented in controlling hemorrhage from around the femoral or hip area, the shoulder, and the chest are not so simple. Intrathoracic hemorrhage and its control are described in more detail in Chapter 21. Major injuries to vessels of the trunk may occur without obvious signs of bleeding, and it is important to realize that these occult injuries are usually associated with the absence of the pulse distal to site of injury, perhaps with a large hematoma, and even with a neurologic deficit. Several thousand milliliters of blood can be lost in the thigh alone.

The emergency transfusion of whole blood can, indeed, be lifesaving. Whether or not the use of the universal donor or unmatched whole blood is ever justified is open to argument, since the instance of severe complications is high and because colloid as a blood substitute is especially effective as a volume expander. It is almost always desirable to use carefully cross-matched blood. Whole fresh blood also has the advantage of combating some of the coagulation abnormalities commonly present in cirrhotic patients.

Rapid transfusion of whole blood can be hazardous, particularly if it is cold blood that has not been rewarmed. Rapidly administered cold blood can have a very decided adverse effect upon myocardial contractility. Ideally, blood should be warmed by allowing it to pass through tubing immersed in a warm water bath.

Arrest of hemorrhage is usually best accomplished by means of pressure dressings applied manually to the wound or by circumferential bandaging of the extremity. Deep wounds usually require broad pressure areas to arrest hemorrhage, while superficial wound hemorrhage can usually be controlled by more localized pressure. In most accident situations, formal dressings and bandages are not readily available; therefore, direct manual pressure applied over reasonably clean clothing material is most effective. When circumferential bandaging is used, care must be taken in order to avoid interference with the remaining arterial supply to, or venous drainage from, the distal extremity.

A tourniquet should be used if direct wound pressure does not give satisfactory control of hemorrhage. A tourniquet is applied to the thigh or the arm; it is not applied to the leg or the forearm. The rationale involved in this application of tourniquets becomes obvious when one considers the fact that the two bones of the forearm or the leg will act to prevent ordinary tourniquet pressure from compressing arteries that lie between the bones.

Easily available tourniquet material, such as ropes or belts, is usually too narrow. When tourniquets must be made from such materials, they should be applied over strips of clothing or other padding material in order to prevent tissue damage. Common mistakes in using tourniquets include:

1. Failure to try to control bleeding by application of pressure dressings before turning to this more dangerous method
2. Loose application, which results in increased venous bleeding from increased venous pressure during continuation of arterial flow to the wound and to the extremity
3. Failure to evaluate peripheral pulses and appearance of the extremity both prior to and during tourniquet application
4. Failure to record tourniquet time and to effect 5-minute periods of release at regular 45-minute intervals

Again, it should be emphasized that tourniquets are to be used only when pressure, elevation, and immobilization are unable to control hemorrhage. Successful arterial reconstruction may be seriously handicapped by tourniquet application, with amputation an unfortunate sequel.

Careful arrest of hemorrhage and proper splinting of extremity fractures are the prime essentials of peripheral vascular first aid. Following institution of these measures, and prior to the time that definitive care becomes available to the patient, observation is essential. Only careful observation can prevent detrimental results of first aid treatment. Every effort should be made to provide reconstructive arterial surgery as soon as possible to enhance the chance of success.

chapter 25

Emergency eye care

Richard O. Coe, Jr.

GENERAL CONSIDERATIONS

There is but a handful of true ocular emergencies that require the proper treatment within 30 minutes to several hours after onset. These include orbital cellulitis, gonococcal conjunctivitis, *Pseudomonas* corneal ulceration, acute iridocyclitis, acute closed-angle (congestive) glaucoma, retinal detachment (prior to macular involvement), central retinal artery occlusion, and various types of trauma to and about the eye. These cases are serious; however, it is equally important to manage other types of eye conditions that the patient terms an "emergency." These patients are usually prompted to seek help at all hours whether they experience a simple redness of the eye or more profound ocular discomfort. Mismanagement of a so-called emergency may create a serious ocular problem at a later date.

In management of an unconscious patient, even without ocular problems, two things must be done: search for the possibility of contact lenses, and annoint the eyes of the patient with an ophthalmic preparation.

Topical anesthetics and ointments delay epithelial regeneration. Except in the actual removal of a superficially embedded corneal foreign body, topical anesthesia should not be used in the treatment of acute ocular pain. In a patient with welder's kerato-conjunctivitis or sunlamp keratoconjunctivitis, one is tempted to make use of these agents; however, it should be remembered that this delays corneal epithelialization. Icepacks with sedation constitute a superior form of treatment. For the physician who occasionally deals with acute ocular disease, the antibiotic-steroid ophthalmic preparations should be avoided. Herpetic and fungal keratitis have been increasing since the widespread promiscuous use of these preparations. Often the patient develops a sensitivity with the first administration of an antibiotic preparation. Later, when antibiotics are prescribed during a true infection, the patient develops an allergic blepharoconjunctivitis.

Occasionally, a patient with a mildly infected eye with tearing presents himself for treatment. This is mistakenly taken for a "simple" conjunctivitis, when in actuality it is the beginning of a viral (usually herpes simplex) keratitis. This condition progresses rapidly in the presence of steroids. If one is in doubt and if the patient demands treatment, one should dispense or prescribe one of the nonspecific zinc eyedrops (Zincfrin). If the case is diagnosed as mild mucopurulent conjunctivitis after taking a culture and sensitivity, one of the 10% to 15% sulfacetamide preparations should be prescribed. The ever-popular antibiotic eyedrops should be saved for a real need.

History

A precise history, brief but to the point, must be recorded for every patient who is seen on an emergency basis.

Visual acuity

An initial, best visual acuity must be taken on each eye. If the glasses are not available or if a refraction problem is suspected, a simple pinhole punched in a card or piece of plastic through which the patient can view the chart will suffice. If a standard visual acuity chart is not available, the examiner may hold any print (for example, a newspaper) at a distance and record the size of the print and *maximum* distance at which that particular type could be recognized by the patient.

Technique of examination

Gentleness should be stressed. A thumb placed on either the upper or the lower orbital rim can retract a lid with a rolling maneuver. Absolutely no pressure should be applied on a globe suspected of having a perforating injury. No child suspected of a serious perforating ocular injury should be wrestled with. It is best to examine this type of patient under general anesthesia in the operating room, and the examination should preferably be made by a qualified ophthalmologist.

A strong, focal bright light is an essential for satisfactory gross examination. Shining it from one side and varying the angle will create less of an ordeal for the patient and will provide a better technique for the examiner, particularly in identifying corneal abrasions or lacerations and in estimating the all-important anterior chamber depth, since the transparent cornea domes forward from the flat iris diaphragm.

Binocular magnification of some sort is extremely desirable.

Ophthalmoscopy is essential. Ten percent phenylephrine (Neo-Synephrine) is a rapid mydriatic that should be used on every ocular injury where intraocular penetration is suspected and not frankly evident.

Orbital x-rays should be made on any and every eye injury caused by a foreign body, particularly a missile-like injury (for example, history of a sudden sharp pain while operating a lathe, hammering a nail, or running a lawn mower).

TRAUMA
Orbital injuries

The real danger in orbital injuries lies in failure to recognize their presence. Since the paranasal sinuses virtually encompass the orbits, meningitis or orbital cellulitis may result from trauma about the face. X-rays should include not only the facial bones but also the orbital foramen. When penetrating injuries are discovered, the possibility of retained foreign bodies within the orbit should also be considered.

Although there are many signs of orbital fracture, some of the more important findings are described here.

1. Diplopia may occur, particularly when the orbital contents sag into the maxillary

sinus. These orbital floor fractures may be produced by a baseball or fist-type of blow. The absence of diplopia in a "fresh" contusion about the face should not make one dismiss the possibility of orbital fracture with displacement. As the associated swelling diminishes, the patient's diplopia may appear as much as 1 week later.

2. Anesthesia is another important finding. Fractures of the orbital roof may create pressure on the supraorbital nerve, resulting in anesthesia above the eyebrow. Fragmentation in the area of the infraorbital foramen produces anesthesia over the cheek and ala of the nose and upper lid.

3. Rhinorrhea may be the hallmark of a torn dura in the anterior fossa, associated with fractures of the prominent supraorbital rim and frontal sinus. The sharp crista galli may penetrate the dura mater and arachnoid in medial orbital wall fractures.

4. Diminished vision must create suspicion of a fracture of the posterior orbital roof where the bony optic foramen encases the optic nerve.

Lid injuries

Ecchymosis. Blood seepage under the loose areolar tissues of the eye is commonly termed a "black eye." This in itself is no real emergency; use of an icecap will suffice. The physician will find it his responsibility to proceed in an orderly manner and to rule out orbital fracture and contusions to the globe.

Burns. Aside from general supportive treatment to the patient as a whole, only cleansing is necessary for first- or second-degree burns. Third-degree burns are another matter and should be referred immediately to an ophthalmologist. No debridement should be done by the physician initially attending the emergency; this should be left to the discretion of a specialist.

Lacerations. Although it is important to initiate prompt repair before lid swelling occurs, adherence should be made to the general principles of surgery such as antitetanic measures, irrigation, and hemostasis. In extensive lid lacerations without corneal involvement, the cornea should be protected from exposure by instilling a sterile antibiotic ophthalmic preparation prior to the referral. An apparently simple puncture type injury to either lid may, in actuality, also involve the intraocular structures.

Simple suturing is usually adequate when less that one fourth of the eyelid is missing. Margin involvement and severance of one or both canaliculi must be considered. Lid margin repair by direct suturing should be the procedure of choice for the occasional operator when referral to an ophthalmologist is an impossibility.

Injuries to the globe

Contusions. Blunt trauma to the globe is almost a study within itself. No intraocular structure is "safe." Tears and ruptures can occur in almost any of the eye's component parts. It may not be noticeable objectively, yet severe edema may develop in the macular area, resulting in a visual acuity of 20/200 or less. Most ruptures occur in the upper nasal quadrant, concentric to and adjacent with the limbus. Hyphemia may be either immediate, delayed, or both. Hemorrhage can occur as late as 10 days after the injury. Eyes have been lost between the time of thoughtless "discharge" from treatment for a so-called tiny clot in the anterior chamber (or just a smoky appearance in the anterior segment) and the patient's next visit 7 days later. Any blood in the anterior chamber may be the hallmark of more severe hemorrhage. Observation in a hospital and binocular patching are essential. It is best for the general physician to refrain from the instillation of any miotic or mydriatic, leaving this to the discretion of a specialist. The so-called secondary hemorrhage is usually more severe than the initial one, thus making it quite necessary for the patient to be under an ophthalmologist's care at the time.

Foreign bodies. Most small, penetrating intraocular foreign bodies remain undetected because insufficient time was taken in eliciting a history or because the scope of the ocular examination was narrow. The only sign of such an injury may be a tiny area of cornea edema, a "spot of subconjunctival hemorrhage," or a slightly eccentric pupil. Injuries sustained from air guns, sand blasting, hammering of nails, metal chips from lathes, or chipping of stone are all subject to this suspicion.

It is unfortunate that greater pain results from the presence of a foreign body near the limbus of the cornea than from one nearer the center, because central corneal lesions heal more slowly and produce more serious permanent visual disability. Also, administration of tetanus toxoid (or TAT) should not be neglected following an injury that is exclusively corneal. Tetanus has been recorded 10 days following a "simple" corneal injury.

Corneal injuries resulting from a fleck of sand, metal, or splinter embedded in the superficial cornea should be irrigated initially. If this does not dislodge the foreign body, a drop of 0.5% tetracaine or 5% proparacaine hydrochloride (Ophthaine) is instilled, and the patient should be made comfortable in a supine position. A sterile 20-gauge needle on a syringe (used as a handle) can be brought in from the side and the foreign body can be gently lifted from the cornea. Binocular magnification is necessary, along with good oblique focal illumination. It should be remembered that the degree of corneal injury is proportional not only to the depth of the foreign body and the time elapsed until its removal but also to the amount of trauma inflicted in attempts to remove the foreign body. It is desirable to place even these simple problems in the initial care of an ophthalmologist. Corneal penetration deeper than Bowman's membrane should always be referred immediately to an ophthalmologist.

Lacerations. Nonperforating lacerations of the cornea should be thoroughly irrigated, preferably with sterile physiologic saline. This treatment should be followed by the instillation of some broad-spectrum antibiotic drops or ophthalmic ointment. Referral is urgent. A penetrating corneal laceration with various degree of anterior segment involvement should be treated mainly by binocular patching (after instillation of topical ophthalmic antibiotics). No attempt should be made to remove any visible foreign bodies or blood clots. At times the iris may resemble a blood clot, and the attempted removal by forceps would produce more dangerous results than gentle irrigation with sterile saline.

Abrasions. "Clean" abrasions of the cornea should be gently irrigated, following which frequent instillation of antibiotic drops (or 10% to 15% sulfacetamide) should be undertaken. Small abrasions can be left unpatched. Larger ones are extremely painful and should be carefully patched, using two or three eye pads in thickness and enough tape to keep the lid from opening. Patients with such injuries should be seen again, within at most 24 hours and preferably 12 hours later. If the abrasion is obvious, staining with fluorescein is not only unnecessary but hazardous, since fluorescein itself is an excellent culture medium for *Pseudomonas aeruginosa.*

Irradiational burns. Snowblindness, sunlamp conjunctivitis, and the more severe welder's keratoconjunctivitis are all caused by injurious exposure to ultraviolet light. The initial symptoms usually begin 12 hours following exposure. No condition is more frequently mismanaged, usually by the unwise multiple instillation of topical anesthetics. If any instillation is indicated it is usually only at the time of initial examination. The severity may range from a chemosis of the bulbar conjunctiva to a diffuse corneal epithelial desquamation. Ice compresses, head elevation, analgesics, and sedatives are the accepted forms of treatment.

Chemical burns. The emergency treatment of chemical burns of the eye (whether acidic, alkaline, or refrigerant) consists of immediate, profuse, and prolonged irrigation with water (sterile physiologic saline, ideally). Acidic burns are not quite as serious as the others, because of stoppage by an action in which the acid combines with and coagulates the superficial tissues. Alkaline burns soften and penetrate in a relentless fashion; in these cases, irrigation for at least 30 minutes should be performed, followed by instillation of 1% atropine drops to prevent the iris from adhering to the lens or cornea (secondary iritis). Some potentially dangerous refrigerants are oil soluble; therefore, instillation of olive or mineral oil should be used in irrigating them from the eye. If the conjunctiva is involved, an ophthalmic ointment should be instilled to help deter symblepharon formation.

Thermal burns. Thermal burns from an open flame are usually not very serious. Boric acid ophthalmic ointment instilled several times daily, along with 2% homatropine, usually suffices.

MEDICAL CONSIDERATIONS
Acute conjunctivitis (purulent)

Neisseria gonococcus can produce the only real emergency situation of the conjunctival diseases. The condition in the adult is usually unilateral, with a copious discharge of pus almost literally pouring from a beefy red, tremendously swollen conjunctiva. Corneal perforation is always a hazard. Scrapings must be taken from the raw conjunctiva for immediate fixing and staining, along with culture and sensitivity studies for later information. *Neisseria catarrhalis* and *Meningococcus* are also gram-negative, intracellular diplococci; however, they present a much less severe clinical picture.

The cornea should be carefully examined, preferably after irrigation. Any loss in inherent luster (and in uptake of fluorescein dye) is the first evidence of corneal involvement. If a penicillin ophthalmic ointment is not immediately available, one of the chlortetracycline (Aureomycin) ointments should be immediately sought.

Treatment of ophthalmia neonatorum is essentially the same.

Corneal ulcer

Any corneal ulcer is an urgent case; however, when the causative organism is *Pseudomonas aeruginosa*, it is an ocular emergency in the truest sense. An eye can be lost because of this organism in 48 hours. Presumptive evidence is the appearance of a blue-green cast. Any corneal infiltrate should undergo immediate culture and sensitivity studies, delicately scraping the edge for pathogenic material. The appearance of a clear center in an ulcer is usually not a sign of healing but more than likely will eventually be identified as the herniation of Descemet's membrane through the necrotic stroma. Some of these patients have had an eye saved by a lamellar keratoplasty, if referred to the ophthalmologist in time.

The red eye

Most physicians have seen at one time or another, a chart showing the salient points in differentiation of acute conjunctivitis, acute glaucoma, and acute iridocyclitis. The important thing is for the attending physician to recognize and know the significance of a deep ciliary infection. It is the hallmark of serious intraocular disease. Referral should be immediate. Both acute iridocyclitis and acute glaucoma have this sign. It is a radial spoke-like sunburst type of infection, is most intense where clear cornea joins white sclera, and fades in intensity peripherally from the limbus. Some describe a purplish hue; however, the pattern is the important feature. A cross-like pattern may also be present, created by engorgement of the penetrating anterior ciliary vessels at the insertion of the four rectus muscles. In acute iridocyclitis, the pupil is miotic as a result of spasm and irritability of the iris sphincter, and the pupil may be slightly irregular if portions of its margin adhere to the lens. The pupil is large in acute glaucoma because the iris is paralyzed by the extremely high intraocular pressure.

Acute iridocyclitis should be treated with cycloplegics. If early posterior synechia are present, they may be broken with 10% phenylephrine (Neo-Synephrine). The crucial danger point is attempting to dilate an "irritable" eye where acute glaucoma is already present. This is more likely to happen by mistake if the patient arrives for emergency treatment at the time a self-limited remission of an acute attack is taking place. The treatment for acute (angle-closure) glaucoma is primarily surgical and the patient should be placed immediately in the hands of an ophthalmologist, if possible. Otherwise 2% to 4% pilocarpine drops should be instilled every 15 minutes. There are cases in which these measures fail. Osmotic agents must then be resorted to—Osmitral is a good example.

Central retinal artery occlusion

Sudden blindness in any eye should instinctively make the physician reach for an ophthalmoscope. In cases of central retinal artery occlusion, the posterior pole of the eye will appear blanched and the macula will stand out as a "cherry-red spot." The arterioles will be thread-like and no amount of digital pressure will create a venous pulsation that can be seen with an ophthalmoscope. Paracentesis of the anterior chamber or retrobulbar injection (accepted treatment by an ophthalmologist) is not to be attempted by anyone else. Inhalation of amyl nitrite, nitroglycerine administered sublingually, and inhalation of carbon dioxide alternating with oxygen and ocular massage can all be resorted to by the general physician. The prognosis in most cases is extremely poor, even if detected within the first 30 minutes; however, the accepted methods of treatment should be faithfully executed.

Retinal detachment

Any patient who complains of a curtain blocking his field of vision, coupled with light flashes or black spot, should be carefully examined (with dilated ophthalmoscopy) for a detached retina. The red reflex may be absent in one or more quadrants; and ophthalmoscopy, particularly for the occasional observer, may be puzzling. A large, grayish, wrinkled curtain may be evident. All efforts should be directed toward evaluating macular involvement. If the macula is intact, the case is definitely an emergency. Prior to calling the ophthalmologist, bed rest (flat on the back) and binocular patching should be performed. It ceases to be a real emergency if the macula is detached, although here the case is urgent. Surgical treatment has improved in the past 10 years, and no case should be slighted. Even a slight haze in the media (early vitreous hemorrhage) may actually be caused by an undisclosed retinal break. Cases of so-called iritis have later been identified as unsuspected retinal separation.

chapter 26

Initial care of head and spinal injuries

John T. Bonner

When the traumatized patient has sustained central nervous system injury, two primary modalities become particularly important: maintaining the airway and maintaining adequate blood volume.

MAINTAINING THE AIRWAY

As with other organ system injuries, the initial concern is the maintenance of an airway. This is not only necessary for survival of the individual in overall terms but is especially critical to the central nervous system, since it requires adequate oxygenation for survival. An inadequate airway may actually aggravate the neurologic injury and not allow neural tissue survival because of the lack of oxygen availability. Airway obstruction may not only decrease available oxygen but may also increase expiratory pressure, resulting in increased venous pressure and worsening any cerebral edema that may exist. Also, airway inadequacy may obstruct venous drainage within the intracranial cavity, thus allowing an increase in carbon dioxide content that may aggravate cerebral edema. Physical obstruction such as vomitus and blood may often be easily removed by adequate suctioning, but usually a more dependable airway mechanism is needed in the comatose individual to allow assurance of an airway and to permit attention to the care of other injuries. Recently the technique of placing endotracheal tubes has been mastered by most physicians and it is an expeditious and satisfactory means of maintaining the airway. Tracheostomy is the other method of choice. It should be familiar to all physicians and may become necessary in such situations, especially where extensive oral or facial injuries may not allow adequate placement of an endotracheal tube. Possibility of a neck fracture in traumatized individuals specifically precludes excessive movement of the neck in placing an endotracheal tube. Under most situations this can be done safely, but occasionally tracheostomy may be the procedure of choice.

As mentioned before, in the patient who is comatose from a head injury, the possibility of cervical fractures must be given paramount consideration so as to avoid aggravating any spinal cord neurologic injury or causing one to occur. This consideration is especially important in extracting injured individuals from places such as damaged automobiles and may require great care. One is very rarely justified in dragging an injured individual through apertures such as windows, which often requires twisting and manipulation of the body on its axis and the great possibility of spinal cord or root damage in the presence of spinal fractures.

Adequate care will involve removing the individual with a seat or on special extraction boards that are carried by most ambulances, thus allowing the head and neck to stay in alignment with the axis of the body, probably the most important principle involved in such situations. In transporting an individual with a possible spinal fracture, especially cervical, it is sometimes useful to assign one individual the task of assuring that the head and neck are properly positioned. Cervical halter traction is quite useful in this situation, especially if mandibular injury is not present. Even in the presence of such injuries, care in manually controlling the head may be time and energy well spent in protection of the spinal cord.

Unless endotracheal tubes are satisfactorily placed at the site of injury and adequate suctioning is available, one is rarely justified in transporting the injured, comatose individual in the supine position. Transportation on the side in the so-called decubitus position or in the prone position is better, since these positions assure a better airway and also less likelihood of aspiration if vomiting does occur. Again I emphasize the importance of keeping the head and neck in proper traction and alignment and preventing neck flexion, which can also be satisfactorily done in these positions.

MAINTAINING ADEQUATE BLOOD VOLUME

Shock and low blood pressure cannot, for practical purposes, be attributed to head injuries. Only in the infant, who has a relatively small circulating volume and an expandable intracranial cavity because of the lack of suture closure, can an intracranial hemorrhage be sufficient to occasionally cause shock. In the adult, intracranial pressure from hemorrhage or other cerebral injuries usually results in hypertension. Thus when shock is present in the traumatized individual, one must look for blood loss in other areas, such as pelvic fracture and intraabdominal or thoracic hemorrhage. Only in the terminal phase of brainstem decompensation does shock occur with neurogenic loss of vasomotor tone. Coma may be secondary to hypotension itself, and it is not an uncommon experience in the emergency room to see an individual awaken upon replacement of an adequate circulating volume, demonstrating that he may have only a minor head injury or perhaps none at all.

Adequate replacement of circulating volume, especially blood, is important in minimizing cerebral injury and allowing adequate oxygenation of the brain. In replenishing circulating volume, one must remember that in the presence of significant head injury, especially one involving the possibility of cerebral edema, excessive fluid replacement should not occur nor should excessive amounts of sodium be given. Aggravation of the cerebral edema may occur and thus worsen the intracranial pathology. In the absence of loss of significant circulating volume, fluids should be restricted and any saline given should not usually be greater than one-half normal in concentration. During a 24-hour period, 2,000 ml of fluid with a very limited amount of exogenous sodium is usually more than ample for an adult with a head injury, to avoid worsening cerebral edema. Steroids such as dexamethasone (Decadron), 10 mg intramuscularly or intravenously as a loading dose, followed by 4 mg every 6 hours, or methylprednisolone (Medrol), 40 mg intravenously as a loading dose and 40 mg every 4 hours are often quite beneficial initially for cerebral edema in a contused brain.

Steroids do not seem to be as efficacious in this situation as they are in treating the edema surrounding brain tumors; they should not be given as a routine but only when clinically indicated. Hypertonic fluids, such as mannitol intravenously, should be given only for specific indications, such as to decrease cerebral edema to allow one to buy time while evaluating the patient for possible operative intervention in such lesions as acute epidural, subdural, or intracerebral hematomas. I favor 1 gm/kg of weight of mannitol intravenously as a bolus, although many favor 0.5 gm/kg.

One must be careful that a Foley catheter is in place to handle the hoped-for diuresis. Because of the possible rebound phenomenon with such agents, initially reducing cerebral edema but then aggravating it, these agents can act as a two-edged sword. Also, by reducing cerebral edema they may allow a hematoma to enlarge proportionally and thus if rebound does occur, it may extremely compromise the situation. Thus hypertonic fluids do have their indications in buying time for evaluation, including diagnostic procedures when operative intervention is a distinct possibility, but because of the rebound side effects, they should be used in only strict clinical indications and certainly not as a routine. When necessary, mannitol seems to be more desirable than urea, since experience indicates that there is less rebound with it.

As anyone knows who has handled extensive scalp lacerations, the scalp is extremely vascular and a very significant blood loss may occur. Control in hemorrhage is usually relatively easy, using digital compression along the scalp edge and then placing mosquitoes or other hemostatic instruments on the galea and turning the instruments back, thus tamponading the bleeding vessels. It is usually a worthless, time- and blood-wasting exercise to attempt to clamp individual bleeders or to tie off individual bleeding scalp arteries.

INITIAL TREATMENT

In head and spinal injuries, evaluation and treatment are designed to appropriately treat the patient. There are no *routine* procedures as such. This especially true in the consideration of lumbar puncture, which is certainly not a routine item in the evaluation of the nervous system. There are very few situations where lumbar puncture is needed or indicated in the acute evaluation of trauma, and in many situations it is extremely deleterious and dangerous to the patient. In the presence of a mass, lumbar puncture may hasten herniation once it is started by upsetting the dynamic balance of pressures that exist. Information gained in the acute evaluation of trauma may be not worth the risks involved. Obviously such manipulation is contraindicated.

Control of seizures

Fortunately, seizures are infrequently seen in acute trauma, but if seizures are occurring, adequate control by the intravenous route is necessary. Dilantin has little effect or place in stopping acute seizures, but its use is appropriate for long-term seizure control. Initially, intravenous barbiturates such as amobarbital (Amytal) can be given, which I favor because of the ability of Amytal to control seizures for an adequate time without exceedingly long depression, which may mask any progressive consciousness deterioration. Intravenous diazepam (Valium) is often also useful, especially with a focal seizure pattern. Intravenous paraldehyde is also useful for seizure control, especially if appropriate amounts of other medications have not been successful. One must remember that pulmonary hemorrhages may be a complication of using intravenous paraldehyde, but this is infrequent. Paraldehyde is also well absorbed rectally and thus is especially useful in infants when there is difficulty in obtaining intravenous routes.

The important feature in obtaining seizure control is in using adequate medication. No exact dosage amounts or limits can be given, since this varies according to the clinical situation, which is determined by the relative refractoriness of the seizure disorder. One must be prepared to support respiration if that much anticonvulsant is needed to control the seizures; but, on the other hand, one does not carry the initial intravenous medication past a safety margin after seizure has stopped, in order to prevent unnecessary respiratory depression. One must not forget the initiation of long-acting anticonvulsants such as diphenylhydantoin (Dilantin) for continued control.

Open skull fracture

If an open skull fracture is present with perhaps dura exposed or dural lacerations and brain exposed, one should remove and irrigate away the grossly evident foreign material and cover the exposed brain area lightly with sterile sponges. This is the one situation in which induction of general anesthesia may be acutely justified immediately after admission in the emergency room, so as to not allow the patient to fight, buck, or cough, which progressively herniates more cerebral tissue from the skull defect and results in a greater loss of brain substance than would otherwise be necessary.

THE EXAMINATION

When one has attended to the immediate lifesaving procedures, attention should then be given in a more detailed and ordered fashion to the patient as a whole. A general physical examination is necessary, including an adequate neurologic examination, which need not be complicated but which does require accuracy. The important aspects are the level of consciousness, orientation in the verbally responsive patient, and especially whether the patient is improving or deteriorating. If scalp lacerations are present, careful exploration should occur both visually and with a sterile gloved finger to determine whether skull fractures are present in this region. Often fractures may be noted that would not be visible on x-ray. One must take care that subgaleal or subperiosteal hemorrhages are not mistaken for fractures. They are commonly misinterpreted as depressed skull fractures.

Examination of the eyes

The pupillary size and response to light should be noted, as well as the ability of the eyes to move, and, in the comatose individual, the vestibuloocular reflexes (doll's eyes) to limited head rotation. Such examination can occur without putting the neck in jeopardy. The corneal response is seldom checked in the emergency room but should be, since it often gives valuable information as to the level of the patient's neurologic injury and often gives hints of possible lateralization. Funduscopic examination should not be neglected, but the presence of papilledema is seldom seen at an early stage of increased intracranial pressure, thus the funduscopic examination is often normal. There are situations in which increased intracranial pressure may be present and retinal vein pulsations preserved, although this is not the usual siutation. Examination of the head in neurologic injuries includes noting the condition of the nose, ears, and other signs.

Examination of the nose and ears

The presence of hemorrhage from the external auditory canal in the absence of an obvious superficial ear laceration is presumptive evidence for a basal skull fracture. Additional support would be given by escape of cerebrospinal fluid. When there is blood in the external auditory canal, most physicians believe that appropriate antibiotic coverage should be given as partial treatment for the basal skull fracture. Irrigation of the blood from the external ear canal for further examination is not indicated, since it could introduce retrograde infection that may not otherwise occur. Allowing bloody fluid from either the ear or nose to drop upon a sponge or pillowcase is often informative, since the double ring sign formed by the quick migration of cerebrospinal fluid circumferentially from the drop around the central blood spot may often verify the presence of cerebrospinal fluid. In the absence of hemorrhage from the external auditory canal, the tympanic membranes should be carefully visualized, since the presence of blood or fluid behind them is also evidence for a basal skull fracture, as is its identification in the pharynx. The clear fluid can be further verified as cerebrospinal fluid by obtaining a positive result with a glucose stick. Nasal secretions, except during an upper respiratory infection, usually test glucose-negative. Blood in the fluid negates the validity.

In addition there are other external manifestations of basal skull fracture, such as the well-known "battle sign." This is ecchymosis over the mastoid region reflecting the dissection of cerebrospinal fluid and blood into the mastoid air cells and overlying tissue. Bilateral periorbital ecchymoses or the initial development of such by discoloration medially around each eye in the absence of direct injury to the eye is also indicative of basal skull fracture. There is dissection of blood and cerebrospinal fluid through the ethmoid air cells and into the loose areolar tissue around the eyes to produce the colloquially identified "coon's eyes" because of the similarity to the periorbital markings of the well-known raccoon.

Examination of the neck

In the comatose, disoriented, or irrational individual or one presumed to be under the influence of drugs such as alcohol, attention must be given to prevention or aggravation of a neck injury by maintaining the axial orientation, which has been mentioned before, by adding either halter traction or sandbags around the side of the head to prevent head turning. In the awake and rational patient, ability to voluntarily move the neck with little or no discomfort is reassuring. Significant neck injuries usually elicit enough paravertebral muscle spasm to make neck motion uncomfortable and thus are self-protective. An awake or rational individual who is able to and wants to move his head around does not need such protective measures and is unlikely to have a significant neck injury.

Examination of range of motion and reflexes

Other important points in the neurologic evaluation are the ability of the individual to move his extremities and whether he moves them equally and symmetrically. This may be ascertained in the comatose patient by his response to noxious stimuli such as pressure over the supraorbital nerve or squeezing the clavicle, thus eliciting periosteal pain. Any difference in ability to move extremities is an important observation concerning possible lateralization. The tone of the extremities should also be determined since difference of tone, such as suggestion of spasticity, is also important lateralizing evidence. One must interpret extremity examination in light of possible local injuries or fractures. Change of tone and paresis can often also be easily elicited, although this is not done as often as it should be, by noting the difference in the rate or direction of fall of extremities when elevated and, especially in lower extremities, the amount of rebound the leg has after being dropped from a height against the mattress. The side with more paresis will have less tendency to bounce on rebound and thus gives important lateralizing information. The deep tendon reflexes should be carefully evaulated for possible asymmetries, ankle and knee clonus, presence of Babinski responses, and symmetry and lateralization of responses. The ability of the individual to respond to noxious stimulation of the extremities should also be noted. Paresis will often be uncovered by difference in withdrawal ability, remembering that differences in sensation reception can also aid in laterality and modify response. The superficial reflexes, abdominal and cremasteric reflexes in males, and abdominal reflex in females should also be examined or asymmetry noted, thus obtaining important possible lateralizing information. The examintation of superficial reflexes is one that often offers valuable information, yet it is one that is most often neglected. The activity of the superficial reflexes can be considered to some extent the "neurologic sedimentation rate" in that it gives some indication of the severity of injury.

Notation of change of state

An important facet in evaluating the patient with head injury lies in noting whether he is static or whether he is changing in level of consciousness or in other parameters of neurologic function. When the patient is improving, it is unlikely that he has a mass of significance that would need acute treatment. One who shows progressive improvement is highly unlikely to have a mass at all. Even with the improving patient, close observation is important, since it is possible that he may start to deteriorate, in this manner reflecting either a progressive extrinsic or intrinsic lesion or progressive cerebral edema, usually secondary to contusions. But a general rule is that while a patient is improving, it is inappropriate to manipulate him by performing diagnostic procedures such as arteriography.

On the other hand, the patient who is deteriorating is of great concern, especially if he is showing lateralization in his clinical picture. This is the individual who needs accurate and appropriate diagnostic measures to treat a mass when brainstem compression has not progressed to the point where the individual cannot be salvaged.

Recording an adequate history

By now it should be clear that detailed examination and observation of the neurologic function are important, are easily and quickly accompiished, and are not overly complicated. One of the more important details is to accurately record significant findings at the time of initial examination and also during subsequent examinations, so that judgment as to whether the patient is changing clinically should not be left to memory. Under the stress of the situation, especially where multiple-system trauma is present or where many traumatized individuals arrive at the same time, clinical confusion is quite common. Right-left disorientation is especially common among observers. Jotting down significant details is certainly not time wasted and may be the factor allowing appropriate judgment to be made on patients, saving much time and morbidity in the long run. One is often amazed at the dearth of records on traumatized individuals and the subsequent confusion and lack of clinical information even in the better emergency rooms. This attitude is completely inexcusable.

Roentgenographic evaluation

The most important factors in initially evaluating trauma, as in other aspects of medicine, are the combined product of history and physical examination, with clinical appraisal being the paramount source of information. Other examinations such as x-rays, although they do often add further significant information, are in a true sense ancillary, with a clinical appraisal being most important. Roentgenograms *should not* be obtained until the patient has been sufficiently stabilized for movement, and most modern hospital emergency rooms have x-ray facilities present or available on a portable basis that are of good quality and adequate for initial evaluation. Because of the high incidence of neck injuries associated with head injuries, at least a single lateral cervical spine film should be obtained with the skull films of such patients.

SPINAL INJURIES

The handling of spinal injuries is an especially critical consideration in the initial care of acute trauma. It must be reiterated that such injuries often accompany head injuries. Evaluation for spinal injuries is essential in both the history and the physical aspects to prevent aggravation of these injuries (with neurologic consequences) during transportation and care of other systemic injuries. Spinal fractures do not of necessity involve nervous system injury, but there are many examples where the initial trauma did not cause neural damage while subsequent evaluation and handling resulted in such damage, a tragic situation. The fact that the head and neck should be kept in the same axis as the remainder of the body has been emphasized before. Torsion of the thoracic or lumbosacral areas must be avoided by utilizing the log-rolling technique in comatose individuals to protect against neural damage. In positioning such patients, a degree of hyperextension of any of the involved areas is certainly much more desirable than any flexion, and, at times, it is more desirable than the neutral position.

Initial care

Use of conservative therapy versus the value of open operative decompression in the various injuries is a long and complex one and need not be gone into in detail in discussion of initial care. This subject may be summarized by stating that the general experience is that the individual who is improving should be allowed to improve on his own and not be considered at that time for an operative decompression. The conservative treatment involves traction and attempted closed reduction of the fracture, especially in the cervical region, by such methods as on-arrival cervical halter traction while initial evaluation is occurring. Then, as early as possible, one places more permanent skeletal traction, such as the well-known Crutchfield tongs or other appliances such as Barton tongs. Individuals with spinal cord injury should have a Foley catheter placed in their bladder as soon as possible after admission to allow bladder decompression, preventing overdistension that may, in itself, add months in the rehabilitation process. After the initial evaluation in such patients as paraplegics and quadraplegics and the placement of tongs in cervical fractures, the patient should be placed on equipment such as a Foster frame or circle bed during the initial care period to prevent compromise over skin pressure points and the development of decubiti.

As with head injuries, a complete review of the various types of pathology in spinal injuries is beyond the scope of the discussion but one of the more common injuries is the musculoligamentous injury of the neck and low back, the initial care of which is often unfortunately poor in the emergency room situation. Musculoligamentous (myofascial strain) injury of the neck is often termed *whiplash injury,* a term of dubious medical background and out-of-proportion medical-legal litigation overtones. After determination that cervical fracture is not present, appropriate care usually involves using adequate analgesics. Muscle relaxants are often benefical to the patient. Cervical collars are often of temporary usefulness for paravertebral muscle spasm for a few days until this phase has passed. After that time they should be removed, since continued immobilization often causes spasm to continue and also causes joint degenerative changes in the cervical spine. In addition, these collars become, to many patients, severe psychologic crutches.

Examination

Examination of the back itself, the most obvious maneuver, is often neglected, and there is loss of significant information that could be gained. Swelling or prominence of frank hematoma over the spinal area is certainly suggestive of local injury, which is likely to involve bony fracture. In the conscious patient, local tenderness may often be elicited over the area of injury by mild percussion up and down the spinal axis. The location of paravertebral muscle spasm that is made apparent by local scoliosis or tilt is suggestive of local injury, and it is manifested not only by discomfort of the patient in that area but by actual palpation of the paravertebral muscle spasm by the examiner. The spinal processes may often be quite prominent as a gibbus at the area of fracture. Often there will be a frank fracture dislocation as a result of a flexion or torsion injury or a compression fracture of the vertebral body. Open injuries involving the spinal column, whether they be by sharp or blunt trauma or by gunshot wound, obviously need care to control local hemorrhage and temporary sterile tamponade dressing to avoid retrograde infection, especially if spinal fluid communication exists.

Neurologic deficit may be gross and unmistakable or it may be quite subtle; nevertheless, it is usually demonstrable, even in those patients who are comatose. The ability to voluntarily move extremities may show deficits, or asymmetries, or both. Observed deficits in reflex response to noxious stimuli are also important observations that may imply neural damage. One must remember that in acute cord injuries, spinal shock may be present for variable lengths of time, minutes to months, and thus flaccid paralysis may be present, although one does frequently see varying degrees of spastic paralysis in acute trauma. There will be the usual spasticity to passive and involuntary movement of the extremities; hyperactive, deep tendon reflexes combined with ankle clonus and up-going toes; and absence of superficial reflexes. The presence of priapism is always suggestive of spinal cord injury above the sacral area. In the awake, cooperative patient identification of the injury level is usually quite accurately done by examining the extremities for specific root deficits and, in the case of the trunk, with a pinwheel or usual safety pin, bilaterally eliciting the sensory level. In the awake patient this sensory examination should be done with care since both an upper and lower sensory level may frequently be elicited, with the upper level occasionally exhibiting dysalgesia as well as hypalgesia and, at times, hyperesthesia. The upper sensory level, which is the one most suggestive of the level of pathology, is called the primary sensory level and the lower is the secondary. When the level is up to the region of the clavicles, one then examines the upper extremity in detail for root distribution sensory loss, as well as doing specific muscle testing and reflex eliciting to determine site of lesion. A discussion of the neurologic findings representative of the various lesion levels is beyond the scope of this initial care discussion and can be found in most good neurology and neurosurgery texts, correlated with one's knowledge of the anatomy.

Information may also be gained by examining the patient for sweat level, which is another useful but neglected technique. One may determine such a level by sweeping one's hand lightly up the trunk of the patient and noting the position where additional "drag" occurs, identifying the region where moisture represented by perspiration begins, or one may use starch. One may occasionally visualize the discrepancy of moisture that exists above and below this level by using an ophthalmoscope with a bright light and actually visualizing beads of sweat above the level and noting a relative or absolute absence below the level. Cord injury in the thoracic area (or above) often results in a sympathectomy with relative hypotension that is quite sensitive to postural change. Again may I repeat: completeness of examination is important but is only useful for evaluation if properly recorded, even if in an abbreviated, shorthand fashion. Repeat evaluations are necessary and, as in the situation with head injuries, the patient's course when initially seen is of paramount importance. The patient who is improving will be of less immediate concern than that patient who is deteriorating in neurologic function.

PERIPHERAL NERVE INJURIES

Plexus and peripheral nerve injuries are also frequently seen in acute injuries, more often in a wartime environment. Brachial plexus injuries especially often result from a stretch mechanism and not infrequently include avulsion of the brachial roots themselves from the spinal cord. With direct injury to the brachial plexus area, neighborhood injuries are also often present, such as subclavian artery lacerations or aneurysms. Tenderness or fullness on palpation high in the axilla is often present, as is tenderness on palpation in the supraclavicular area and bruits on auscultation of the proper areas in associated subclavian artery injuries. Such injuries and associated neighborhood injuries are less frequent in the lumbosacral plexus region. Peripheral nerve injuries are frequently present in orthopedic injuries of the extremities and will be discovered only if proper neurologic examination of such extremities is done. There are obvious medical-legal connotations.

It is usually agreed that laceration of peripheral nerves is best repaired after a waiting period of 3 to 6 weeks, but many good and valid arguments can be proposed for the acute repair of such injuries. I believe that delayed repair is usually preferable so that the limits of the central neuroma and central scar may be apparent; thus there is somewhat more assurance of a successful repair at the first procedure. In acute situations the nerve ends should be identified and approximated so that they do not retract and may be more easily anastomosed in the future. Small wire sutures are valuable tagging devices for the nerve ends in the acute situation, since they not only have the tensile strength to keep the ends in approximation but they serve as satisfactory radiographic and palpable surgical aids in the future procedure. Delayed repair of peripheral nerve injuries is also more easily done since the epineurium is thicker and thus stronger for suturing. Furthermore, in the cleaner, secondary wound, under elective circumstances, the surgeon is less likely to make the well-known error of suturing a nerve to a tendon.

The initial care of injuries is only partially considered unless one reflects on some of the mechanisms of trauma and their prevention. It has been widely publicized and it is apparent in most hospital emergency rooms that alcohol is a major contributor to severe and fatal automobile crashes. Alcohol and other drugs do alter and influence the clinical picture. It must be remembered that a portion of the depression in a head injury may be secondary to the alcohol in an intoxicated individual. It is all too easy, however, to write off such presentations as intoxication. This is a diagnosis of exclusion only. For medical-legal reasons one should be hesitant to make a firm diagnosis of alcohol intoxication unless one is prepared to support it by such means as blood alcohol levels. This is often impractical, and the best course is to enter an impression of "possible alcohol intoxication" and to be certain not to underestimate the degree of head or spinal injury present.

chapter 27

Esoterica: hiccups, fishhooks, rings, and such things

There are a few well-known yet little-discussed emergency situations that challenge the writer of an emergency care textbook at least as much as they disturb the patient or those who are responsible for his initial—and in these cases perhaps definitive—care. They are ill adapted to fit comfortably into the usual chapters of either a topographically organized text or one oriented by emergency situations or by specialties. Therefore they are not frequently discussed, except by those who have suddenly found themselves solely responsible for their immediate care at inconvenient times and in "faraway" places. Then these situations rapidly cease to appear esoteric, merely lacking in the aura of drama that characterizes many major emergencies.

HICCUPS

Hiccups, hiccoughs, or singultus may appear ludicrous or unimportant, at best, to one who has never experienced a protracted or even intractable episode. The treatment, however, has taxed the ingenuity of the medical, paramedical, and nonmedical practitioner for as long as one man has tried to help another.

Hiccups are defined as abrupt, intermittent, involuntary, purposeless, jerky diaphragmatic contractions resulting in sudden inspiration opposed by abrupt closure of the glottis. The phenomenon is frequently unilateral, the left side being most commonly involved. Most persons experience transitory episodes of hiccups at some time or other with little inconvenience; however, cases lasting as long as several years have been reported. Such cases prevent adequate eating and sleeping and may be accompanied by severe weight loss and extreme discomfort. At least one patient has been described in the literature in whom transient heart block was triggered through the vagal nerve stimulation involved in hiccups. Remedies have ranged all the way from quite colorful examples of folk medicine, through the perhaps physiologically and psychologically sound techniques of scaring or startling, down to the ultimate expedient of crushing either one (usually the left) or both phrenic nerves for permanent relief. (The efferent limb of the hiccup reflex arc is apparently the phrenic nerve. The center is located at cervical cord levels between the third and fifth cervical segments. The afferent limb is the vagus nerve, phrenic nerve, and the sympathetic chain from the sixth to twelfth thoracic segments.)

Several recently published aids to hiccup control stop short of this rather drastic nerve-crushing procedure, however, and they appear worthy of brief consideration here.

Stimulation of the pharynx. Stimulation of the proper area of the pharynx by means of a nasally introduced catheter was found to stop hiccups. A plastic or rubber suction catheter is introduced through the naris to a distance varying from 3 to 4½ inches, and stimulation by a "jerky, to-and-fro movement" interrupts the reflex and effectively abolishes the hiccuping. Occasionally suction may need be applied simultaneously to clear mucus from the pharynx. Orally introduced catheter stimulation, while found to be equally effective, is less well tolerated by the conscious patient. The catheter may be left in place for restimulation if needed.

The area of the pharynx to be stimulated is that just behind the uvula and opposite the body of the second cervical vertebra.

Use of methylphenidate. Various drugs, including amyl nitrite, inhaled ether, intravenous atropine, sedation with narcotics, barbiturates, chlorpromazine and other central nervous system depressants, quinidine, procaine given intravenously or instilled into the abdominal or thoracic cavity, methamphetamine hydrochloride, and large doses of edrophonium chloride (Tensilon) all have been variously recommended in suppressing singultus. Currently, however, more favorable results are being reported with the use of methylphenidate (Ritalin), administered intravenously in the amount of 20 mg. Considerably smaller doses may be effective in certain patients, and as much as 30 mg has been used in one patient. The method is apparently more effective with the conscious patient than in the unconscious or anesthetized patient, and its success—like other modalities in this area of treatment—is not universally endorsed.

Pulmonary inflation. While its successful use has been reported primarily in the surgical patient where hiccuping may have been occasioned by visceral manipulations (particularly if the anesthetic used was either nitrous oxide or tubocurarine), brief hyperinflation of the lungs bears an obvious relation to one of the favorite folklore remedies—holding the breath. Increasing airway pressure by manual compression of the reservoir bag for 10 to 20 seconds is effective; the apparent threshold pressure required ranges from 30 to 40 cm H_2O.

Regardless of the approach used, it should be pointed out that all of the methods referred to are actually the treating of a symptom rather than a cause; the multiplicity of the suggested forms of treatment is exceeded only by the variety of possible etiologies.

REMOVAL OF FISHHOOKS

A common minor emergency in coastal areas or those adjacent to the large lakes is the problem of the accidentally embedded fishhook. In addition to the usual precautions of wound treatment and tetanus prophylaxis, there is the problem of removing the hook from the skin with minimal tissue damage.

The usual method of choice has been the simple push-through technique. Under local anesthesia, the shank of the hook is grasped firmly and held at such an angle that the point with its barb can be forced out through the skin by the most direct route. Care should be taken that the direction of movement is, as much as possible, at right angles to the plane of the skin, since any needless motion in the plane of the skin will cause unnecessary tissue damage. After the barb has been brought through the skin, it is cut off and the hook can be easily withdrawn. The method is particularly applicable when the point of the hook is nearly through the skin.

When the point is rather deeply embedded, a recently reported technique may best be used. After proper cleansing, a local anesthetic is introduced into the entrance wound itself in relatively small amount. Remembering that a fishhook barb is unilateral and located to point across the U of the hook toward the shaft, one grasps the hook and moves in such a manner as to disengage the barb. The first motion is a slight one in the direction of the point; then, pressing sidewise so that the unbarbed outside of the hook bears upon the subcutaneous tissue, the hook is backed out as far as possible. This maneuver, perhaps repeated a time or so, will usually bring the barb out to just below the dermis.

A No. 11 Bard-Parker blade is then introduced alongside the shaft of the hook and carefully made to contact the point of the barb. The blade is used to incise the few fibers engaging the barb and the blade is then rolled over and held firmly against the point of the barb. With the point thus covered, the hook can be brought through the skin without further enlarging the entrance wound.

Alternately, an 18-gauge disposable needle may be introduced along the barbed side of the hook with the bevel toward the inside of the hook curve. Slight pressure upward on the hook shank disengages the barb from the flesh; the needle is pushed gently inward and rotated until the lumen locks firmly over the barb. Both the hook and the needle can then be maneuvered out through the entrance wound.

Another technique, described as having originated with native fishermen of Australia, involves the use of only 3 or 4 feet of string or fishline. A loop of the line is made around the curve of the embedded hook, and both ends are wound several times around an index finger in preparation for pulling it out. First, however, gentle pressure is applied to the hook in such a direction as to disengage the barb. Then, holding the hook in this alignment with the free hand, the string is carefully aligned in the plane of the hook's long axis—and a quick yank brings it out.

Some small time spent in the consideration needed to master one or more of these techniques may well be worthwhile for several reasons: simplicity, minimal distraction of tissue, less discomfort to the patient, small area of anesthesia needed, no need for cutting the shank of the hook, absence of a second wound and resulting scar, and possibility in some cases for handling situations where the shank has multiple hooks. The methods are not, of ocurse, applicable where the point of the hook is already through or nearly through the skin.

THE RING-STRANGULATED FINGER

One can, of course, merely cut the ring off the finger with any one of several implements that may be handy, including—surprisingly enough until we reflect upon the relative softness of the gold and silver alloys usually involved—a sturdy pair of ordinary scissors. But one not infrequently meets deeply emotional entreaties regarding the sentimental import attached to the ring. Such considerations may not be unimportant in the overall patient evaluation, particularly in the aged person who frequently presents this problem as a seemingly minor manifestation of a serious problem that may be causing the edema.

If there is time—and one must remember that gangrene may result within 4 or 5 hours, certainly within 10 to 12 hours if there is complete obstruction of the circulation—the following maneuver with a piece of string or suture may easily preserve the ring and make a significant emotional contribution to the patient's stability.

Starting at approximately the most distal joint, string is wound smoothly around the finger, with one strand touching. the next, and tightly enough to compress the swollen tissues as much as possible. One should not skip areas that will leave edematous projections between the rounds of string. One continues winding smoothly and tightly right up to the margin of the ring. (It has been recommended by some that winding start at the ring and proceed distally, but this procedure has a "milking" action that tends to merely push the swelling further along the finger rather than compressing it.) The end of the string is slipped under and through the ring. If this proves to be difficult, any small, rounded object such as a matchstick or the end of a clamp may be slipped beneath the ring and then the string run through beside it. The string is then slowly unwound on the proximal side of the ring. The ring is gently twisted downward over the spiraled string as it is unwound from beneath the ring, thus providing a sort of leverage to help move the ring along the finger.

HEMATOMA BENEATH THE FINGERNAIL (SUBUNGAL HEMATOMA)

Bruised fingers can be excruciatingly painful. Mere analgesic treatment of the pain is unsatisfactory. Drainage of the hematoma is usually done by either making an incision from underneath the distal end of the nail or by drilling through the nail. Either of these procedures is usually traumatic in an already painful situation.

An alternative method of draining the hematoma involves the use of a straightened end of an ordinary paper clip. The clip is held in a hemostat, the straightened end is heated red-hot in any suitable flame, and it is used to melt through the nail. Immediate relief of pain occurs. The nailbed is protected from injury by the hematoma itself, and almost none of the pressure required for drilling need be applied to the painful area. The nail should be painted with an antiseptic solution before burning through. Any remaining blood may be easily expressed after penetration, and a light dressing is applied to absorb further drainage.

ACUTE ARTERIAL OCCLUSION

The sudden onset of an acute arterial occlusion may present a dramatic sort of an emergency. For some reason, an acute arterial occlusion frequently goes unrecognized. The sudden onset of an excruciating pain in the extremity associated with numbness and inability to move the limb should certainly point toward the possibility. The six P's of acute arterial occlusion may well be kept in mind; they are pain, pulselessness, paresthesia, paralysis, pallor, and prostration.

In most instances, the immediate or emergency management of such a lesion prior to hospitalization is primarily to recognize that an urgent situation is present and that probable surgery is indicated. The rapidity with which the embolus is removed often determines the eventual outcome. Initial treatment should include protection of the limb from injury and avoidance of local application of heat.

■ part four

Poisoning

chapter 28

Poisonings

Georgia B. Nolph

APPROACH TO THE PATIENT

One should find out as soon as possible the "3 W's"—who, what, and when. *Who* includes the patient's name, age, approximate weight, and telephone number. If a telephone caller states that someone has been poisoned, the above-mentioned data can be obtained at the time of the call, records can be obtained, and everything can be prepared by the time the patient arrives. Time is important; therefore, it is important that the patient be brought to the place where the necessary equipment for treatment is at hand. While talking, one should find out *what* has poisoned the patient (if one is not familiar with the symptoms of toxicity and the treatment, this gives an opportunity to look it up), *when* the patient was poisoned, and how long a period of time has elapsed. Finally, have the container, plant, or other involved object brought in along with the patient.

INGESTANTS (ANTIDOTES)

Antidotes are used to delay absorption of the poison and to buy added time to get the patient to where further emergency treatment and then definitive treatment can be given. Unless contraindicated, the use of oral antidotes should be followed by gastric lavage. In the past, many physicians considered a universal antidote as necessary to every household medicine cabinet as syrup of ipecac. Universal antidote consists of activated charcoal, magnesium hydroxide, and tannic acid in proportionate parts of 2:1:1. Activated charcoal should however be used in preference to universal antidote because magnesium in solution binds sites on the charcoal, making the universal antidote only 40% as effective on a weight-for-weight basis. The recommendation is to give bone charcoal, 1 tablespoon in 30 ml water.

Table 28-1 lists some of the more common antidotes. In using an antidote more harm than good may accrue unless extreme caution is used.

SURFACE-ACTING POISONS

The patient should be drenched immediately and thoroughly with a steady stream of water while his clothing is being removed; the skin should then be cleansed with water. Eye contamination also requires immediate washing of the eyes with a gentle stream of running water while holding the eyelids open. Do not use chemicals in washing the eyes!

153

Table 28-1 Antidotes

Poisons	Antidotes	Dosage	Side effects
Acids	Milk | Water ∫	For patients 1 to 5 years, give 1 to 2 cups; for those over 5 years, give up to 1 quart	
	Milk of magnesia	1 Tb/cup water	
Alkalis	Milk \ Water } Vinegar / Orange or lemon / juice	For patients 1 to 5 years, give 1 to 2 cups; for those over 5 years, give up to 1 quart	
Organic phosphate insecticides (Parathion, TEPP, HETP)	Atropine		
Morphine	Nalline	5 to 10 mg intravenously	Blocks central nervous system depressive effects
Alkaloids, atropine, strychnine, nicotine, quinine, morphine, physostigmine	Potassium permanganate 1:10,000 Tannic acid, 0.5%	For gastric lavage	
Heavy metals	Sodium thiosulfate	15 gm/2 liters	
Mercury, copper, gold, arsenic, antimony, lead	BAL (2,3-dimercaprol, British anti-Lewisite); less effective for silver; ineffective if extensive tissue damage; **do not use for cadmium or iron**	For severe intoxication: 3 mg/kg every 4 hours for 2 days, every 6 hours on third day, then every 12 hours for 10 days or until recovery For mild intoxication; 2.5 mg/kg every 4 hours for 2 days, every 12 hours on third day, then daily for 10 days	Lacrimation, salivation, nausea, vomiting, increased temperature, decreased blood pressure, pulmonary edema (these may be diminished by previous administration of ephedrine)
Snake bites	Antivenin		

INHALANTS

Open all doors and windows and carry the patient to fresh air immediately. Loosen any tight clothing, wrap him in blankets, and keep him quiet. Again, do not give alcohol to the patient. If convulsions occur, keep the patient in bed in a semidark, quiet room. Watch the patient's respirations; if they should become irregular or stop, begin artificial respiration.

EVALUATION

The evaluation of the patient must be tendered with consideration of how much time has elapsed since the ingestion or exposure. With this in mind the classification suggested by Teitelbaum is most useful:

	Asleep	Can be aroused	Will answer questions	Comatose	Does not withdraw from painful stimuli	Reflexes absent	Respiratory or circulatory depression
Class 0	X	X	X				
Class 1				X			
Class 2				X	X		
Class 3				X	X	X	
Class 4				X	X	X	X

TREATMENT

Emergency care consists of the basic triad of maintaining an airway, emptying the stomach, and giving a cathartic. In any patient, an airway must be maintained by one means or another. Thick or profuse secretions may require suctioning. An oral airway or an endotracheal tube may be needed to assist the patient in breathing. Be sure to check for cough or gag reflexes in all patients, even those who are awake. Avoid anoxia; give oxygen under pressure for pulmonary edema, and treat the shock, which results mainly from an increased venous space caused by dilation, not myocardial failure. Place a central venous pressure catheter, and restore the effective circulating blood volume.

Emesis

You must decide *whether* emesis should be induced. If it is, place a finger or the blunt end of a spoon at the back of the patient's throat, after having taken precautions to prevent the patient from biting the finger. A second method is to give the patient 2 tablespoons of salt in a glass of warm water. The best and most-recommended method is the use of syrup of ipecac, 20 ml with 2 to 3 glasses of water for a child and 30 ml with 2 to 3 glasses of water for an adult. (This corresponds to 4 teaspoons for a child and 2 tablespoons for an adult.) Syrup of ipecac should be in the armamentarium of every household with children. A patient in whom emesis is being induced should be in a face-down position with the head lower than the hips to prevent aspiration of vomitus.

Anything that will cause more damage on the way up and that can be neutralized in the stomach should be left there. Contraindications to emesis include an unconscious or comatose patient; convulsions; ingestion of petroleum products such as kerosene, gasoline, or lighter fluid; ingestion of corrosive poisons with symptoms of severe pain, vomiting, or burning in the mouth and throat; acids and acid-like products such as toilet bowl cleaners (sodium acid sulfate); rust removers (hydrofluoric acid); iodides; silver nitrate (styptic pencils); alkalies and alkali-like substances such as drain cleaner (sodium hydroxide, lye); washing soda (sodium carbonate); ammonia water; and household bleach (sodium hypochlorite).

Gastric lavage

Gastric lavage allows some quantitation of the material removed plus an entry for antidotes and cathartics. Lavage should be performed within 3 hours of ingestion unless large amounts of milk, cream, or enteric-coated drugs have been taken. These delay absorption and therefore make lavage feasible after a longer period of time has elapsed. Small nasogastric tubes may be easier to put into place but they limit the amount and particle size of the material that can be removed. Therefore, select a No. 28 French tube for children and No. 32 to 42 French for adults. Chilling and application of lubricating gel to the tip facilitate its passage. Position the end of the tube under water; if air bubbles are seen leaving the tube, reposition it to make certain it is in the stomach and not the bronchus. The patient should be on his left side with his head lower than his hips to increase drainage and minimize aspiration.

Table 28-2 Lavage solutions

Solution	Concentration	Effective against
Activated charcoal	15 to 30 ml/250 ml water	All chemicals except cyanide
Tannic acid	0.5%	Alkaloids, certain glucosides, many metals, apomorphine, hydrastine, strychnine, veratrine, cinchona alkaloids, and salts of aluminum, lead, silver
Potassium permanganate	1:10,000	Alkaloids, atropine, quinine, strychnine, nicotine, morphine, physostigmine
Magnesium oxide or magnesium hydroxide	25 gm/1,000 ml water	Acetylsalicylic acid, oxalic acid, sulfuric acid, and other mineral acids
Sodium bicarbonate	5%	Iron sulfate
Calcium lactate or calcium gluconate	15 to 30 gm/1,000 ml water	Fluoride and oxalates
Calcium chloride	4 gm/1,000 ml water	Fluoride and oxalates
Ammonium acetate or dilute ammonia water	4 ml/500 ml water	Formaldehyde
Normal saline	0.8% or 4 ml/500 ml water	Silver nitrate
Iodine	15 drops tincture/125 ml water	Lead, mercury, silver, quinine, and strychnine
Starch	75 to 80 gm/1,000 ml water	Iodine (lavage until no blue returns)
Milk	Fresh or evaporated	Copper sulfate, croton oil, chlorates, thioglycolic acid

In general, tap water or normal or half-normal saline may be used. Activated charcoal will increase absorption. As important as the choice of a specific lavage solution is the manner in which it is used. Use small amounts (50 ml) repeatedly rather than larger amounts less often, in order to decrease the passage of poison into the intestine. Table 28-2 lists specific lavage solutions. When the return is clear, give activated charcoal in water and a saline cathartic via the tube to promote rapid passage of the poison through the intestine. Cathartics are contraindicated when the poison causes dehydration secondary to severe diarrhea and shock.

SPECIFIC CARE

Substance categories include foods, plants, heavy metals, drugs, and household products.

Food poisoning

Food poisoning can be traced to either a chemical or a bacterial source. Two variables are the dosage of the toxin or organism and the resistance of the individual. Some of the common food poisons are analyzed as follows.

Chemical	Source	Symptoms	Incubation
Antimony	Gray enameled utensils	Vomiting	Minutes to 1 hour
Cadmium	Acid liquids placed in cadmium-plated ice cube trays, pitchers, etc.	Cramps, diarrhea	15 to 30 minutes
Sodium cyanide	Silver cleaner	Weakness, coma, respiratory failure	Few minutes
Sodium fluoride	Cockroach powder (mistaken for baking powder or soda)	Gastrointestinal upset, convulsions, paresis	Minutes to 2 hours
Zinc	Acid foods cooked or stored in galvanized iron utensils	Pain in mouth, throat, and abdomen; diarrhea	Few minutes
DDT	Animals exposed to it	Unknown	Unknown

Poisonous plants

Poisonous plants or parts of plants so completely surround us in our everyday living that we tend to minimize their dangers, often through indifference or ignorance.

Among the inedible mushrooms or toadstools, *Amanita muscaria* produces muscarine poisoning within minutes to 2 hours of ingestion. The symptoms are lacrimation, miosis, salivation, sweating, dyspnea, abdominal cramping, diarrhea, vomiting, and circulatory failure followed by mental disturbances, coma, and convulsions. Onset of intoxication by phalloidin from *Amanita phalloides* frequently appears 6 to 24 hours after ingestion and has a higher morbidity and mortality than the muscarine poisoning. The symptoms of gastrointestinal upset are the same as with muscarine intoxication. Liver and kidney damage, circulatory failure, and coma are usually seen within 1 week. The treatment of muscarine and phalloidin poisoning are the same: gastric lavage with 1:200 tannic acid or

Table 28-3　Bacterial sources of food poisoning

	Botulism	Staphylococcus	Salmonella
Source	Home-canned vegetables, preserved meats and fish	Airborne droplets or skin infection, especially in milk, mayonnaise sandwiches, cream, salads, custard, cream-filled pastries, mincemeat, salted meat and chicken, cured and tenderized ham	Rat and mouse urine and feces, infected meat, duck eggs, unpasteurized milk and cheese, housefly and human carriers
Incubation period	2 hours to 8 days, usually 12 to 36 hours	2 to 3 hours; may be from 1 to 6 hours	Usually 12 to 24 hours; can be 7 to 72 hours with 6 to 8 hours minimum
Symptoms	Headache, dizziness, diplopia, constipation, vomiting, diarrhea, abdominal pain, drooping lids, difficulty in swallowing, aphonia, or respiratory paralysis	Nausea, vomiting, diarrhea, cramps, acute prostration, recovery within 1 to 3 days	Septicemia versus intestinal; abdominal pain, chills, fever, diarrhea, vomiting
Treatment	Treat respiratory failure; botulism type A, B, E antitoxin, cleansing enemas	Nonspecific; maintain hydration	Maintain hydration and electrolyte balance; paregoric or morphine for pain and diarrhea
Comments	Two thirds of cases in USA are fatal; prevent by properly canning foods in pressure cooker; boil foods for 15 minutes before eating; smell the toxin when opening a container	Toxin is heatstable; has no odor or taste, is not destroyed by boiling for 30 minutes or by refrigeration for 67 days	

with 1:10,000 potassium permanganate, followed by a saline purgative. Overstimulation of the parasympathetic nervous system by muscarine can be antagonized specifically with atropine sulfate, 0.1 to 0.5 mg (1/640 to 1/120 grain) subcutaneously. Peritoneal dialysis or hemodialysis is useful in treating the renal tubular necrosis that may develop. General supportive treatment includes steroids and vasopressors for shock, anticonvulsants, dialysis, maintenance of an adequate airway, antiemetics, kaolin or similar antidiarrheal medications, and fluid replacement.

The leaf blades of rhubarb plant are very toxic. With the exception of good tubers, the entire plant of the potato, including raw sprouted potatoes, are in the same category. Among the poisonous garden flowers are the foxglove (flowers, leaves, and seeds);

lily-of-the-valley (leaves, roots, fruit, and flowers); delphinium, larkspur, and staggerweed (seed and young plants); monkshood (flowers, leaves, and roots); and the bulbs of the narcissus, daffodil, and jonquil. Elderberry and black locust are among the poisonous trees and shrubs, while the rhododendron, rose bay, azalea, oleander, mountain laurel, and yellow jasmine are poisonous plants that are considered ornamentals. One should be wary of the leaves and roots of the caladium, the seeds and leaves of the castor bean, the stems and leaves of the dumbcane, and the berries of the lantana. Perilous wild plants include the bloodroot, baneberry, Jack-in-the-pulpit, marsh marigold, water hemlock, false hellebore, nightshade, poison hemlock, pokeweed, and jimsonweed. The number of plants mentioned illustrates the necessity of identification of any plant eaten, the part of the plant ingested, and the amount. Symptoms usually occur within 4 to 12 hours after ingestion of plants, with mushrooms being the exception, since onset may be greater than 12 hours. If you see the patient within 4 hours of ingestion of a plant, if there are no symptoms, and if you question the toxicity of the plant, give 15 ml of syrup of ipecac; repeat in 15 minutes if the patient has not vomited, and observe the patient for 12 hours. Jimsonweed and other plants containing atropine produce the symptom complex of increased temperature, dilated pupils, decreased respirations, and shock.

Heavy metals

Heavy metal poisoning is usually caused by ingestion of bichloride of mercury or by ingestion, inhalation, or absorption of lead via the skin. Symptoms of mercury poisoning include a metallic taste, gastrointestinal upset including bloody diarrhea, foul breath, sore gums, excessive salivation, progression to circulatory and respiratory failure, and severe renal tubular degeneration. The earlier the treatment, the more effective it will be. Therefore, first have the patient ingest raw eggs or milk to inactivate the mercury. (This can be done before the patient is brought to the physician.) Copious lavage is followed by the administration of BAL (British anti-Lewisite), according to the dosages recommended in Table 28-1, or Cuprimine (a penicillamine derivative), which is an oral antidote and very effective against mercury. The dosage of Cuprimine is 250 mg three to four times per day for adults and children and 250 mg per day in fruit juice for infants.

Symptoms of lead poisoning include anorexia, vomiting, abdominal pain, constipation, irritability, drowsiness, incoordination, convulsions, coma, weakness, or paralysis. Signs include an increased blood pressure, papilledema or optic atrophy or both, and paralysis of one or more cranial nerves. Treatment is begun with gastric lavage using warm water or a 1% sodium sulfate solution followed by administration of a saline cathartic such as 30 gm of magnesium sulfate. Milk or a demulcent may be given as needed for the colic that follows; severe pain may be treated with morphine sulfate, 15 to 30 mg subcutaneously for adults; the maximum dose for children is 1 mg/10 pounds of body weight. Further treatment should be done to remove lead from bone tissue, but only on hospitalized patients.

Drug intoxication

Symptoms of salicylate or aspirin intoxication are rapid, deep, pauseless breathing secondary to a direct central nervous system effect that decreases the carbon dioxide content of the blood, producing a respiratory alkalosis. Bicarbonate is then excreted by the kidney in a compensatory action. In addition, the patient may vomit and thereby lose chloride and water. Other symptoms include extreme thirst, profuse sweating, fever, and confusion or delirium followed by peripheral circulatory collapse, coma, convulsions, oliguria or anuria, and hemorrhage. Salicylate increases metabolism and prothrombin time and blocks utilization of ketones. Therefore what began as a respiratory alkalosis progresses to a metabolic acidosis. Children under 3 years of age develop the ketosis so rapidly that the respiratory alkalosis is rarely seen.

Treatment of salicylate poisoning is aimed at correcting the metabolic imbalance as quickly as possible. Thus the first step is to give syrup of ipecac (preferably at the site of ingestion, before the patient is moved), 15 to 20 ml, followed by a large amount of water for a patient over the age of 1 year. This may be repeated in 30 minutes if emesis has not occurred; if this too is ineffective, gastric lavage should be done. The half-life of salicylate in serum is 200 hours at urine pH 5.0 but is 4 hours at urine pH 7.5. The rate of salicylate excretion in alkaline urine (pH greater than 7.5) is ten- to twentyfold that in less alkaline urine. Use of potassium citrate of acetazolamide (Diamox) may be preferred to sodium bicarbonate as a means of alkalinizing the urine. Potassium and fluids will help overcome dehydration and increase urine flow. Fever may be lowered with cold or tepid sponges. Vitamin K decreases the bleeding tendency. Glucose decreases ketosis and increases blood sugar, which tends to fall (by an unknown mechanism). Oxygen may be needed. When starting the intravenous therapy, blood should be drawn to determine the serum salicylate level. Six hours after ingestion, if the serum salicylate level is 40 mg/100 ml or less, the patient may be discharged. If the level is 40 to 50 mg/100 ml, there is mild to moderate intoxication; if 60 to 80 mg/100 ml, moderate to severe intoxication; and if more than 80 mg/100 ml, severe salicylate intoxication.

Ammoniated mercury ointment, camphorated oil, methyl salicylate (oil of wintergreen), and boric acid are all dangerous and useless drugs and have no place in the family medicine cabinet. One teaspoon of methyl salicylate is equivalent of the salicylate found in twelve 5-grain ASA tablets. Boric acid intoxication is often the result of its indiscriminate use over large areas of broken skin or mucous membranes. Symptoms are erythema and exfoliation of skin (the "boiled lobster"), vomiting, inanition, dehydration, and convulsions. Treatment consists of the removal of as much boric acid as possible, intravenous fluids, barbiturates to decrease convulsions, and peritoneal dialysis in critically ill children.

Overdosage of headache remedies such as acetanilid or acetophenetidin produce methemoglobinemia, while the pyrazolon analgesics (for example aminopyrine) occasionally produce an agranulocytosis and aplastic anemia. Symptoms include cyanosis, chocolate-colored blood, severe anemia, and renal damage resulting from precipitation of methemoglobin in kidney tubules. The decrease in hemoglobin causes respiratory difficulties, and vascular collapse ensues, secondary to anoxia and central nervous system depression. One should lavage with water or 1:10,000 potassium permanganate, leaving 60 to 90 ml in the stomach at the end of the lavage. One should also give enemas and laxatives, keep the patient warm, administer 5% dextrose in water intravenously, and place the patient in the oxygen tent or use artificial respiration as needed. The use of methylene blue, intravenously or orally, has been recommended in the past, but it must be used with extreme caution, and only under the direction of those who are qualified and experienced in this matter.

Sniffing of glue, gasoline, and Freon is usually treated with fresh air or oxygen and a

5% carbon dioxide mixture. Alcohol taken with other drugs can produce an intoxication of the mixture and may present as too much of either component. Digitalis intoxication is usually caused by therapeutic measures but may result from intentional overdosage. It presents with symptoms of anorexia, nausea, vomiting, abdominal pain, drowsiness, dizziness, visual disturbances, mental confusion, emotional disturbances, hallucinations, delirium, tremors, and convulsions. Cardiac signs vary from sinus bradycardia to ventricular tachycardia and on to ventricular fibrillation, cardiac arrest, and death. Treatment includes lavage and keeping the patient warm and sedated. The cardiac disorder should be monitored and treated with the appropriate medications. Diphenyl-hydantoin is effective in correcting some arrhythmias, but its use has been recently questioned, and at this time the matter is unsettled. Intravenous sodium ethylenediamine tetraacetic acid (EDTA), a chelating agent, obviates the toxic symtons of digitalis by decreasing serum calcium.

Iron poisoning is seen more frequently in recent years since more and more women are taking iron preparations. As little as 1 gm is dangerous, and 2 gm can be fatal to a small child, since it diffuses through the gastrointestinal tract so quickly that it overwhelms the iron-binding capacity, which then leads to shock, in 20 to 48 hours, with corrosion of the gastrointestinal tract and hemorrhagic periportal necrosis of the liver. Vomiting, epigastric pain, diarrhea, a weak rapid pulse, pallor, cyanosis, and finally coma and respiratory damage may occur. Milk, magnesium oxide, or bismuth subcarbonate should be given immediately and followed with gastric lavage using a sodium phosphate solution. Plasma, blood, and glucose-saline intravenous solutions may be needed for shock and dehydration. Desferoxamine (Desferal), a chelating agent, has been used. British anti-Lewisite (BAL) should not be used, since it is harmful in this situation. Lipotropic agents and B-complex vitamins are recommended for prevention of liver damage. Although iron is reported to be nondialyzable, dialysis does seem to help at times.

Atropine, belladonna, and stramonium (found in jimsonweed, stinkweed, or thorn apple) all present symptoms and signs of burning and dryness of mouth, flushing, fever, intense thirst, visual disturbances, widely dilated pupils that do not react to light, weakness, giddiness, staggering gait, mental confusion, excitement, and delirium. Treatment consists of withdrawal of the causative agent and, in severe cases, lavage with 4% tannic acid solution with a residual of activated charcoal to absorb the atropine left in the stomach at the end of the lavage. Along with other symptomatic treatment, pilocarpine, 10 to 15 mg, or methacholine, 10 to 30 mg, may be given to relieve the oral and visual symptoms.

Patients with morphine intoxication have a decreased rate and depth of respiration, pale and cold skin that becomes cyanotic, and then circulatory failure. Central nervous system depression is usual, although with meperidine (Demerol), codeine, and thebaine, excitement and convulsions may occur. Pupils are initially constricted and dilute potassium permanganate or tincture of iodine, 15 drops/100 ml water, is given. Strong black coffee may be given if the patient is conscious. Nalorphine (Nalline) or levallorphan (Lorfan) aids respiration. Diphenoxylate hydrochloride (Lomotil) and dextropro-poxyphene hydrochloride (Darvon) are antagonized by the narcotic antagonists and are treated with nalorphine, 0.5 mg intravenously, to aid respiration, decrease seizures, and decrease cardiac arrhythmias. Symptomatic treatment may also be required.

Successful drug suicides are most often accomplished with barbiturates (80%). The symptom complex of barbiturate intoxication includes excitement and hallucination going to mental depression, stupor, coma, decreased respirations and blood pressure, decreased renal excretion, and shock. These signs and symptoms are treated by supporting the respiration and circulation by the use of artificial respiration using 95% oxygen and 5% carbon dioxide if needed, pressor amines, blood transfusion, Trendelenburg position, and hydration with 5% to 10% glucose solutions for shock. When the vital signs are stable and renal function is adequate, osmotic diuresis with intravenous urea, large amounts of fluids, and alkalinization of the urine may be undertaken. If the serum phenobarbital level is 20% or if the intermediate barbiturate serum level is 7%, dialysis should be performed.

Ataractic or tranquilizing drugs are safer than the barbiturates when taken in too great an amount, but they need to be recognized and treated in a specific manner. The symptoms are a deep sleep or coma or extrapyramidal signs such as motor restlessness, parkinsonian syndrome, or some types of dyskinesias. The phenothiazine derivatives produce an initial sedation, then restlessness followed by tonic-clonic convulsions, deep respiratory depression, and a precipitous drop in blood pressure. These patients should be lavaged at once and intravenous fluids begun. Methylphenidate (Ritalin) (not amphetamines) and norepinephrine (not other pressor amines, since they further decrease the blood pressure) may be used. **Do not use epinephrine.** Glutethimide (Doriden) intoxication causes ataxia, nystagmus, mydriasis, drowsiness, and coma. The respiratory rate is normal but the ventilation is poor, the pulse is increased, and the blood pressure is decreased. Treatment includes thorough gastric lavage, leaving 30 to 60 ml of castor oil in the stomach, and supporting the respiration. One should use caution in the administration of fluids to these patients, since they can easily be overhydrated. If the blood level of glutethimide is 1.0 to 2.5 mg/100 ml, the patient should be treated with adequate ventilation, pressors, and central nervous system stimulation. If there is no response to this treatment or if the blood level is more than 3 mg/100 ml, the patient should be dialyzed. The dialysis equipment should be kept in place until the blood level fails to rise during a period of several hours during which no dialysis has taken place.

Household agents

With the categories of household products and insecticides, the best source is a current textbook of toxicology and the annual review of poisons and their dialyzability in the *Transactions of the American Society for Artificial Internal Organs.*

In treating patients with intoxication from one of the chlorinated hydrocarbon insecticides (benzene hexachloride [Lindane], chlordane, chlorophenothane [DDT], difluoro-diphenyl-trichloro-ethane [DFDT], dieldrin, heptochlor, methoxychlor, and Toxaphene among others), from phosphorus in rat or roach poisons or fireworks, and from moth repellents. One should recall that oily or fatty substances such as milk, cream, oil purgatives, or demulcents should not be given becuase they increase the absorption of these substances.

REFERENCES

1. Teitelbaum, Daniel T.: Initial management of poisoning, Emergency Med., February, 1970.
2. Arena, Jay M.: Clin. Symp. 18:1, 1966.
3. Coleman, Allen B.: Current concepts, accidental poisoning, N. Engl. J. Med. 277:21, 1967.

chapter 29

Immediate care in the drug scene

George R. Gay

We have seen innumerable "O.D.'s" (overdoses) at the Haight-Ashbury Free Medical Clinic. These unfortunates have often been dumped on our doorstep, or sometimes an actual call for help from several doors or streets away may reach us. Resuscitation bag in hand, then, we make the 100-yard dash to help.

As our experience has broadened, we have found several rules of thumb to be particularly valuable and often lifesaving.

1. Don't look for *pinpoint pupils.* This is a time-wasting activity that will not actively help anything, and this is the sign of the amateur. Hypoxia or mixed drugs may mask this sign of opiate intoxication.
2. Don't look for intubation equipment. First *oxygenate* this patient, *breathe for him!* ("pink him up"), and leave the more exotic job of intubation to other experts. Call for them as time allows, but don't waste precious moments in "on-the-job training."
3. Don't waste other precious moments looking for needle marks. (They may be anywhere from the feet to the penis and other places you'd never think of looking.)
4. *Do* expect *multiple drug abuse* to have produced these cases of respiratory depression. Only the true opiate-using novice or the patient who has been "clean" (such as in jail or involuntarily detained by the military for "detoxification purposes") will be in danger of respiratory depression and death from the poor grade "stuff" (heroin) available on the streets of San Francisco (which may be 1% or less in purity) *or* the individual who is using multiple respiratory depressants concurrently.

Pure heroin overdose patients classically present with pinpoint pupils (unless anoxia has caused dilation), areflexia, marked respiratory depression (from apnea to two or three shallow gasping breaths per minute), and a cyanotic, clammy pallor. *Always* suspect that a young comatose patient with a questionable or nonexistent history may be a heroin (or other sedative hypnotic) overdose case.

INITIAL TREATMENT

Treatment, then, to be effective, must be prompt, and proper measures are essential. Here, in simple outline form, is the method of emergency therapy we've developed at the Haight-Ashbury Free Medical Clinic.

Remember—*in this order*—the ABCD's of resuscitation.

A. Clean the mouth and establish the *airway*.

B. *Breathe* for the patient if he is apneic or not breathing for himself or *assist* his respirations if they are inadequate.

C. Assess the *cardiovascular system* and give support where necessary (from a vigorous slap on the chest to external cardiac massage to intravenous or intracardiac stimulating drugs).

D. Give the *drugs* necessary to maintain your patient—cardiac stimulants, bicarbonate to reverse acidosis, steroids, or *whatever*—but *only* after A, B, and C, are fully managed and under definite control.

Establish an airway

Clean the patient's mouth. (We use a quick wipe with a towel, handkerchief, or shirttail, and at the same time we pull his tongue forward.) Mucus, blood, vomitus, gum, or tobacco may be found with surprising regularity.

With the patient in the supine position, tip the head slightly up and back. Grasping the jaw at the angles of the mandible and at the point of the chin, draw his head back, chin high, to a "sniffing-like" position, being careful not to hyperextend his neck. Pull his tongue forward, making sure it isn't occluding his posterior oropharynx. A flaccid tongue is in every way analogous to a quarter-pound of hamburger occluding the airway. (If reflexes *are* present, he'll protect his *own* airway, so watch your fingers!) If his oropharyngeal reflexes are *absent*, insert an oropharyngeal airway; if an airway isn't available, hold his tongue forward with your fingers.

Provide air to the lungs

Breathe for the patient if he is apneic or if he is breathing inadequately—mouth-to-mouth, or mouth-to-nose, or use Ambu bag if one is handy—don't wait! If we consider room air to be composed of 20% oxygen, we can expect your mouth-to-mouth respiration to get at least 15% oxygen into the patient. Make sure that air is entering his lungs and that his chest (not his stomach) is expanding. Listen for breath sounds with a stethoscope over both sides of the chest and over the stomach.

Quickly assess the cardiovascular system

Check the pulse for rate and rhythm. Check the precordial, femoral, temporal, and radial pulses. Don't be lulled into complacency by the strong, full pulse of hypoxia, for this may be the premonitory to terminal arrhythmia and cardiac cessation. Remember: *if the patient arrives with a heartbeat,* you have a good chance of saving him!

If hearbeat is absent, give a firm, full-handed "slap" over the precordium. If there is no immediate response, then begin external cardiac massage, placing the palms of your hands over the patient's lower sternum and depressing firmly sixty times per minute. Determine the cardiac status and rhythm pattern with an electrocardiograph (if available). Institute appropriate action such as defibrillation or pacing, if possible.

In severe cases of narcotic and other drug overdose, especially if long neglected, the patient's cardiovascular system may be so depressed that pulmonary edema may develop.

In this case, intubation or tracheostomy—plus continuous positive pressure respiration—may be lifesaving.

Administer drugs

Administer such drugs as may be considered necessary but continue treatment as in a heroin overdose.

Utilize the Narcan, Lorfan, or Nalline (or narcotic antagonist) test, which is diagnostic for narcotic overdose. Even if other drugs are involved, respiratory depth and rate will improve following this simple procedure. Give 1 ml (4 mg) naloxone hydrochloride (Narcan), 1 ml (1 mg) levallorphan tartrate (Lorfan) intravenously, or 1 ml of nalorphine (Nalline) (5 mg). Narcan is presently believed to be the drug of choice in overdose cases, since no additive narcotic depressant effects are seen with its use. These dosages will bring the victim of "pure" heroin overdose back to consciousness in seconds (almost literally one circulation time). The same drug given intramuscularly may take up to 20 minutes to act, and then not as dramatically.

If the patient has "collapsed" veins, as many addicts do, try the external jugular or the femoral veins—they may be poking right out and make more of an expert of you than you'd imagined. You may repeat the dosages of these drugs *one time* within 10 minutes. If there is no response after this time, however, you are probably dealing with more than a *pure* narcotics overdose, and further doses of Lorfan and Nalline may contribute to respiratory depression. If, however, you stick to the doses recommended, you have utilized a *true* narcotic antagonist test, and the chances of contributing to respiratory depression are *absolutely* minimal.

If you have good reason to suspect a *recent* overdose of respiratory depressant drugs, consider giving 3 to 5 ml (1 ml=20 mg) doxapram hydrochloride (Dopram) intravenously. If, however, some time has elapsed and if in *any way* a metabolic acidosis is suspected, this drug is *definitely contraindicated.* Dopram must *always* be given with great care; it generally has a high safety margin but it *does* create a temporary hypertensive effect and an increase in metabolic rate that may contribute to a preexisting acidosis. In any case, it is only a "stop-gap" aid. When used in the manner described, however, this is an extremely *safe, powerful, temporary* (lasting 3 to 5 minutes), *nonspecific* respiratory stimulant. It usually has immediate and dramatic effect, so by all means be sure the patient's mouth is clear and his airway is open, and *never* turn your back on the patient. In the presence of a "pure" narcotic depression deep, spontaneous respirations will appear and then "wear off" after several minutes. In addition, Dopram has temporary but definite cerebral arousal effects. In brief Dopram should be regarded as only a temporary aid, and certainly as one *not* completely free of danger.

Stay with the patient until he is fully responsive. Observe him for several hours. If he has used a long-acting narcotic, such as methadone hydrochloride (Dolophine), he may lapse back into coma and die a respiratory death as the relatively short-acting narcotic antagonist wears off. This is where you can utilize the services of the friend or friends (if any) who brought in your overdosed patient. (These are "friends" in a very real sense, because being sophisticated in drug lore, they realize the chance they take in bringing him to you. They can be held legally responsible for their unfortunate companion's condition or for his possible death.) If present, however, and if handled properly in a nonpunitive, nonjudgmental manner, these friends can be utilized as the most knowledgeable and practical private duty nursing service available.

If your patient fails to respond, follow routine and established emergency procedures. First, secure a route for administering intravenous fluids, preferably with a large-bore cannula. Begin the administration of a glucose-electrolyte solution. If moderate to severe acidosis is suspected, administer sodium bicarbonate in appropriate amounts. Draw blood for chemistries. Search for any possible nondrug etiology such as evidence of head trauma, blood loss, diabetes, acute infectious process, or increased intracranial pressure.

If long-standing drug depression is suspected (for example, when a patient is discovered unattended), be on guard for atelectasis, pulmonary edema, or pneumonia. In this event avoid the Dopram and initiate immediate hospitalization, vigorous pulmonary therapy, and aggressive antibiotic treatment.

What we see increasingly is the "smack-head" who professes to disdain "downers" (or "reds" or "yellows") and alcohol ("juice is for rednecks . . . rednecks and straights!") but who increasingly takes these drugs along with the poor grade "street junk" both to help him "get off" and alleviate symptoms of withdrawal or carry him over until he can "score" again.

SPECIFIC PATTERNS IN COMMONLY MISUSED DRUGS

With the emergence of the new widespread use and abuse of multiple psychotropic drugs, the physician must, to "keep up with the times," educate himself in an entirely new sphere of psychologic and medical therapeutics.

Marijuana

To our knowledge no one has as yet died of marijuana overdose. Overdose may result in an occasional case of nausea and vomiting. When a person with a very structured (rigid or inadequate) personality (or psychologic "set") experiments with the drug in an improper physical setting, he may not be able to cope with feelings of "spaciness" or "depersonalization" (losing control) and may thus experience an acute anxiety reaction. This has been seen several times in middle-aged people who ate "Alice B. Toklas" ("hash") brownies. That is, they are unable to adequately "titrate" their degree of intoxication. The more experienced user will take just what he feels he needs as the "roach" is passed around a communal circle. Indeed, he may experience a "social high" ("contact high") in proper company without *any* drugs.

Usually a calm and sympathetic counselor is all that is needed in these cases. Sedatives such as chlordiazepoxide (Librium) or diazepram (Valium) may prevent recurrence of panic or anxiety reaction.

When calm, the marijuana smoker and the LSD user appear strikingly similar: "cool," nonviolent, often offering "vibrations" of brotherhood and love to all who are in attendance. The marijuana and the LSD users are *not* violent individuals—with one exception—when trapped with the drug that can mean a prison record and long years of criminal indoctrination for them.

LSD and the "mind benders"

A similar calm and sympathetic therapeutic atmosphere is vital in the emergency care of the LSD-induced anxiety or paranoia. The patient should be taken to a supportive environment (this area is called the calm center at the Haight-Ashbury Free Medical

Clinic) and should be talked to in a quiet, sensitive, reassuring voice. Physical contact (holding hands) should be employed if it is not uncomfortable to the patient.

It is truly amazing how rapidly a rational and sympathetic individual can calm the severely agitated LSD user. By all means avoid crowds and noises; do not employ nurses or other attendants in uniforms; and do *not* attempt to pass a nasogastric tube ("they're trying to put a snake in me!").

Again, the LSD "bummer" is probably caused by an improper environmental setting, or the person may possess too rigid or inadequate a "set" for a "good trip."

Our "talk-down" technique has proved to be very successful. We firmly believe, as well, that chlorpromazine hydrochloride (Thorazine) and other phenothiazines are almost always contraindicated. Aside from the psychologic implications of the needle, the LSD trip will be pharmacologically "aborted" and subconsciously will be subverted. This material may later reappear (in the form of flashbacks) and severe anxiety and even suicidal impulses may appear. So with an adverse LSD reaction, be gentle, be rational, be sympathetic. *Do not* be overly clinical.

When LSD "flashbacks" occur after a "bummer" (or after mismanaged medical intervention), again best management is by reason and reassurance. If the patient is acutely agitated, a mild oral tranquilizer (Valium, 10 mg, or Librium, 25 mg three times a day) may be of value. Chloral hydrate (1,000 to 1,500 mg) may also make sleeping easier. Avoid needles and syringes whenever possible!

Occasionally you may be called upon to treat a baby or a child (yet unable to talk) for LSD ingestion. The treatment here is to love and fondle the child. Offer it physical contact and love for at least 8 hours. The child is in no physical danger and will often respond immediately to your close attention.

Amphetamines ("speed")

As a physician, you will probably not be called upon to treat a "speed freak" during a "run." Should this occur, however, he is *not* hard to spot. He looks like Rasputin: wild-eyed and woolly, undernourished. He looks as if every nerve ending in his body were raw and being stimulated. Acute amphetamine psychosis, full-blown with paranoia and auditory and visual hallucinations, may require hospitalization.

The paranoia attendant to large-dose amphetamine abuse will invariably keep the patient away from the doctor's door. Be happy of this, too; for the amphetamine abuser (who has rewritten the pharmacology books by sometimes "shooting" up to 5 gm per day) may develop a paranoid psychosis and is often prone to violence, so make sure you have the proper "muscle" around before you take on an aroused "speed freak."

Not physically addicting in itself, "speed" will eventually "burn itself out"; that is, the user will "crash." The pattern is then one of prolonged sleep, followed by ravenous hunger and then deep depression—at which time he will either initiate another "speed run" or will turn to barbiturates, heroin, glutethimide (Doriden), meprobamate, or alcohol or other "downers" to allow his body some rest.

Your fear as a physician is, first, is he violent and paranoid? Then, is he near an exhaustion phase? Then, is this problem compounded by other drugs (barbiturates, heroin, and so on)? The classic treatment for the *"pure"* "speed freak" is chloral hydrate (1,000 to 1,500 mg) and a mild tranquilizer, but *not* if the water is muddied by the other medications noted previously.

Barbiturates (Doriden, dopers, or downers)

The pure "doper" is easy to spot. He dresses sloppily, has poor personal hygiene, burns holes in his clothing with his cigarettes, and talks at 33 1/3 rpm. If he is in this toxic state, there is little to do but observe him for proper respiration and try to get him committed. As he "comes off" barbiturates, convulsions are liable to occur, or even hyperpyrexia and death. However, few "barb freaks" take barbiturates alone, so beware of the superimposed pharmacology of additional drugs.

Many of our sophisticated young drug users accept convulsion as part of "coming down" off barbiturates. If possible, however, hospitalization should be arranged. As few as six secobarbitals taken over a 30-day period can cause convulsions upon withdrawal.

Grouped pharmacologically with the barbiturates are glutethimide (Doriden), methaqualone (Quaalude), meprobamate, diazepam (Valium), chlordiazepoxide (Librium), and alcohol. Watch for a combination of these.

Scopolamine and its derivatives

In addition to the standard depressant, stimulant, or hallucinogenic drug problems, the physician may be challenged by a variety of miscellaneous adverse drug reactions such as scopolamine delirium, since these and other similar drugs are widely available in nonprescription, over-the-counter medications such as Compoz and Sominex. Treatment of belladonna delirium may be a high-risk task, for if the physician administers the wrong medication (such as a phenothiazine tranquilizer), he may produce an additive reaction that can kill the patient. We recommend supportive treatment for the scopolamine intoxication, although some investigators advocate the use of physostigmine in anticholinergic drug-induced delirium and coma.

Diacetylmorphine ("smack")

For $15 to $25 the "junkie" buys a 350- to 400-mg "bag" or "balloon" of "junk" as he aptly calls it. Of this material, 2% to 10% may be pure heroin. The remainder is probably milk sugar, powdered coffee, quinine, or other gritty white powdery material—or, if he is marked for a "death hit" ("hot shot"), strychnine or arsenic. He "shoots up" three to four times a day. His average habit costs between $50 and $75 per day.

Aside from the hepatitis of the dirty shared needle, he may show up in your office with the racking chills of "cotton fever" (either acute septicemia or an allergic response to the multitude of foreign material that he injects into his veins daily).

Cocaine

Systemically, cocaine stimulates the central nervous system from above downward. The first recognizable action is on the cortex. In man, this is manifested in definite euphoria, garrulousness, restlessness, and excitement. (There is some evidence that perceptual awareness and cognitive speed are increased.) There may also be an increased capacity for muscular work, probably because of a lessened sense of fatigue. Headache may be reported. After small amounts of cocaine, motor activity is well coordinated, but as the dose is increased stimulation of lower motor centers causes tremors and convulsive movements.

If overdose occurs, the victim may report depression, confusion, dry throat, and dizziness. Hyperreflexia is noted, and eventually clonic-tonic convulsions appear. Such acute reaction, when accompanied by cardiovascular and respiratory collapse, constitutes the prototype "caine reaction" and demands immediate supportive medical intervention.

Cocaine potentiates the responses of organs supplied by sympathetic nerves to epinephrine and norepinephrine and appears to slow the normal uptake of these "neurohumors." A direct effect of this is increased gastrointestinal motility with a cathartic response and an occasional explosive result.

The action of cocaine on the medulla results in an initial increase in respiratory rate; the depth of respiration is then soon diminished to a rapid and shallow pattern. As depression follows stimulation, irregular or Cheyne-Stokes respiration may appear, and death may then occur as a result of central respiratory depression. The vasomotor and vomiting centers may also share in a stimulation, and sweating and vomiting are not uncommonly noted. A central effect on the heat-regulating center in the diencephalon, as well as vasoconstriction, increased muscular activity, and reduced heat radiation, may contribute to a dangerous elevation in body temperature. (Hyperpyrexia plus hyper-metabolism may contribute directly to convulsion.)

Other than purely supportive respiratory measures, resuscitative efforts should be carried out *only* in *controlled situations* (ambulance, hospital), and *by experts*, along these lines:

1. Administer oxygen, by positive pressure and artificial respiration if necessary. First, be *assured* that an open airway is present.
2. Use the Trendelenburg position (head down). Wrap arms and legs if needed.
3. Inject *small amounts* of short-acting barbiturates (for example, thiopental [Sodium Pentothal] 25 to 50 mg) *if* convulsions are present. This may be repeated but *gently* (do *not* force general depressant effect to point of no return).
4. Administer intravenous stimulants for cardiotonic effect (phenylephrine, 10 to 20 mg).
5. Keep patient cool and keep crowds away.
6. Give general muscle relaxants if necessary (curare, succinylcholine) to facilitate administration of positive pressure oxygen.
7. Continuously monitor vital signs.

Cocaine is the prototype of the stimulant drug that is capable of producing euphoric excitement and, in high dosage, hallucinatory experience. These properties rank it high in the esteem of the experienced drug abuser and lead to the highest degree of psychic dependence.

In the current drug subculture, cocaine has become the "champagne of drugs" because of its expense and scarcity. The "coke" user looks down on the other drug types and indeed represents the "upper" class. The "rich man's" drug, cocaine may be purchased illegally for from $500 to $1,500 an ounce. (This is usually diluted or "stepped on" by the street peddler.) Pure wholesale cocaine sells to medical institutions for $20 an ounce. Recently, with the influx of cocaine into the Hollywood elite and other upper economic classes, the practice of "snorting" or "sniffing" (in which a "line" of cocaine is inhaled into a nostril, often through a rolled high denomination bill) has been revived and has to some extent supplanted intravenous use. Wavy Gravy has called cocaine "the thinking man's Dristan." One of the complications of sniffing, however, is the frequent perforation of the nasal septum by necrosis secondary to the vasoconstricting effects of cocaine.

"Sniffers," "snorters," or "snarfers" are also prone to infection of the mucous membranes. In addition, a "reactive hyperemia" (or clogging of nasal airways by engorged membranes) occurs as the vasoconstriction wears off, accounting for the dyad seen carried by chronic cocaine sniffers: (1) the paraphernalia (spoon, snuffbox, and so on) and (2) the nose drops.

Cocaine is the drug of "special occasions," both social and sexual, hoarded and then doled out like champagne or rare old brandy.

TREATMENT OF "PURE HEROIN" OVERDOSE OR MIXED ADDICTIONS

Follow treatment as detailed in the opening section of this chapter.

THE BATTERED FLOWER-CHILD SYNDROME

These overdose victims may be dumped at your doorstep like the morning paper, or they may be accompanied by one or two frightened and reticent friends. They can be *your* best friends in this case, as well, for they can provide an all-important history of what has occurred and can serve private nurse duty in sitting with their friend as he is recovering, *after* your ministrations. The vital point is *not* to turn these young people away or to underestimate their street knowledge.

Remember that you, as a physician (not to be trusted) and as being over 30 (certainly not to be trusted), are the court of last resort for these young people. They will have previously instituted their *own* street methods of resuscitation before consulting you. Not only must you then deal with narcotic reversal (Narcan, Lorfan, or Nalline, 1 ml intravenously) or with multiple drug depression—perhaps a combination of alcohol, barbiturates, tranquilizers, and heroin or methadone (respiratory augmentation and support)—but you must further deal with the possible adverse consequences of these methods of street resuscitation. Briefly, your problem may be any of the following.

"Boxer's mouth"

"Stimulation" is the common form of street resuscitation, and this may consist of walking the overdose victim around, putting him in a cold shower, applying ice to his testicles, vigorous slapping around (hence possible blood, mucus, or broken teeth in the mouth), or squeezing sensitive areas such as the testicles or nipples.

"Speed" reversal

The pharmacologic knowledge of the street recognizes that depressant overdose may respond to amphetamines. Hence, your client may have recently been "shot up" or "dosed" with "speed." This *really* muddies the waters, and in the hypoxic, comatose patient, it may cause convulsions.

"The heavy salt trip"

The mythology of the street says that table salt will "take up" or "bind" heroin, hence nullifying its depressant effects. Therefore, a like volume of salt to the amount of heroin used (for example, 1 spoonful) is diluted with tapwater and injected intravenously. This strongly hypertonic solution, in the presence of an already severely depressed cardiovascular system, may well contribute to pulmonary edema. Perhaps some basis for perpetuation of the salt injection theory is the not uncommon occurrence of "missing" the sclerosed junkie's veins and injecting subcutaneously. The intense pain attendent to such a procedure certainly has an arousal effect on the overdose victim.

"The milk run"

The "street-wise" (although not necessarily "smart") drug user also nurtures a common myth that milk given intravenously will "reverse" the overdose. In actuality, a lipoid pneumonia may be the sad result of this practice.

"Cotton fever"

Acute septicemia or allergic reaction ranging upward to anaphylactic shock and death may follow injection of unknown foreign material by infected "outfits."

Less immediate problems such as malaria or syphilis transmitted by unsterile syringes, abscesses, bacterial endocarditis, or bacterial emboli may be watched for, but these complications are within the concept and experience of the emergency physician. It is rather the hidden, self-inflicted injuries of the criminalized drug-using counterculture—the battered flower-child syndrome—of which we must be increasingly wary.

CHANGING PATTERNS IN DRUG ABUSE

Drug patterns, particularly among adolescents and alienated youth, have changed dramatically in the last 10 years. In the accepting and somnolent 1950's, patterns were relatively constant and predictable. "Illegal" drugs were confined to certain racial, ethnic, and philosophic minorities, most often submerged within black, Puerto Rican, Mexican-American, and Oriental urban ghettos. The dominant culture (our great "silent majority") confined itself to relatively traditional (and "legal") agents of abuse such as alcohol, cigarettes, and certain prescription psychotropic drugs. Through the dissatisfied, violent 1960's, however, and into the vocal 1970's, contemporary drug patterns have shifted so dramatically that at the present time the only thing that we can predict for sure about the drug scene is that it will change. This changing problem presents disturbing new challenges to the physician at every level, particularly in the management of acute drug reactions. The physician must keep abreast of the dynamics of our drug-oriented society, which first heeded Tim Leary's proselytizing of "turn off, tune in, drop out." Its current philosophy of "better living through chemistry" is reinforced through a variety of channels from physician overprescription of amphetamine diet pills to television ads that say "take 'Compoz' so you can listen to the riot news."

Along with increasing availability of psychoactive drugs, we see a growing youthful contempt for years of misdirected "scare" drug education (analogous to the old venereal disease movies of World War II). Potential drug experimenters mistrust traditional sources of drug education given by parents, church groups, or the family physician. Unfortunately, much of this drug information gap was created by the dishonest presentation of facts on marijuana by those who have for generations espoused the "killer weed" philosophy. We have created our own credibility gap by intimating that the good guys are still *us* and the "bad" guys are still *them*. We have our puritanical lists of "good" drugs and "bad" drugs: aspirin and penicillin are "good" (unless, of course, an overdose of aspirin promotes gastric bleeding or penicillin produces an allergic response and possibly death); alcohol and cigarettes are, if not good, at least legal; while marijuana and LSD are "bad."

In truth, drugs are neither "good" nor "bad." "Drugs can make sick people healthy and healthy people sick." By varying doses, drugs can produce neutral, beneficial, or adverse psychopharmaceutical effects on different individuals in different sets and in different settings.

Through a mixture of miseducation and our ever-present puritanical reliance upon law, order, and punishment to legislate morality in medical situations, the individual drug user has come to be viewed (and, not coincidentally, to view himself) as a "criminal" and not as a "patient." Further, there is a romantic element involved here. The criminal aspects, the "hustling," the paraphernalia, and the almost semireligious ethic of this underground life style are at first exciting and invigorating to the adolescent. Whatever the new wide-ranging sociologic patterns, a large percentage of youth will experiment with illegal drugs because of now almost universal drug availability and peer group pressure.

These two variables have interacted in coordinated lock-step. Peer pressure has always been with us, but never before has there been available the astonishing assortment of drugs, manufactured both legally and illegally, that is now to be found on every street corner and in every schoolyard. As a result, the youthful drug user is mistrustful of physicians in general. The authoritarian and in general frustrated physician has contributed directly to this mistrust by his often punitive and moralizing manner. The youthful drug user is often reluctant to seek help in traditional in-patient medical facilities until his physical or psychologic pain becomes almost unbearable, and often only after experiencing an acute drug crisis.

part five

Evaluation and treatment of psychiatric emergencies

chapter 30

Immediate care of the apparently disturbed person

James M. A. Weiss

Psychiatric emergencies are those in which the patient demonstrates a disorder of thought, mood, or action that is likely to result in dangerous, self-destructive, or socially disturbing behavior.

Often in psychiatric emergencies either the patient, his family, or even casual onlookers will demand immediate action. This insistent pressure probably results in more mistakes than any other single factor, since hasty action will generally make the situation worse. In very few so-called psychiatric emergencies is there actual immediate danger to the life or health of the patient or those around him. The main factor that makes a psychiatric emergency an "emergency" is usually anxiety or fear on the part of the patient, his family, or both.

Almost all disordered behavior, no matter how disorganized or noneffective it may seem, represents an effort to adapt to internal ("psychologic") or external ("environmental") stress. The type and severity of a person's reaction to external stress depends upon his personality and the internal tensions already existing. For example, in wartime some soldiers react even to the mention of combat with panic, whereas other soldiers withstand many days of combat without demonstrating deviant behavior.

All human beings have psychologic defense mechanisms that generally operate to produce emotional homeostasis. Therefore the "emergency" nature of most psychiatric disorders is transient and temporary and not infrequently self-limited. Even the most acute emergency may be transitory; even the most bizarre, grotesque, and socially disruptive behavior may be short-lived. The important point is to recognize that most patients with such disorders—even violent patients—are usually frightened, anxious, and uncertain and that the nature of change in such disorders is often toward improvement, self-control, and more socially acceptable behavior.

BASIC PRINCIPLES OF EVALUATION AND TREATMENT

In evaluating a patient with a psychiatric disorder, the first step is to uncover as rapidly as possible the answers to four questions: (1) *What* are the symptoms and signs? (2) How *severe* are the symptoms and signs? (3) To what problems or stresses do the symptoms

175

and signs represent a reaction—*why* have they occurred? (4) What is the general nature of the *disorder* manifested by the symptoms and signs?

Only after determining at least tentative answers to these four questions should one ask the last question: "What should be *done*?" Rational treatment (even first aid) must be based on rational evaluation. In dealing with psychiatric emergencies, however, proper evaluation is in itself often therapeutic and is in fact the beginning of any more prolonged treatment. In this respect, there are three fundamental principles to remember.

1. *Be as calm, confident, direct, and purposeful as possible.* Panic is communicable, and often the patient's relatives are themselves anxious, fearful, agitated, or panicky. This is understandable, but unfortunately such attitudes and feelings are usually conveyed to the patient, who then himself becomes more disturbed, producing a vicious circle of disorder. If you are calm, confident, direct, and purposeful, both the patient and the family will often react with improvement. On the other hand, if you appear to be upset, tense, hurried, or in a dither, the patient will react either with more anxiety or with more manipulation of those about him, since he will then believe that his disorder must be a severe one.

2. *Begin evaluation and, if possible, treatment at the home or wherever the emergency occurs.* Don't rush the patient off to the hospital until you have made some initial attempt to evaluate the situation. Just as the surgeon tries to follow the precept "splint them where they lie," so in dealing with a psychiatric emergency one should attempt to evaluate the situation where it occurs. This gives the frightened, stunned, or confused patient the chance to recover some emotional balance in familiar surroundings. It often helps the patient and his family to realize that at least this emergency phase of the disorder may be transient and reversible. And, finally, it permits simple and brief methods of treatment to be effective before maladaptive behavior patterns have become fixed by time, repetition, or "secondary gain" (the superimposed and usually obvious advantage that the patient can derive from "being ill").

3. *To be effective, emergency treatment must be based on brief and relatively simple methods.* Such methods will not remove fearful or traumatic experiences, alter basic personality traits, or provide magical solutions for all of the patient's problems. The more lengthy and complex procedures should be reserved for the psychiatrist. But experience has indicated that a brief, sympathetic, noncritical interview, with measures to relieve hunger, pain, and minor physical symptoms, in an atmosphere suggesting that recovery is expected, provides the most favorable condition for rapid improvement. Such an interview serves both a diagnostic and a therapeutic purpose, providing psychologic support, alleviating the patient's basic anxiety or fear as well as his secondary symptoms and signs, and supplying an atmosphere in which more definitive treatment, if necessary, can be planned and arranged for.

PRINCIPLES ON INTERVIEWING AND BRIEF PSYCHOTHERAPY IN EMERGENCY SITUATIONS

Size up the problem as accurately and as quickly as possible. Interview the patient *alone* if possible. Relatives can wait outside—you can obtain their stories later. Try to find out why the patient is behaving as he is. Frequently, simply asking what happened to him will give you the answer. Let the patient reply in his own way. Let him "ventilate," tell *his* account of the problem and his feelings about it. This allows the patient to express anxiety, depression, anger, or other emotions and to feel better by just being able to talk about these emotions. Such a procedure helps the patient to reestablish communication and to feel that someone is trying to understand and to help him.

Do not attempt to direct the flow of conversation. Do not interrupt to ask routine "medical history" questions. You can't let the patient ramble on endlessly, but you should allot 15 to 45 minutes for the interview. This time belongs to the patient and should not be shared with other distractions. Even 15 minutes in which the patient can talk freely will often markedly relieve some of his feelings of helplessness and despair.

Be interested but not maudlin or oversympathetic. Treat the patient as a person you expect to improve. If you overwhelm him with pity, he will only feel more helpless, since your attitude will confirm his worst fears about himself. Sometimes, if the patient is excessively anxious or rather withdrawn or hostile, a cigarette or a drink of coffee, soup, or warm milk will be enough to calm him and to establish rapport. Asking relatives to prepare coffee or soup may also divert *their* anxious fluttering about into purposeful activity.

Accept the patient's limitations and his right to have his own feelings. Do not blame, ridicule, judge, or criticize him for feeling as he does. Your job is to help him cope with his feelings, not to tell him how he *should* feel. Remember that each person has had certain unique experiences that can strongly affect his emotions in relation to subsequent events in his life. If a man's leg is shattered, no one expects him to stand up and walk. But if his ability to deal with his emotions is shattered, many (often including the patient himself) are inclined to expect him to function normally again almost immediately. It does not help to resent the patient's problems, to scold him, to tell him to "snap out of it," or to reassure him that he is "normal" when you yourself don't believe it.

Accept your own limitations in an emergency situation. Do not try to solve all the patient's or the family's problems. Many such problems require specialized psychiatric treatment, and your main job may be simply to calm the patient and his family so that you can get him to a psychiatric facility. The primary goal in psychiatric first aid is to establish effective contact with a disturbed, overwhelmed patient who has lost some degree of self-control, or ability to communicate, or capacity to evaluate the world as it is. Once such contact is made, it becomes relatively easy either to help him return to adaptive living or to arrange for more definitive professional care.

With some patients, the simple ventilation of their feelings to you will be sufficient treatment. When the problem seems to be situational ("environmental"), you may often be of most aid by serving as an objective auditor, one who is essentially not involved emotionally, in a discussion that helps the patient (or his relatives) to clarify the situation, to consider alternative courses for action, and to make a realistic decision. With more helpless patients, direct advice or honest reassurance may be useful. Sometimes a patient will insistently demand some article or action that has not been given him because it is inconvenient (but not dangerous) to do so. For example, a patient may want to telephone a distant relative in another city, but his family will not allow him to do so because they consider his request "silly" or inappropriate. It is frequently reassuring if the patient is allowed his wish.

At some point before, during, or after the interview, it might become apparent that the patient's symptoms may be related to organic disorder, especially if the patient appears confused or disoriented, has memory loss, or is delirious. Emotional or behavioral disorders can be mimicked by or related to a variety of organic disorders ranging from cerebral abscess to thyroid dysfunction, from impending diabetic coma to heroin intoxication. A brief but reasonably comprehensive physical and neurologic examination will most often rule out at least the most obvious organic disorders. Have someone (perhaps the calmest relative) stay with you and the patient during the physical examination. Explain what you are doing as you perform the examination, and reassure the patient in direct and simple language if the findings are negative (even if the patient does not seem to be attending to your words). Omit for the time being the more intimate portions of the physical examination, such as investigation of rectal, pelvic, and genital areas.

The course of the patient's behavior during this relatively brief period of evaluation will usually soon make it clear whether he is having reasonable success in overcoming his initial internal turmoil or whether he will require more specialized care. Remember that most patients—even those who appear confused or disoriented—will respond in some degree to the kind of communicative attempt outlined above. Do not assume that it is impossible to interview *any* patient until you have tried.

SPECIAL PROBLEMS IN PSYCHIATRIC EMERGENCIES

Psychiatric disorders are not clearly categorized as black or white but tend to range on a continuum from the least to the most severe disorganization of behavior. A simple classification system expresses disorganization as mild, moderate, or severe, with symptoms or signs classified in one of six groups. *Affective* symptoms express mood disturbance (as elation, depression, or agitation). *Anxietal* symptoms express anxiety consciously perceived (as fright, fearfulness, or worry). *Behavioral* signs express disturbance manifested by overt action patterns (such as destructiveness or violence). *Mentational* symptoms express disturbance pertaining to intellectual functions, memory, orientation, or judgment. *Reality distortional* symptoms express gross failure in evaluating external reality ("seeing the world as it really is"), as evidenced by hallucinations, delusions, or bizarre or paranoid thinking. *Somatic* symptoms express a disturbance that the *patient* usually considers to be at least partly physical in origin. Within this classification, certain syndromes stand out as common or especially important psychiatric emergencies.

Mild reactions

The *mild affective reaction (elated type)* is usually manifested by euphoria and overactivity of speech, thought, and movement. The patient may be restless, interfering, sleepless, and too distractable or too "busy" to pay much attention to food. He often seems rather similar to the man who becomes expansive after a few drinks. Although an interview is important to evaluate the situation, this reaction usually represents an early stage of a severe manic-depressive psychosis, and the biggest problem is to convince the patient and the family that prompt referral to a psychiatrist is of great importance.

The *mild affective reaction (depressed type)* is manifested by dejection, discouragement, self-accusation, tearfulness, and slowing of speech, thought, and movement. Such a depressive reaction may be hidden under a smiling "front," but the patient will usually admit to "the blues" if he is asked. This reaction is perhaps less serious if the patient is reacting to an obvious external stress, such as the loss of a loved one. Unless suicide is a concern (see Chapter 32), brief psychotherapy will probably be adequate treatment.

The *mild affective reaction (agitated type)* is manifested by irritability, hyperactivity, and overdistractability. The basic mood is usually either elation or depression, and once this is determined in the interview, the patient can be treated as a primary elated or depressive type of reaction.

The *mild anxiety reaction* may be manifested by apprehension, worry, increased muscular tension, gross trembling of any or all parts of the body but especially of the hands, temporary speech difficulties, sweating of the palms of the hands, poor appetite (sometimes with nausea or even vomiting), occasional abdominal discomfort, urinary frequency and urgency, diarrhea, rapid heartbeat, giddiness, or breathlessness. Such reactions are very common and are most often transitory, and the patient is helped by ventilation and reassurance in the interview situation.

The *mild behavioral and mentational reactions* only very rarely occur as emergencies and, if they do, can usually be easily treated on the basis of the principles already established.

Reality distortional symptoms are, in my opinion, always indicative of a serious disorder.

The *mild somatic reaction* often may involve symptoms that are "organized" so that they appear as part or parcel of a syndrome of organic disease (such as a heart attack, stomach disorder, cerebral concussion, and many others). A supportive interview and a physical examination will usually provide the solution to at least the emergency problem.

Moderate reactions

The person suffering with moderate to severe psychiatric reactions may demonstrate some impairment of verbal communication and will usually appear sick or disabled to some degree. The *moderate affective reaction (elated type)* is manifested by a flurry of activity, rapid and often somewhat incoherent talk, inappropriate jokes, marked distractibility, and usually some grandiosity of plan or behavior. Since there is the danger of a sudden switch to assaultiveness or to suicidal depression, immediate hospitalization is indicated. Do not be taken in by the easy rapport one achieves with such persons—their high spirits may be contagious and their jokes may be funny, but they can rapidly become dangerous to themselves or to others.

The moderate affective reaction (depressed type) is manifested by marked dejection or apathy and retarded speech and action. A person suffering from this disorder often seems overwhelmed, with a vacant gaze, answering in monosyllables or not replying at all when spoken to, and perhaps suddenly breaking into tears. Unless such a person responds rather well in the interview situation, and unless one is quite certain that this person is *not* suicidal, immediate hospitalization is generally required to avoid self-destruction.

The *moderate affective reaction (agitated type)* is usually manifested by tremulousness, choked speech, excessive sweating, a startled reaction to noise, wringing of hands and pacing up and down, and sometimes an appearance of great fearfulness. A brief interview will not infrequently calm such a patient and allow you to determine whether the basic affect is one of elation, depression, or anxiety.

The *moderate anxiety reaction* will usually present with these same symptoms and can often be treated with brief psychotherapy; but if elation or depression of this degree is suspected, the important thing is not to leave the patient alone (even for a moment while you step out to call the hospital) and to get the patient to a psychiatric facility. The *moderate anxiety reaction* may be seen also in the person who shows no evidence of depression, elation, or overt anxiety but who seems stunned, puzzled, or confused. Such a person may answer questions in monosyllables and make little or no effort to respond to any stimuli. The chances are that this syndrome represents a "stun reaction" to some sort of environmental catastrophe or to what the patient interprets as a catastrophe (which may not be obvious to the onlooker), or else the syndrome may be a serious depressive reaction. If the patient does not respond rather rapidly to brief psychotherapy, treat him as having a serious depressive reaction until further evidence indicates otherwise.

The *moderate behavioral reaction* may be seen in the person who is angry, hostile, and threatening violence. If no alleviation of his behavior occurs after a psychotherapeutic interview, the emergency would appear to be more social and legal than medical and should probably be referred to the police or similar authority. However, if the interview reveals any bizarre thoughts or actions on the part of either the apathetic or the angry patient, a schizophrenic (reality distortional) break may be impending.

The *moderate reality distortional reaction* may be manifested by inappropriate apathy or anger, as well as by vague somatic symptoms, increasing withdrawal from occupational and social activities, eccentric or odd behavior or verbal expressions, feelings of outside control of thoughts or emotions, attributing special significance to irrelevant events, silly mannerisms and laughter, or excessive jealousy or suspiciousness. It is often very difficult to empathize with such a patient, that is, to "put yourself in his shoes." A person with such symptoms is frequently aware that something is very wrong and will accept hospitalization voluntarily, but in any event immediate psychiatric treatment is necessary.

The *moderate* (or even *severe*) *mentational reaction* is manifested by confusion, disorientation, memory defects, and anxiety, fear, or shallow or quickly changeable emotions. Such a patient may be frankly delirious and may hallucinate. (Remember that all patients who hallucinate are not necessarily schizophrenic.) The condition tends to be exaggerated at night. Technically termed the organic brain syndrome, this reaction is commonly associated with an organic disease process. The first step in treating the patient in such an acute delirious or confused state, then, is to ascertain the cause, which may be uremia, coronary thrombosis, fluid or electrolyte imbalance (especially after trauma or surgical operation), cerebral neoplasm, pneumonia, drug intoxication, or a variety of other disorders. Basic treatment in this condition must be directed to this underlying cause.

The patient should have continuous nursing attendance in a room with a night light (which decreases liability to hallucinations and helps the patient orient to his surroundings). Friends or relatives of the patient should be about. If fluid, salt, or vitamin balances are disturbed, they should be corrected. Drugs should be avoided until the cause of the reaction is known; then if there are no contraindications, thioridazine hydrochloride or chlorpromazine may be administered. If the patient is quite disturbed, hospitalization may be necessary. The patient should be prevented from harming himself, and the possibility of suicide should be kept in mind.

The *moderate somatic reaction* is usually manifested as psychologic blindness, deafness, loss of voice, or weakness or paralysis of one or more extremities. Multiple aches and pains or loss of touch sensation in an unusual distribution may be present. Such symptoms usually involve the sensory or voluntary motor system and may include a sudden collapse, convulsive-like seizures, or attacks of extreme pain. The patient is usually not agitated but rather presents a characteristic bland indifference.

A thorough physical examination to rule out organic disorder is a must, of course; but if the examination is negative, one is sometimes tempted to believe that the patient is malingering or "faking." Most of these patients, however, are completely unaware that no physical basis for their symptoms exists, and they are just as disabled as if they had a physical injury. Furthermore, the person who *is* malingering is emotionally ill in another way. Such patients, as well as those who present with the psychologically related symptoms of amnesia, should be referred for thorough psychiatric evaluation and treatment.

Severe reactions

The *severe reactions* are generally manifested by symptoms and signs that are similar to but exaggerated forms of those in the moderate reactions. These tend to involve either marked overactivity or marked underactivity. Such persons are more or less out of contact with or dissociated from reality. For all practical purposes they have lost much of their ability to communicate rationally with others.

The *severe affective reaction (elated type)* is manifested by extreme euphoria, excitement, and even manic delirium, which may closely resemble the *severe mentational reaction. Schizophrenic excitement,* on the other hand, usually involves random impulsive activity or continuous unorganized hyperactivity, as well as rage, uncontrolled and seemingly purposeless destructiveness, sometimes incontinence or smearing of excretory material, and often response to hallucinations ("listening to" or "answering" an unseen person). Speech, if present, is incoherent, bizarre, or wild.

The *dissociated reaction* ("panic" or "blind flight") is somewhat similar, manifested by purposeless, undirected, uncontrolled motor behavior that may lead to self-destruction. Such a person runs about wildly and may weep or laugh uncontrollably. A severe dissociated or panic reaction can result when a person with obsessive or phobic thoughts is forced into an untenable situation—for example, the mother who has obsessive thoughts about killing her child and is left alone with that child, or the patient who has a phobia about being in small rooms and is trapped in an elevator.

When dealing with the excited, panicky, hyperactive patient, it is worthwhile to at least try first a calm yet firm interview approach. If this fails or if you can't even get the attention of the patient to begin communication, tranquilizing drugs may be most helpful. If they are used, however, explain to the patient why you are using them, even if he doesn't seem to understand. Otherwise, on awakening in a strange hospital, the patient may suffer increased confusion, anger, or even a paranoid hatred for you.

Such a patient must, of course, be taken to the nearest psychiatric inpatient facility as quickly as possible. You will need two or three others to help get the patient there, even if he is sedated (for he may suddenly become violent). If only one or two persons attempt to transport such a person, even by force, the patient will probably break away and become even more disturbed. For the same reason, mechanical restraints (such as leather cuffs) should be used only in a dire emergency, for patients so restrained often become more excited or combative or develop extreme physical exhaustion and sometimes cardiovascular collapse. It is better to "crowd" the patient with three or four people. It should go without saying that, contrary to popular belief, slapping an emotionally disorganized patient or dousing him with cold water usually makes things worse and may indeed provoke extreme assaultiveness.

The *severe apathetic reaction* ("stupor") is manifested by marked retardation in thinking, speech, and motor activity. A patient suffering from this reaction may be, in fact, mute and immobile. He may appear completely withdrawn and may not react at all to external stimuli. He may be incontinent or dribble saliva. He may seem very depressed or without any apparent overt emotion at all. Sometimes such a patient can be led, like a small child. In *schizophrenic apathy,* the posture may be fixed, with muscle rigidity; the patient will sometimes demonstrate repetitious movements or mannerisms or will appear negativistic, and he may act as if he is responding to hallucinations. Often such patients do not eat and refuse food when it is offered to them.

The severe apathetic reaction may also be a variant of the "stun" reaction or may be related to organic etiology. In any case, prompt hospitalization is necessary. Precautions should be taken, for as such patients begin to recover from their apathy they may become suicidal; or, if the basic process is a schizophrenic one, the patient may suddenly switch to a state of homicidal excitement.

Finally, the *severe delusional reaction* is characterized by false and bizarre beliefs, most often relating to sinfulness, worthlessness, persecution by God or by a certain person or group (often by organizations such as the Federal Bureau of Investigation), and sometimes to gradiosity. Such distortions of reality always indicate severe psychiatric disorder and are best treated with immediate psychiatric hospitalization.

FINAL NOTE

Frequently a well-trained psychiatrist takes a calculated risk designed to benefit both the patient and society and, for example, follows as an outpatient someone who might conceivably be dangerous to himself or others. The psychiatrist takes this chance, however, on the basis of his special knowledge, knowledge of the probabilities and prognoses in similar cases, and knowledge of this particular patient based on intensive interviews, psychologic tests, social histories, and similar data.

The person who, without specialized training, attempts to take similar risks in dealing with psychiatric emergencies is providing only irresponsible disservice to the patient and to those around him. Thus the rule for the person who would render first aid in psychiatric emergencies should be: in case of doubt, get the patient to a psychiatrist or to a hospital. If possible, ascertain what psychiatric facilities are available in advance. Many general hospitals now provide psychiatric service. Even where such a service is not available, many psychiatrically disordered patients can be treated with brief psychotherapy and drugs, as well as with good nursing care, on the nonpsychiatric services of such a hospital. Finally, remember that the local or state police or sheriff may be called upon for assistance in an emergency; such officers are legally responsible for, and often equipped to deal with, the psychiatrically disturbed patient who may be dangerous to himself or others.

In psychiatric emergencies, however, the *attitude* of the person providing aid is likely to be the most important factor in the original contact with the patient and often makes the difference between success or failure in handling the situation. The basic features of this attitude include calmness, confidence, empathy, and the willingness to listen to the patient's problems. In these cases, perhaps the best medicine the "first-aider" has is himself.

chapter 31

Chemotherapy in psychiatric emergencies*

James M. A. Weiss

Because many new psychoactive drugs have been introduced in the past decade and because new pharmacologic agents are continuously being made available, it is a great temptation in dealing with psychiatric emergencies to use chemotherapy as *the* first aid, even before any attempt at competent evaluation has been made. There are, however, many reasons why drugs should be used only after as thorough an evaluation as possible has been obtained and after brief psychotherapy ("interviewing") has been attempted. The psychoactive drugs can be useful in alleviating undesirable symptoms and signs in certain patients, but they do not act against specific known etiologic agents. When given in sufficient doses to control a disordered patient, they may cloud his symptoms, making correct diagnosis difficult or impossible, may modify the disorder temporarily so that definitive treatment or disposition becomes more complicated, or may even be toxic in their effect.

The psychiatrically disordered patient is one who does not think clearly. However calming a sedative or tranquilizing drug may be, it will often add to his confusion and make him even more inaccessible to evaluation and treatment. It does seem that chemotherapy is simpler than other techniques when dealing with a wild, panicky, or severely agitated patient. But such a seriously disorganized person often requires very large and dangerous doses of even appropriate drugs. These drugs may, in fact, produce paradoxic responses, in which an agitated patient becomes even more excited or sometimes suicidal when given a drug that usually has a sedative or tranquilizing effect. Sometimes so-called antidepressant drugs will precipitate an excited, violent panic.

Frequently the psychoactive drugs will be prescribed in quite small doses, in which case they are especially liable to produce a paradoxic effect or to have little or no effect at all. In such a situation, one is tempted to try another and yet another drug and may end up giving the patient a series of drugs, all of inadequate dose but cumulatively dangerous. Even in small doses, the effects of these drugs cannot always be predicted. Except in special situations, it is therefore preferable to leave the chemotherapeutic approach in psychiatric emergencies to the qualified psychiatrist or to use such drugs only in the

---

*Dr. Widad E. Bazzoui, Associate Professor of Psychiatry at the University of Missouri, Columbia, Missouri, assisted in preparation of this chapter.

hospital situation. If you do administer drugs and then send the patient on to a psychiatrist or a hospital, be sure to indicate clearly what drug was given, what the dosage was, and when it was administered. Otherwise, the patient may be given additional amounts of that or a similar drug that could be most harmful in combination with the first dose.

Chloral hydrate, 0.5 to 2 gm, or *paraldehyde*, 3 to 15 ml in orange juice, is still used in the treatment of excitement, mania, delirium, and severe anxiety. These drugs often have the desired quieting effect on motor behavior but produce in addition an undesirable somnolence and lethargy and may have other side effects. Chloral hydrate must be given orally or rectally (in olive oil) and will not take effect as quickly as a drug that can be injected intravenously or intramuscularly. Chloral hydrate is also dangerous in patients with liver or kidney damage and should never be administered simultaneously with coumarin anticoagulants.

In mild or moderate agitation or anxiety, *phenobarbital* or some of the newer sedatives are sometimes used. Recent research involving extensive clinical studies with hypnotic, sedative, and minor tranquilizing drugs has indicated that in most cases the oral barbiturates and *gluthethimide* (Doriden), *methyprylon* (Noludar), *ethchlorvynol* (Placidyl), *methaqualone* (Quaalude), and *meprobamate* (Equanil, Miltown) all lack efficacy, or interfere with REM sleep, or tend to produce habituation or addiction, or have dangerous side effects or high toxicity. The benzodiazepine derivatives appear to be superior in almost all ways. Orally administered *chlordiazepoxide* (Librium), 25 mg, and *diazepam* (Valium), 10 mg, are useful minor tranquilizers, and *flurazepam* (Dalmane), 30 mg, is the hypnotic drug of choice. However, none of these drugs is really appropriate for emergency treatment; their administration is usually not necessary (psychotherapy is generally more effective) and their use can lead to the masking of important symptoms or may produce unwanted psychologic and physiologic side effects.

In more severe agitation, *thiopental* (Pentothal Sodium), 0.5 gm in 20 ml at the rate of 1 ml/minute until sleep occurs, or *amobarbital* (Amytal), 0.05 to 0.2 gm, possess short-acting sedative action and can be administered intravenously, but these drugs may depress respiration and vascular tone, may precipitate laryngospasm, may produce a paradoxic response, and may increase an underlying depressive affect in an agitated person. Such drugs are also dangerous in the presence of undetected liver, kidney, respiratory, or cardiovascular disorders.

In the emergency treatment of severely agitated states, however, the more potent tranquilizing drugs can be of great help. The route of administration of any psychoactive drug must depend on the patient's state. Oral administration is probably best if you or a relative can persuade the patient to take the medication. Many emotionally disturbed patients are frightened by an injection or regard it as some sort of an attack, but if necessary, the injectable form of these drugs can be used.

Therefore adequate doses by mouth of some major tranquilizer—specifically chlorpromazine (Thorazine), 100 mg repeated in 1 hour if necessary, trifluoperazine (Stelazine), 5 mg, haloperidol (Haldol), 5 mg, or thioridazine hydrochloride (Mellaril), 100 mg—are the most helpful in the severely agitated patient. If the patient is so disturbed that parenteral therapy is required, the same drugs (except Mellaril) may be administered intramuscularly, but the recommended oral dosage should be cut in half and should be repeated only after 2 hours for Thorazine and 4 hours for Stelazine and Haldol. (When using Thorazine, keep in mind the danger of a sudden drop in blood pressure.) In cases of delirium tremens, chlordiazepoxide (Librium) intramuscularly in doses up to 100 mg has been found very useful.

Of course, all the dosages recommended in this discussion are ranges or averages and must be varied in relation to the patient's size, general physical condition, and degree of behavioral disorder. It should be remembered that the tranquilizing drugs are neither specific nor curative, that their effects vary from patient to patient, and that their *continued* use should generally be under the direction of a psychiatrist, who is specifically trained to evaluate the indications for and the effects of these medicines.

A comparatively new group of drugs is the antidepressants (sometimes called "psychic energizers"). Currently, however, the action of these drugs is so variable, and undesirable side effects are so common, that they are *not* recommended for emergency use.

Other specialized somatic treatment (such as electroshock therapy) may also be very useful and even lifesaving in certain psychiatric emergencies, but such treatment almost always requires a physician with advanced specialized training in psychiatry for administration and in general should be administered in a psychiatric inpatient setting.

chapter 32

The suicidal patient

James M. A. Weiss

The suicide of a patient, because of its finality, is perhaps the most devastating experience that can occur when one is dealing with psychiatric emergencies. Furthermore, suicide is the prime cause of death among psychiatric patients. Whether or not any individual human being will commit suicide appears to depend upon the group attitudes in his particular society, the adverse environmental pressures that he must meet, and the interaction of these with the character and personality of that person.

The clinical problem is to determine which patients are actually suicidal. In evaluating suicidal danger one must remember that suicidal thoughts or ideas, considered in more than a passing manner, have been found in as many as half of so-called normal persons by some investigators. Some apparently suicidal persons make attempts that are simply suicidal gestures, because persons in this group do not intend to end life and are certain that they will *not* die as a result of their actions, although the action is performed in a manner that other persons might interpret as suicidal in purpose. Such attempts seem to be made in many or most cases to gain attention or to influence other persons, and the individual often takes considerable precaution to make sure of remaining alive by making the attempt with other persons present, informing someone of the attempt, or initiating his own rescue. Other persons who attempt suicide are quite sincere in their intention to end life, expect to die, and, indeed, are often successful in achieving their aim. Finally, there are many persons who attempt suicide in such a way that death *might* result from their action but, again, might not—their action, in fact, has the nature of a gamble with death.

One study indicates that suicidal attempts are most likely to be serious or successful if the individual is over 40 years of age, if he attributes his difficulty to "mental illness" or the fear of same, if he himself describes or admits his intent as serious, or if he appears to be clinically psychotic. Suicidal attempts are much less likely to be serious or successful if the individual is under 30 years old, if he attributes his difficulty to "family troubles," if he does not appear to be severely disturbed psychiatrically, and if his admitted intent is anything other than certain death. Serious or successful suicidal attempts are more likely to occur among older persons than among younger, among men rather than women, among whites rather than blacks, among persons isolated socially, among those who appear depressed, and among persons who have made prior suicidal attempts.

Such information only provides a guide to probabilities; the fact remains that any emotionally disturbed person who indicates suicidal intent should be evaluated by a

187

competent psychiatrist. Every depressive reaction carries with it some danger of suicide, and no suicidal talk should be considered lightly. Several studies have indicated that a large majority of persons who successfully commit suicide communicate their intent to someone prior to the act. A depressive reaction involving feelings of futility, loss of appetite or loss of weight, insomnia (especially early waking with inability to fall asleep again), or distortions of reality must be considered as particularly dangerous. The important thing is to gauge the intensity of the patient's distress, but remember that people who talk about suicide often *do* kill themselves.

If there is any suspicion at all of suicidal intent, one should not be afraid to question a patient about it. When the patient makes some mention of his distress, one might ask: "Do you feel so depressed (upset, disturbed) that life does not seem to be worth living?" If the patient answers "Yes," one should then ask, "Have you though about suicide (or about killing yourself)?" Such a procedure will *not* give the patient any ideas of suicide that he did not already have, and his response will often help you to determine his intent. If his response is bizarre or illogical or delusional, includes ideas of worthlessness, or indicates a preoccupation with thoughts of suicide and with actual concrete procedures for carrying out the act, one should consider that the danger of a serious or successful suicidal attempt is great. Remember also, however, that suicidal desire may hide behind the reassuring words of the patient apparently recovering from a severe depression.

If suicidal intent is suspected, immediate hospitalization of a patient on a psychiatric inpatient service is indicated. It is most important that such patients not be left alone, even to go to the bathroom. A careful vigilance must be maintained until the patient is transferred to definitive professional care and treatment.

part six

Immediate care germane to certain selected specialties

chapter 33

Effective early efforts in dental emergencies

Hugh E. Stephenson, Sr.

Of foremost importance in the consideration of dental emergencies is observation of the signal precaution that referral of the patient to the appropriate dental specialist should always be made in any case where the mode of treatment is in any way debatable. It is frequently of particular significance to make far deeper considerations than those involved in the immediate medical emergency. In cases of fracture of the jaw, for instance, mere setting of the bony separation itself is a relatively minor consideration as compared to others that will be pointed out.

The purpose of this section is to discuss several of the more common dental emergencies that may be encountered on a first-aid basis and to point out measures that may be used in the conservative handling of all except the most minor injuries until such time as expert dental aid may become available. Injuries to the mouth are quite often involved in the general problem of today's accident victim. Emergency care of these injuries may present a real challenge to most practitioners who are relatively unfamiliar with dental problems.

CHIPPED OR BROKEN TEETH

The problem of chipped or broken teeth is one of the most frequently encountered dental emergencies and is particularly prevalent in the upper central and lateral incisors of children with mesioversion. Immediate handling of the emergency depends upon the degree of involvement, particularly upon whether or not the pulp is involved.

Examination should be made immediately for visibility of the pulp cavity at the broken edge of the tooth. The presence of bleeding is indicative of pulp-cavity involvement; however, bleeding from injury to the gum is not to be confused with bleeding from the pulp. Gentle removal of blood with a pledget of cotton may serve to distinguish bleeding of the gum from that of the pulp. Once the field is cleared, the severely chipped tooth will show a distinct cavity containing the artery, the vein, and the nerve in a sheath from which the tooth is fully calcified and sealed off at between 8 and 10 years of age. If the pulp is not involved, the dentist will usually place a thin stainless steel crown on the immature tooth, which will, in any event, eventually be replaced by a permanent porcelain jacket.

191

Deciduous teeth, again the upper incisors in particular, may occasionally sustain a blow that will literally drive them up into the gum line. In administration of first aid, it is most important that this type of injury be carefully distinguished from that involving broken teeth. Again, identification of the pulp cavity at the broken edge will serve to identify a broken tooth.

In no case should any mechanical effort be made to bring such embedded teeth back into normal position. Such manipulation may easily injure the bud of the permanent tooth. Experience has shown that the embedded deciduous tooth will gradually make a spontaneous return to its original position within approximately a month's time.

MISSING TEETH

Upon administering first aid to a patient who has lost one or more teeth, the importance of their replacement should be made clear to him. Several points of dental hygiene dictate that any missing tooth should be replaced in some manner. Professional treatment should be urged for these reasons:

1. The remaining teeth will spread apart, leaving a space in which food will lodge, thereby causing a pyorrheatic condition.
2. Malocclusion of the opposing tooth will occur.
3. Constant attempts by the patient to force occlusion while chewing will occasionally result in the even more serious matter of a misshapen jaw.

The use of bridges must, of course, be avoided in cases of missing teeth in developing mouths. The use of a partial plate until the mouth has matured will preserve the alignment of adjoining teeth.

The accident victim, particularly if injuries are generalized, may tend to minimize the importance of losing a tooth unless the underlying dental principles are impressed upon him as they are discussed here.

BROKEN JAW

In examining an emergency patient for a broken jaw, it is wise to keep in mind the fact that the break will almost always be bilateral. This fact is particularly true as applied to the mandible, as will be self-evident if one considers the physical principles involved in the application of a traumatic force to any part of an arch whose ends are relatively fixed.

The physician should not attempt to set the broken jaw. A dental surgeon should see the patient so that most careful attention may be given to the matter of occlusion of the teeth. While apparently excellent setting of the fracture may be made in the physician's office—and occlusion may appear to be perfect—experience has shown that, upon healing, jaws have had to be broken again and reset to proper occlusion. In many of these cases, it is particularly difficult to properly evaluate relative anteroposterior occlusion, a problem that may well lead to the situation in which occlusion of only the back teeth is possible in the healed jaw. Severe attrition results, and only extensive dental surgery will salvage the back teeth.

Furthermore, use of currently available techniques by the dental surgeon may make the jaw almost immediately usable, thereby adding greatly to the comfort and general well-being of the patient while knitting is taking place. For instance, by making plaster cast models of the lower jaw, as broken, and by then cutting and setting the pieces of the model back to proper occlusion, an aluminum casting may be made for cementing onto the teeth as the bones are forced back into proper alignment. The aluminum casting acts not only as a splint but provides a chewing surface that may be utilized almost at once. Hooks at the ends of the casting hold tissue in place.

Gauze wrappings should be applied to hold the fractured jaw closed while the patient is being transported for treatment by the dental surgeon. The possibility of severe hemorrhage is rare. Fracture of the upper jaw is considerably more rare but requires much more complicated treatment.

TOOTHACHE

The toothache is a not uncommon minor emergency for which first-aid treatment is requested. If a nerve is exposed or protruding, eugenol (active principle: oil of cloves) may be applied with cotton and gauze. Care should be used in such application in order to minimize the possibility of "burns" to adjacent oral tissues.

In case of any marked looseness of a tooth, it should be suspected that the pulp may be destroyed; professional dental aid should then be sought. In cases where death of the pulp is suspected, the tooth is particularly susceptible to the application of heat in any form because of the simple physical principle of pressure from expanding gas volume.

Occasionally a patient may falsely describe the existence of pain in a tooth located adjacent to a maxillary sinus. Referred pain from a maxillary sinusitis is frequently elusive and may masquerade quite effectively as "toothache." So-called pain in an apparently sound tooth in this area should occasion radiologic visualization for darkness of the maxillary sinus and referral to an otorhinolaryngologist.

Referred pain is a frequent problem in the entire oral area because of the neurologic implications involved in the union of the superior and inferior maxillary nerves with the ophthalmic nerve at the gasserian ganglion.

FOREIGN BODIES OF DENTAL ORIGIN

In the general picture of emergency care and first aid, it is important that the mouth of the injured patient be inspected, not only because of the dental considerations pointed out above but because of the distinct possibility that a tooth, bridge, or plate—or a broken part thereof—may become a foreign body in the esophagus, trachea, or other part of the airway. Careful administration of first aid must include locating all the dental fragments.

A POINT OF MEDICODENTAL PHILOSOPHY

In urging that the accident victim be made aware of the extreme importance of seeking expert dental aid for any problems that may appear comparatively minor at the time, and in urging that the physician avoid all dental treatment except first aid, we are brought to the fundamental philosophy of this section. There is, today, a rapidly growing emphasis upon dental rehabilitation rather than upon mere immediate repair. Fortunately passing into oblivion is an age-old tendency to ignore dental problems because they won't kill the patient. The dentist no longer simply fills one cavity at a time because it is causing toothache; he finds the cause, taking the mouth as an entity and seeking a balance. He sees the importance of properly functioning teeth in the picture of total health. He knows, for example, that malocclusion—as from an improperly set jaw fracture—may cause a condyle to wear down to the extent that the eustachian tube may be occluded, causing a serious hearing impairment. The dentist is interested not just in maintenance for today but in looking toward a comfortable old age for the patient.

chapter 34

Emergency care and first aid in obstetrics and gynecology

Russell E. Hanlon

While the vast majority of births in the United States today occur in hospitals under medical supervision, occasionally an expectant mother is faced with impending delivery under suboptimal conditions, without the benefit of attendance by trained medical personnel. Hemorrhage either during pregnancy or in the first few hours following delivery may, on occasion, constitute a serious problem. Some infants do not initiate respiration spontaneously. In these cases, proper resuscitative techniques may prevent irreversible brain damage and may indeed be lifesaving.

With these thoughts in mind, this chapter stresses the basic principles of diagnosis and immediate management of obstetric and gynecologic difficulties under adverse conditions. In all cases, the best medical personnel and facilities available should be obtained as quickly as possible.

MANAGEMENT OF LABOR AND DELIVERY

When a patient in labor is encountered, the first question concerns the availability of trained medical personnel. Under most circumstances this simply means telephoning the physician and transporting the patient to the hospital where she has been previously scheduled for delivery. If the patient has received no prenatal care, a police officer can usually give directions to a hospital where care will be provided, and many times he will provide transportation. Moreover, in some areas, policemen have received training in emergency delivery. Unless delivery is imminent, as signified by signs of the second stage in a multipara or actual "crowning" (presentation of the head) in a primipara, it is probably best to transport the patient to a hospital if one is reasonably available. If this is not feasible, her physician, if she has one, or any physician if she does not, should be notified immediately. Any patient in advanced labor should be transported in a reclining position, either in an ambulance or, lacking this, the rear seat of an automobile. It is best for the patient to remove any underclothing that might obstruct delivery during the trip. Under no circumstances should any attempt be made, either mechanical or medical, to delay delivery.

On rare occasions, precipitate delivery may occur in public places or crowds. When this occurs, it is best to place the patient in a reclining position in an area where maximum privacy can be obtained with minimum dust contamination and maximum cleanliness. No attempt should be made to provide analgesia or anesthesia unless one is experienced in the management of labor. Pain relief is rarely essential to successful labor and, indeed, may prove harmful if unskillfully administered.

Occasionally in isolated areas or, potentially, under emergency conditions, it becomes obvious that birth will occur without the benefit of trained medical aid. Fortunately, the majority of labors and deliveries are completely normal, and a successful outcome can be anticipated even in the absence of trained personnel and modern facilities. This is particularly true if the attendant has some basic knowledge of care.

A calm, reassuring attendant is probably the best sedative possible even under ideal conditions, and when labor and delivery are to be conducted by a first-aider, this may be even more significant. Early in labor certain preparations should be made. The mother will need a clean, flat surface upon which to lie. The bed should be protected with waterproof sheeting. If this is lacking, six to eight layers of newspapers placed beneath the sheet will provide some protection. In addition, clean, folded sheets or mattress pads may be placed beneath the buttocks, since they can be changed intermittently when, as invariably happens, they become soiled with amniotic fluid, mucus, and fecal material.

Materials to be utilized during the actual delivery should be prepared. A knife, scissors, or other sharp instrument that has been thoroughly cleansed, along with two strips of fabric measuring approximately 10 inches in length, to be utilized as a cord ligature, should be boiled in water for 20 to 30 minutes. If ordinary kitchen forceps are available, they should be sterilized in the boiling water with a string attached to the handle to recover the forceps from the solution, after which they may be used to recover other articles from the water. The water and instruments contained therein should be allowed to cool before use. Although presterilized and packaged cord ties and clamps are available, they are unlikely luxuries in the emergency situation. Suitable substitutes may be found in gauze bandages 1 to 1½ inches in width, narrow strips of clean white cloth, or even shoe laces. Narrow caliber ties should be avoided since they will tend to cut into the soft, gelatinous cord.

A second large vessel of water containing several washcloths should be boiled for 20 to 30 minutes and allowed to cool for use in cleansing the perineum.

All attendants should scrub their hands and forearms thoroughly with soap and water, utilizing a rich lather and a liberal, thorough rinse, before handling the perineum or the infant. The fingernails of attendants should be thoroughly cleansed with a nail file, if available, prior to the initial scrub.

If the patient is not in advanced labor, a soapsuds enema is desirable to evacuate the lower bowel and to decrease the risk of fecal contamination during labor and delivery.

It is also desirable to shave the perineum if equipment and time permits. Good lighting, soap, water previously sterilized by boiling, as well as a clean sterile safety razor, are essential items. After the attendant has thoroughly scrubbed his hands, a sterile cotton pledget, gauze sponge, or sterile cloth is placed in the introitus to prevent contaminated substances from entering it. It is essential during this and other cleansing procedures of the vulva that nothing enter the vaginal orifice, including the hand of the attendant. A rich lather is made in the hairy area of the vulva with soap and water. The area is then carefully shaved, working from above downward, then outward to the inner thighs, leaving the area surrounding the anus until last.

After the shaving procedure, the pledget in the vaginal introitus is removed and replaced with a fresh one. The entire vulva and inner thighs are cleansed with soap and water, again working from above downward and from the introitus outward to the inner thighs.

It is advisable that the patient receive no solid foods during her labor, but she should be offered water, tea, or soft drinks in small amounts at intervals. She should be encouraged to empty her bladder frequently during labor; however, she should not use the toilet after the vulva bulge (in a primigravida) or signs of the second stage (in a multipara) have been reached. During the first stage, ambulation is permissible. Signs of the second stage are suggested by strong contractions, 2 to 3 minutes apart, accompanied by a bearing-down sensation as though having a bowel movement, increased bloody show, and bulging of the perineum. At this time, preparations for delivery are made.

The patient should try to avoid bearing down as much as possible. She should assume a supine position in bed. The attendant should again thoroughly scrub his hands with soap and water for 10 minutes, if time permits, and put on sterile rubber gloves, if available. The perineum should again be cleansed as previously described and a clean pad should be placed beneath the buttocks. Once the head is crowning (95% of infants are born head first), the hand should be placed against the presenting head during contractions to prevent sudden expulsion, which may result in severe lacerations. No other assistance is necessary and, indeed, the attendant should let the infant be born by itself. Under no circumstances should the attendant's hand enter the vagina, nor should any attempt be made to pull the infant from the vagina. Birth need not occur in a hurry.

Usually, after the head is delivered, the shoulders will follow with the next contraction, usually occurring within 1 to 2 minutes. If, after the head is delivered, the membranes cover the head, the sac should be torn with the fingers to allow the amniotic fluid to escape and to permit the infant to breathe. A check should be made to be certain that the umbilical cord is not wrapped around the infant's neck. The cord, if wrapped tightly around the neck, may impede the progress of delivery, result in airway obstruction to the infant after the head has emerged but before completion of the delivery, or result in fetal blood loss as a result of tearing of the umbilical cord. If the cord is found around the neck, a gentle attempt should be made to slip the loop over the fetal head. If this fails, then one should attempt to slip the cord back over the shoulders and await the completion of the delivery. After the shoulders are delivered, the remainder of the body will slip from the vagina without difficulty. The sole manipulation by the attendant should be to support the infant as it emerges from the introitus. The attendant should avoid touching the rectum of the mother during delivery.

After the head has emerged, milking the trachea with a gentle stroking motion of the fingers from the base of the neck to the chin will aid in clearing the trachea of secretions.

The newborn infant is slippery and difficult to hold. As the shoulders emerge, by placing the right hand *behind* the neck of the infant with the thumb and index finger around the sides of the neck, the attendant is able to achieve control of the baby without a tight and possibly injurious grip. The body, as it emerges, should be supported with the left hand in order to avoid contact with the bed, which should be regarded as contaminated.

INITIAL CARE OF THE NEWBORN INFANT

After the baby is born, he should be held head down. This is best accomplished by holding him up by his ankles, utilizing a firm grip with the index finger inserted between the ankles, and supporting the shoulders with the other hand. The infant should be held just above the bed or other soft, flat, clean surface in order to avoid injury if he is inadvertently dropped.

The baby should not be spanked, although sometimes gently rubbing the infant's back or slapping the soles of the feet may aid in stimulating respirations. Tension should always be avoided on the cord while it is still attached to the placenta within the uterus. When the infant begins to cry, he should be placed on the bed near the mother, with a clean blanket or sheet beneath him. The nose and pharynx may then be gently suctioned with a small rubber bulb ear syringe, if available, to clean the respiratory passages of mucus and debris.

Infant resuscitation

A newborn infant will normally cry and breathe within 1 minute of birth. While it is normally pink in color after respirations are well established (except possibly the hands and feet), an infant who does not breathe will become cyanotic (dusky bluish in color), or, if anoxia has been present or continues long enough, the infant will be pale and limp. If respirations have not been established within 3 minutes, particularly if cyanosis is progressing, resuscitative measures should be instituted.

The most available and efficient method is mouth-to-nose resuscitation. The infant should be placed on its back with the head extended. This may be facilitated by placing a folded sheet or blanket beneath the shoulders. The airway should be cleared as much as possible by gentle rubber bulb suction. The mouth of the attendant should then be placed to the nose or nose and mouth of the infant and the attendant should then inhale and partially exhale into the external nares of the infant. In general, the mouth-to-nose technique is more satisfactory in newborn infants than the usual mouth-to-mouth technique utilized in adults. If only the nose is included within the lips of the attendant, the mouth should be firmly closed by finger compression to prevent escape of air. It is quite possible to severely damage the infant's lungs by this method, but this risk can be minimized by using a "puffing" technique, utilizing the cheek musculature of the attendant rather than forcibly exhaling. The effect can be gauged by placing a hand on the chest of the infant and observing chest expansion. A short puff about every 5 seconds is sufficient. This effort should be continued until spontaneous respirations are established or until efforts are obviously futile as signified by absence of a palpable or audible heartbeat, absence of corneal reflexes, and complete lack of muscle tone. It is advisable, however, to attempt resuscitation for 5 to 10 minutes in the absence of these signs, since occasionally an infant may be revived who appears lost.

Delivery of the placenta

Following the delivery of the infant, uterine contractions will usually cease for several minutes as the uterus accommodates to its markedly diminished intercavitary volume. The placenta normally separates from its implantation site as a result of decreased area of the site. Soon rhythmic uterine contractions resume and the placenta is expelled. This usually occurs within 20 minutes but may occupy over an hour. Bleeding may be anticipated, and an increase in bleeding as well as a rise in the height of the uterine fundus above the pubic symphysis and advance of the cord from the introitus are signs of placental separation. When any of these signs appear it is well to gently massage the uterine fundus suprapubically to aid in contraction. If bleeding seems excessive, putting the infant to the breast will reflexly stimulate uterine contractions. *Under no circumstances should traction be put on the cord* in an effort to deliver the placenta.

Following completion of the third stage, ergonovine, 0.2 mg, or an oxytocic drug (for example, Pitocin or Syntocinon), 10 units, may be administered intramuscularly to aid in contraction of the uterus, thereby minimizing blood loss. Ergonovine may also be administered intravenously in the same dosage. Following delivery, the perineum should be inspected for tears or lacerations; if they are present with bleeding, pressure should be applied with a sterile gauze pad or sterile cloth for 20 to 30 minutes. This will usually control the bleeding. If bleeding does not occur, no further emergency treatment is necessary, although surgical repair is desirable if facilities are available.

Tying the cord

Attention should now be directed to the umbilical cord, which is still attached to the placenta that has recently delivered. There is no need to rush this procedure; time should be taken, if needed, to ensure sterility of the cutting instrument and cord ties. Contamination during this procedure may be an important source of infection to the newborn infant. The cord should be tied firmly and carefully, about 2 inches from the umbilicus, using a square knot. A second ligature should then be placed approximately ½ inch distal to the first. The cord is cut on the placental side of the two ties, approximately ½ inch from the second tie, with the previously sterilized sharp instrument. Special care should be taken in tying the knots to avoid tension on the cord at its entrance to the umbilicus. The cord is easily torn loose at this point, resulting in blood loss by the infant. If sterile ties and instruments are not available or if medical attention can be anticipated in a relatively short time, it is best to wrap the placenta with the infant, as fetal blood will not flow back through the placenta after delivery. No special treatment of the cord stump is necessary and, indeed, no medication of any kind should be applied to the stump.

SIGNS AND SYMPTOMS OF LABOR

The onset of true labor may be preceded by a "bloody show" occurring within 24 to 48 hours of the onset of labor. Frequently the "show" is not seen until labor is established. This consists of a small amount of thick blood-streaked mucus and is the result of expulsion of the plug of mucus occluding the cervix during pregnancy.

In some patients, labor is preceded by rupture of the membranes (amnion and chorion), signified by a gush of clear fluid (amniotic fluid) from the vagina. The amniotic fluid may be recognized by its characteristic musty odor and colorless, sometimes slightly turbid appearance, which differentiates it from urine, which sometimes escapes from the bladder involuntarily in late pregnancy. Rupture of the membranes most commonly occurs in advanced labor but occasionally occurs as much as 24 hours prior to the onset of labor in the term patient. Rarely, rupture may occur days or even weeks prior to the onset of labor.

ECTOPIC PREGNANCY

An ectopic pregnancy is a pregnancy outside the uterine cavity. The vast majority of such cases are located within the fallopian tubes, the wall of which eventually becomes weakened by invasion of developing placental tissue with subsequent rupture of the tube.

This is usually accompanied by the intraperitoneal bleeding, leading to blood-loss shock. The signs and symptoms include:

1. Amenorrhea of less than 12 weeks' duration
2. Vaginal bleeding, usually small in amount
3. Sudden, sharp, unilateral lower abdominal pain followed by progressively more generalized lower abdominal pain
4. Signs of blood-loss shock

This is a serious surgical emergency. The treatment is that of blood-loss shock with transportation to hospital facilities as rapidly as possible.

ABRUPTIO PLACENTA

One of the most serious complications of pregnancy is abruptio placenta, which is defined as separation of the placenta from its site of implantation in the last 20 weeks of pregnancy. The prognosis for both the fetus and the mother will vary with the degree of separation. Only a small portion of the placenta may be involved or, indeed, the entire placenta. This complication sometimes occurs in conjunction with toxemia of pregnancy, but it commonly has no detectable etiology. It is rarely associated with abdominal trauma. Separation of the placenta leaves the vessels at its base open and bleeding. Since the uterus is still distended by the fetus, that organ is unable to contract and retract to effect hemostasis. As the clot behind the placenta enlarges, the placenta tends to become further separated. Blood may dissect beneath the membranes and present through the cervix into the vagina, or it may actually infiltrate the myometrium and other pelvic structures, or both may occur.

The signs and symptoms of this disorder include:

1. Lower abdominal pain
2. Vaginal bleeding, usually dark red
3. A tender, rigid, sometimes board-like uterus
4. Shock out of proportion to blood loss

Further complications may include loss of the ability of blood to clot, failure of the uterus to contract after delivery (uterine atony) with postpartum hemorrhage, and, rarely, renal failure in the postpartum period.

The keystone of emergency management is recognition of the condition, vigorous shock therapy, and immediate medical aid.

The keynote of the modern practice of obstetrics, as well as first aid management in all areas, is expressed in the dictum "primum non nocere" (first, do no harm). In the vast majority of obstetric situations a minimum of aid is necessary for the health of both mother and infant.

GYNECOLOGIC EMERGENCIES

There are a few gynecologic conditions in which emergency management may be considered crucial.

Trauma

Both the internal and external female genitalia are well protected by their anatomic location against all but the most severe trauma. Occasionally, however, lacerations of the external genitalia may occur, accompanied by heavy bleeding. This may usually be controlled by simple pressure applied at the site of bleeding until more definitive medical care can be obtained.

In the past, attempts have been made to treat nearly all types of bleeding from the internal genitalia with the use of a tight pack of gauze or cloth introduced into the vagina. In most cases this is not only futile but dangerous. There are basically two situations when this procedure may be justified. The first of these is in patients with carcinoma of the uterine cervix, who develops massive, life-threatening vaginal bleeding. Occasionally, serious bleeding may result from vaginal lacerations caused by rape or sexual perversion. A pack should be used only if bleeding is life-threatening and if more definitive therapy is not available. The preferred packing material is sterile, 2-inch gauze. A tight pack inserted under direct vision with good lighting may result in control of hemorrhage under the circumstances described. The pack, however, should be removed as soon as more definitive therapy is available.

chapter 35

Ear, nose, and throat emergencies

James M. Landeen

HEMORRHAGE

Lacerations

Severe lacerations to the face, oral cavity, or neck may injure sizable arteries or veins and may cause exsanguination. A 7-year-old girl stepped from a car with soft drink bottles in her arms, headed for a grocery store. She fell on the curb, breaking the bottles. In resuscitation attempts at the hospital, the last of her intravascular fluid was pumped out a laceration of the left common carotid artery by closed cardiac massage. If pressure had been applied immediately to her neck, it may have saved her life.

Oral cavity lacerations may cause bleeding so severe that only bulky packing with gauze may apply the necessary tamponade. This packing may, however, cause airway obstruction. One must be prepared to place a nasal pharyngeal airway or provide an airway through a cricothyrotomy or tracheostomy.

Unnecessary damage to nerves and intact blood vessels occurs by wildly stabbing into facial lacerations with hemostats, trying to stop bleeding. One should use pressure first, then controlled ligation. Large veins that have been opened in the head and neck lacerations may be a source of an air embolus. Pressure over these areas can help prevent embolization and blood loss. Primary suture may be delayed for hours as long as the wound is cleansed and kept moist with saline compresses.

Laceration of the ear is dangerous because of the possibilities of perichondritis, stenosis of the external ear canal, and tissue loss. If the injured party brings a portion of his ear along with him, it should not be thrown away. Later, if it cannot be primarily sutured in placed, it can be buried in surrounding tissue to keep it alive for future reconstruction. Hematomas of the external ear associated with lacerations and trauma need sterile drainage. This may be done with a needle or small surgical incision that does not cut into the cartilage. A hematoma here, as well as a septal hematoma of the nose, may elevate the perichondrium away from the cartilage, thus robbing the cartilage of its nourishment and leading to necrosis and structural collapse. Blood in the the external ear canal is best left alone. Its source may be an ear canal laceration or the middle ear. Placement of a sterile cotton pad in the concha of the external ear is all that is necessary.

Epistaxis

One of the problems of being a rhinologist is that one acquires the title "nosebleed doctor." The nosebleed problem is created by blood flowing from a "hole," nonvisualization of this "hole," the blood being spewed onto you as it traverses the lips, an excited patient and family, and a disagreeable hour of the night.

Children will bleed spontaneously from the nose. They will also have epistaxis from blood dyscrasias or trauma. Generally this is easily managed since it is anterior in nature: external pressure by pinching the nares together, cold compresses to the bridge, or light intranasal packing of Vaseline gauze or Gelfoam. Severe nosebleeds in young males demand an investigation to rule out a juvenile angiofibroma, a benign but extremely vascular tumor. Control of severe epistaxis is difficult because the measures used in the usual hemorrhage control such as tamponade, suturing, cauterizing, and direct visualization are not easily applied. The adult patient may be diabetic or hypertensive, but one must not forget that multiple myelomas may initially present as a nosebleed.

Besides anterior packing, posterior packs may be necessary. Posterior packing may seem mystical because of the strings and catheters, but more mystical is how the patient can stand it when these packs are placed by an inexperienced physician. It can resemble a medieval torture routine to an observer. The key here is sedation and topical anesthetization. The classic posterior pack is made up of gauze or preferably lamb's wool, which has strings attached to it. Small No. 8 red rubber catheters are placed into the oropharynx via the nose and retrieved through the mouth. One set of strings is attached to the catheters, which are again pulled out the nose, placing the pack securely into the posterior aspect of the nose. These strings are then carefully tied over the columella so as not to cause necrosis. The other set of strings is brought out the mouth, with no tension on the soft palate, and taped to the cheek. Therefore, one string holds the pack, the other retrieves it at the time of removal. When posterior packs are placed, anterior packing is also necessary. Vaseline gauze, ½ inch wide, is carefully layered in. Another means of packing the nose is by inflating a 30-ml Foley catheter balloon while it is in the nasopharynx and pulling it anteriorly until snug. Stevens' nasal balloons are contoured for the turbinates, both left and right, and inflated for pressure. A word of caution here: The pressure from inflation may be so severe as to cause necrosis and subsequent stenosis in the period following removal. Cases have been reported in which inability to control epistaxis by means of nasal packing has necessitated the bilateral ligation of the external carotid arteries in the neck. Though not an emergency room procedure, transmaxillary sinus antrum ligation of the internal maxillary artery has replaced the external carotid artery ligation. The arterial ligation of the internal carotid supply is performed by a curvilinear incision above the medial canthal ligament of the eye, giving access to the anterior and posterior ethmoid arteries.

Postoperative bleeding

Postoperative head and neck cancer patients occasionally develop flap necrosis with carotid artery exposure. This exposure to drying combined with preoperative irradiation makes this artery subject to spontaneous rupture. Large head and neck services ask the family to stay with these patients while the artery is vulnerable. This constant observation for a rupture provides someone who can apply finger pressure while calling for help. The ligation of the artery can take place later in the operating room.

Postoperative tonsillectomy or adenoidectomy patients who are bleeding need to be returned to the operating room immediately. A primary role here is recognition of this potential catastrophe, since more than one child has been found the next morning dead in his bed with a gastrointestinal tract full of blood after swallowing it all night.

The exasperating patient is the one who is bleeding from a dental extraction at 1 AM. Having the patient apply pressure by biting a sterile gauze pad or Gelfoam packing is usually all that is necessary to stop the bleeding.

HEAT AND COLD
Frostbite

Frostbite occurs in the nose, ears, and extremities. Our concern here is with the first two. Some controversy exists concerning the warming rate and temperature at which it should be accomplished. It is more important that the nose and ears not be traumatized. Brisk rubbing and excessive manipulation are mentioned only to condemn them. Frostbite is the effect of the cold on the blood vessels. Vasoconstriction is followed by hyperemia and edema caused by permeability of the capillaries. Regional capillaries filled with clumped red cells cause ischemia, so the prevention of intravascular clotting will be the key factor in determining the final tissue loss. Infected gangrenous tissue should be surgically excised.

Burns

Burns of the head and neck necessitate special attention to the cartilage areas. Burn therapy is a specialty all of its own—the one thing again is do not traumatize! In ingested chemical burns of the deglutition tract, try to identify the agent, start neutralizing fluids, and be sure to inspect the oral cavity. A pleasant surprise is to look into the mouth of a child who is suspected of having drunk lye only to see normal mucosa. Later on this patient, if indeed burned, will need complete endoscopy to determine the condition of the pharynx, esophagus, and larynx.

TRAUMA
Barotrauma

Otitic barotrauma occurs with sudden changes in atmospheric pressure. These pressure changes are not equalized in the middle ear cleft because of eustachian tube malfunction, causing severe otalgia. This is most commonly produced on descent in aircraft or by skin diving. Relief can be gained by pushing air into the eustachian tube by catheterization, Valsalva maneuver, or politzerization. If these are all unsuccessful, a paracentesis of the drum head under strictly sterile technique is necessary. Barotrauma of the sinuses gives acute pain. Cannulation of the sinus ostia is avoided. One should give antihistamines, analgesics, and a nasal spray to shrink the edema around the ostia.

Cosmetic trauma

Medicolegal problems associated with cosmetic surgery are commonplace. If a recent postoperative rhinoplasty patient sustains trauma to his nose, be extremely conservative in your treatment. Notify the surgeon who operated and let him handle the case. By all means do not attempt to shift the nose back where you think it belongs.

Maxillofacial trauma

Patients with severe maxillofacial trauma also sustain cervical spine injuries in a high percentage of cases. Do not overlook this fact in immediate care and transport. Hemorrhage can be controlled with pressure and packings. The mandible and the maxilla can be temporarily immobilized with a Barton's head dressing. This dressing relieves pain and prevents sharp fragments from lacerating vessels. The airway is in danger from the tongue, dislodged teeth, broken dentures, blood, mucus, and associated laryngeal fractures. Laryngeal fractures are diagnosed by the presence of subcutaneous emphysema in the neck, ecchymosis over the anterior neck, and loss of prominence of the thyroid cartilage (the Adam's apple). Definitive care of these wounds may take place hours to weeks later. Intermaxillary fixation is readily accomplished with a healthy set of teeth. If the patient is edentulous, his dentures are used in place of his natural teeth for intermaxillary fixation. If the dentures are broken they can easily be repaired and utilized. A search at the scene of the accident will prove its worth later. When teeth are missing they must be accounted for. If they cannot be found either outside or inside the mouth, x-rays of the abdomen and chest are necessary.

The most common maxillofacial fracture is of the nose. Don't underestimate this fracture. A simple push to realign and a pack for epistaxsis are not enough. Too many people end up unhappy with their crooked noses because time and effort were not made to properly align the fractured nasal bones and nasal septum. Emergency care is usually concerned with the epistaxis, which has already been discussed.

An interesting problem is the dislocated mandible. The condyle of the mandible has slipped out of the glenoid fossa anteriorly. The patient may have yawned widely, screamed as in childbirth, or attempted to get his mouth around too much food. Wrap your thumbs with something to protect against a bite, grasp the mandible bilaterally, and manually apply pressure with the thumbs over the molar teeth, pushing downward and posteriorly. If the patient can shut his mouth you have been successful in relocating the mandible. A patient with chronic dislocation needs the jaw wrapped shut and a preventive medicine lecture given.

Skull trauma

Temporal bone fractures can produce sensorineural hearing loss, vestibular loss, and cerebrospinal fluid otorrhea. Conductive hearing loss is caused by (1) hemotympanum, (2) laceration of the tympanic membrane, or (3) disruption of the ossicular chain. *Do not* apply suction to the external ear canal, wipe it out with Q-Tips, or instill any antibiotic drops or ointment. Place a sterile gauze or cotton ball dressing in the concha of the external ear. Bed rest, sedation, antibiotics, and antivertiginous medications can be started systemically. One of the most important observations and accurate recordings is the fast component of the nystagmus, when present.

INFECTION
Ear

Otitis externa pain is produced by elevation of the pinna. It is distinguished from temporomandibular joint pain, which is anterior to the tragus of the ear. The pain of the mastoiditis is posterior to the auricle over the mastoid portion of the temporal bone. Topical application of antibiotic drops with steroid and placement of a gauze wick in the canal to keep the medication against the canal wall will give relief. Systemic antibiotics and analgesics are sometimes necessary. Once the edema begins to subside, healing is well on its way.

Acute otitis media may rupture the tympanic membrane by fluid pressure in the middle ear. If rupture appears imminent, a myringotomy is performed to relieve the pressure. A poorly visualized, moving tympanic membrane of an irritable child may prove disastrous if a myringotomy is attempted. A dislocated stapes, which allows the infectious material of the middle ear to enter the perilymph, may produce a dead ear, a dead labyrinth, and meningitis. Sedate the child, wrap him securely in sheets, and perform the incision in the posterior inferior quadrant of the tympanic membrane.

Acute mastoiditis is still with us. Some clinicians mistakenly think mastoid problems departed with the entry of antibiotics. The ear is characteristically pushed out and down away from the head. Do not drain it. Refer this patient to an otologist for surgical drainage by a simple mastoidectomy. Chronic drainage from the ears is not a surgical emergency. It should be referred to an otologist.

Nose

The furuncle of the nose is potentially dangerous, since it may communicate via venous channels to cause a cavernous sinus thrombosis. Do not underestimate this "pimple." Treat with systemic antibiotics and moist heat and drain only when "ripe."

Pharynx

Peritonsillar abscesses demand incision and drainage. The diagnosis consists of trismus, drooling, pain, voice change, and shift of the soft palate. Local infiltration by lidocaine (Xylocaine) is ineffective in pain control. Adults under sedation can be drained in a sitting position by placing a hemostat in the proper place and spreading. In this position and awake, the adult can handle the gush of pus and slight bleeding. Children need to be taken to the operating room and placed under general anesthesia. The need for a tonsillectomy in approximately 4 weeks is emphasized.

An enlarged epiglottis can cause airway obstruction, necessitating a tracheostomy. The epiglottis can reach an amazing size when infected. The "hot potato" voice characterizes this problem.

If diphtheria is clinically evident, positive for the bacterial agent on Gram stain, a tracheostomy is indicated. Diphtheria is like mastoiditis—it is still around.

FOREIGN BODIES
Pharynx

Friday night fish fries are notorious for creating the midnight rendezvous to remove a fish bone. Start your search at the inferior pole of the tonsil, base of the tongue, then the piriform sinus of the hypopharynx. In my experience less than 10% of these patients have a bone recovered. The most common physical finding is a small area of erythema and edema where the bone may have been lodged at one time. If the initial examination with a mirror is negative, inform the patient that a direct view with a laryngoscope and esophagoscope will be necessary in the operating room.

Nose

Foul, unilateral nasal discharge in children represents a foreign body until proved otherwise. The objects are rocks, toys, coins, vegetable matter, flowers, and what have you. If the time interval since placement is short, the objects generally remove easily by anterior grasping with a nasal forceps. Do not dislodge the foreign body posteriorly where the child can aspirate the object. Sedate the excited, uncooperative child or schedule general anesthesia for safe removal. It is always a good idea to inspect the ears of these patients. They are fond of all their orifices but play favorites. It is amazing how a child can become a chronic offender even with disagreeable experiences at removal.

Ear

Ear canal foreign bodies can be insects, vegetable matter, toy parts, paper, and beads. Do not attempt removal with suction, curettage, or forceps if the child is fighting. If sedation is unsuccessful, schedule general anesthesia. A tympanic membrane rupture, ossicular chain injury, or otitis media is a high price to pay for carelessness. Be sure the tympanic membrane is intact before an irrigation is attempted to remove insects and the like. A large insect will need ether to kill it before removal. A small insect will wash out with water.

Esophagus

The conventioneer who consumes too much alcohol and steak may lodge a large bolus of meat in the cricopharyngeus, cardiac junction, or midportion of the esophagus where the aorta crosses. Visualization will require esophagoscopy in the operating room. Do not give meat tenderizers, since this may cause esophageal rupture leading to mediastinitis and a possible fatality. Swallowed coins may lodge at the cricopharyngeus only to pass into the stomach with relaxation under general anesthesia.

chapter 36

Immediate care of illness and injury of the genitourinary system

Gilbert J. Ross, Jr.

Most of the acute illnesses and injuries involving the genitourinary system are associated with one or more relatively repetitive features that include severe colicky pain, hematuria, chills and fever, acute urinary retention, abdominal mass, and certain obvious disturbances of the external genitalia.

Basic principles must be constantly kept in mind, particularly the importance of a searching history and careful examination of the urine. Special cognizance needs to be taken of the location and distribution of pain in this area, since it is often as ambiguous as it is severe. The nature of any bleeding, general state of prior health, and the use of various drugs must be critically evaluated.

ACUTE URINARY RETENTION

Acute urinary retention is most commonly seen in conjunction with prostatic obstruction. It is particularly prone to occur in men with incipent prostatism following various surgical procedures or following the use of medication with anticholinergic properties. Other factors that may precipitate acute retention are other forms of urethral obstruction, neurologic disturbances, and bleeding with clot retention. The objectives are clear: to relieve the distension by catheterization without injuring the delicate tissue of the urethra.

In general it is advisable to initiate catheterization in the male with the installation of an antimicrobial ointment into the urethra. A well-lubricated 18 Fr catheter should then be gently passed using firm pressure at the membranous urethral area if required to overcome spasm. If the catheter cannnot be passed and the obstruction appears to lie at the level of the prostatic urethra, an abundant quantity of sterile lubricant should be instilled and an 18 to 20 Fr coude-tipped catheter employed using counterpressure in the rectum, if there is difficulty in negotiating the curve of the bulbous urethra.

In the event that the catheter interrupts in the urethra below the level of the prostate, there is a very real possibility of a urethral stricure. If small (12 to 14 Fr) coude-tipped rubber catheters do not pass through the area easily, the stricture will have to be dilated

208

with filiform and follower catheters. This is a highly specialized procedure, which, although less hazardous than the passage of metal sounds, may easily damage the urethra and should never be attempted by the uninitiated.

In small male infants even the tiniest of the rubber catheters may be too large, but tiny polyethylene feeding tubes in the range of 5 Fr make admirable urethral catheters for short-term use.

BLEEDING FROM THE LOWER URINARY TRACT

Bleeding from the prostatic urethra in the male or from the female urethra characteristically occurs at the beginning and end of voiding, while bleeding arising from the bladder or upper urinary tract always occurs throughout urination. This localization is most important in dictating the nature of subsequent investigation and management.

Bleeding from the prostatic urethra or bladder is often severe enough to require blood replacement and to produce acute urinary retention because of clots accumulating in the bladder. As a general rule, if the bladder can be evacuated and kept decompressed, virtually all prostatic bleeding will stop spontaneously and hemorrhage from the bladder is often, though not invariably, improved or arrested. This is contingent on the nature of the bladder abnormality initiating the hematuria. In any case, as long as clots remain in the bladder, bleeding will usually persist. The major objective in treatment is to render the bladder clot-free.

Catheterization should be performed with a relatively large catheter (22 to 24 Fr), the internal diameter of which is adequate to allow clot evacuation, which is accomplished by copious irrigation with sterile saline. At times in may be advisable to chill the irrigant in an effort to expedite hemostasis.

Not infrequently the decompression of a chronically distended bladder results in profuse bleeding as well as certain undesirable septic sequelae, but again, if the bladder is decompressed, the bleeding will usually stop.

RENAL COLIC

The patient with acute renal or urethral colic building on a background of acute obstruction is frequently in such severe pain that immediate symptomatic measures are often required, provided that certain criteria are met: red cells in the urine, relative assurance that the problem is not that of an acute surgical abdomen, and some confidence that one is not dealing with an attempt to acquire narcotics.

Narcotics in relatively large dosage are needed for adequate analgesia, and there are no admonitions concerning which of these agents may be the most effective or which should be avoided. None of the common narcotics can be clearly shown to have an adverse effect on the smooth muscle of the genitourinary system, and the drug of choice is the one with which the physician is most familiar.

While the use of antispasmodics is subject to some dispute, it is our impression that they are a valuable adjunct in the management of urethral colic. Such anticholingergic agents as propantheline bromide in an initial adult dose of 30 to 45 mg intravenously or intramuscularly may prove to be of distinct value.

It is imperative to obtain an excretory urogram at the time of the pain in the event that the difficulty is caused by an acute and intermittent hydronephrosis, which will return spontaneously to normal following the episode of pain.

SEPSIS

Infection in the urinary tract encompasses a wide range in the severity of the infection episode. The most disastrous complication of urinary infection is gram-negative rod septicemia with septic shock. Perhaps the least hazardous is the localized bladder infection commonly seen in young women.

The usual circumstances that prevail prior to the development of septicemia are the combination of a gram-negative rod urinary tract infection with iatrogenic trauma or obstruction with stasis and residual urine. Clinical circumstances are most frequently traumatic catheterization; lower urinary tract instrumentation in the presence of infected residual urine; upper conduit system obstruction with entrapment of infected urine; and, occasionally, a neglected perinephric, scrotal, or prostatic abscess.

The clinical history is often quite clear. When such a patient is seen with actual or impending shock apparently unrelated to myocardial disease or blood loss, immediate affirmative action should be taken while diagnostic studies are underway.

The bladder should be catheterized to monitor the urine output and to assure that any question concerning residual urine is dispelled. Blood and urine cultures should be obtained concomitantly with the introduction of a venous catheter for monitoring central venous pressure (CVP). My preference is for the use of a long catheter introduced through the basilic vein rather than the subclavian route. If the CVP is low, the extracellular space should be volume-expanded while antibiotic therapy is initiated. In the absence of any prior bacteriologic studies, the choice of antibiotics will necessarily have to be arbitrary.

Because of the necessity for broad antimicrobial coverage, a combination of gentamicin and cephalothin is a reasonable point of departure, taking cognizance of the necessity for dosage modifications in the event of depression in renal function. The use of vasoactive drugs and steroids can be momentarily deferred while response to the initial treatment is evaluated and additional studies are undertaken to categorically rule out the possibility of upper urinary tract obstruction if this is not already abundantly clear.

Even in the absence of a septicemia, the patient with acute bacterial prostatitis, an acute pyelonephritis, or a scrotal or perinephric abscess may be gravely ill. In addition to the usual antibacterial therapy, supportive management often requires parenteral fluids and the use of a cooling blanket. A known or suspected abscess must be dealt with promptly. Categorical assurance that there is no obstruction with incarceration of infected urine along the course of the urinary conduit system must be obtained or if such a situation does exist it must be promptly rectified.

TRAUMA

Most renal injuries can initially be managed conservatively with strict bed rest and blood replacement as deemed necessary. There is relatively little more that can be done in terms of immediate care other than the acquisition of proper urographic studies. The decision to intervene surgically in renal injuries is usually clinical, and it is imperative to obtain a meticulous baseline assessment of the size of any flank mass. This will assure that the repeated physical examination critical to the management of renal trauma can be meaningfully evaluated.

Bladder and urethral injuries with extravasation are true surgical emergencies. The initial management should involve a high index of suspicion following pelvic trauma, treatment of hemorrhagic shock, and examination of the urine (if any is forthcoming) for blood. Catheterization is the preliminary step in obtaining a cystogram to evaluate the nature of the injury.

Frequently, a catheter cannot be passed because of partial or total disruption of the deep bulbous urethra. Occasionally, a catheter passes into the area of the bladder but no urine is obtained because the prostatic urethra has been avulsed from the membranous urethral area and the catheter tip is lying free in the retroperitoneal space. In either instance, a retrograde urethrogram should be obtained to identify the site and nature of the injury.

Contrast media used for cystography and urethrography must always be suitable for intravenous use since there may be rapid absorption from an extravasation into the bloodstream.

EXAMINATION OF THE ACUTELY ILL PATIENT

An order of priorities must be established with attention given first to the most urgent aspects demanded by the clinical situation. Following such fundamentals as assuring patency of the airway and initiating any other resuscitative procedures that may be required, the acutely ill or injured patient should be systematically examined. The scope of the examination should not be unduly conditioned by information obtained through the medical history.

While the stabbing pain of renal or ureteral colic produced by acute obstruction is most clearly perceived over the renal or abdominal area, lower ureteral obstruction may be quite confusing since such pain typically radiates into the scrotum or labia due to overlapping innervation with the genitofemoral nerve arising from L1 to L2. In contrast, acute obstruction of the intramural ureter tends to produce bladder symptoms with straining to void, as well as frequency. Testicular pain is equally ambivalent since, although it is classically visceral with localization in the lower abdomen, there is concomitant local involvement often radiating into the groin.

RECTAL EXAMINATION

Rectal examination in the male is imperative, not only to establish the status of the prostate and lower rectum but also to allow bimanual examination of the bladder, to assess anal sphincter tone, and to evaluate the effect of suspected pelvic trauma on the genitourinary system.

Following pelvic fractures, there is an understandably high incidence of injury to the lower urinary tract. Rectal examination may be most valuable in localizing any bone fragments and in aiding the assessment of a possible injury to the bladder or prostatic urethra. In the event of a shearing injury of the prostate, only a soft, poorly defined mass will be palpated in the area of the prostate, since the urethra has been divided at the triangular ligament and the bladder and prostate have been displaced superiorly.

Only the most infrequent and gentle prostatic examination should be employed in the presence of suspected acute bacterial prostatitis or a prostatic abscess, since it is possible that forceful palpation will instigate a bacteremia or septicemia.

SCROTAL MASS

Despite the accessibility of the area to examination, an acutely painful scrotal mass may present a difficult diagnostic problem. Epididymitis, torsion of the testis, incarceration of an inguinal hernia, torsion of the appendix testis, and testicular tumor are among the most common conditions that must be considered. Helpful diagnostic maneuvers include auscultation for bowel sounds, transillumination if there appears to be an element of free or loculated fluid, and of course palpation. Occasionally, aspiration of hydrocele fluid may facilitate subsequent palpation.

The most pressing problem in diagnosis is to distinguish clearly among torsion of the testis, incarceration of a scrotal hernia, and epididymitis, in view of the radically different treatment employed. Torsion and the incarcerated hernia require prompt operation if a viable testis is to be salvaged or a bowel resection to be avoided. In contrast, the management of epididymitis is essentially medical.

Torsion should be suspected when the testis is noted to be abnormally high in the scrotum, while epididymitis usually shows selective involvement of the epididymis early in the course of the disease. Unfortunately, in both instances a delay in diagnosis (and treatment) may result in a large, tender, confluent mass without any distinguishing features. Less specific ancillary factors must often be relied upon and include the precipitous onset often associated with torsion, the relative rarity of epididymitis in prepubertal children, and the frequent association of lower tract infection with epididymitis. An incarcerated hernia can usually be recognized by hearing bowel sounds over the mass. If there is some dispute concerning whether bowel sounds are present, an x-ray should show bowel gas within the scrotum.

The therapy employed for epididymitis consists of rest, scrotal support, icebags to the scrotum, and antibacterial therapy. If there is a posterior urethritis associated with infected urine, urologic evaluation should be performed after the infection has been asymptomatic for some weeks.

EXTERNAL GENITALIA

Trauma to the external genitalia or urethra may be associated with a variety of findings including obvious loss of penile or scrotal skin, blood at the meatus, hematuria, or evidence of extravasation of urine or blood into soft tissues. Power takeoff injuries are particularly prone to denude the penis and not infrequently they will totally avulse the scrotum.

Damage to the bulbous urethra may produce a rupture with blood and extravasted urine following well-defined tissue planes. The same physical findings occur when extravasation develops in conjunction with a urethral stricture and periurethral abscess or urethral carcinoma. If the blood and extravasated urine are confined by Buck's fascia, the extravasation will present as a swollen indurated penis. If Buck's fascia is not intact, the extravasation will also fill the scrotum and the superficial perineal pouch and extend up the lower abdomen deep to Scarpa's fascia. Tissue reaction and necrosis may be extensive if drainage of the extravasation has been delayed.

Some seemingly minor disorders of the penis may also be responsible for acute and potentially serious difficulty. For example, meatal stenosis or phimosis may be so severe that it produces acute or, more insidiously, chronic urinary retention. Insect bites are quite common in children and should be suspected in the event of sudden, rather painless penile swelling.

Paraphimosis, the fixation of a retracted prepuce, may produce severe swelling and pain. In certain instances the strangulating preputial ring may be sufficient to compromise the blood supply of the glans. Paraphimosis can usually be manually reduced by exerting steady pressure on the glans penis with the thumb and first two fingers of one hand while attempting to slide the prepuce over the corona with the opposite hand. If attempts at manual reduction fail, emergency dorsal slit can be performed by incising the constricting ring after infiltration with local anesthesia.

Phimosis rarely produces acute symptoms unless there is an associated balanitis, in which instance the acute pain and swelling may make it necessary to perform an emergency dorsal slit or circumcision. More commonly, the reaction will subside with the application of warm soaks and systemic antibiotics. A subsequent elective circumcision can then be performed.

chapter 37

Immediate care of common emergencies in infants and children

Gerard J. Van Leeuwen

Most parents and many physicians regard all acute illnesses in children as being emergencies. It is impractical to attempt to present all of these occurrences in a brief chapter. The management of pediatric emergencies is documented adequately in standard pediatric textbooks. This presentation is designed to help one recognize and partially manage some of the more frequently encountered emergencies, with special emphasis on those that are least likely to be discussed in other areas.

FEVER

What is fever? The exact mechanism of the febrile reaction is not clearly understood. An individual, especially the small infant, who has a subnormal body temperature is a greater cause for alarm than is the febrile patient. This indicates that a moderate degree of fever is not detrimental but suggests resistance on the part of the afflicted individual.

Hyperpyrexia, or a rectal temperature of greater than 104° F, has more serious implications. Persistent fever of this degree may be either a result of or a lead to dehydration, and it may result in a "febrile" convulsion and possible brain damage.

There are many approaches to the therapy of pyrexia, when such therapy is deemed advisable. It must be remembered that even though salicylate (aspirin) is primarily considered an antipyretic in children, it is also an effective analgesic. There is little physiologic reason for prescribing aspirin for fever when the hyperpyretic stage has not been reached, but all clinicians and parents will vouch for its efficacy in making the child more comfortable, and aspirin is the most widely used antipyretic. The maximum total amount of aspirin that can be tolerated safely in a 24-hour period is 2.0 grains/kg of body weight. A safe and usually adequate antipyretic dose is 1 grain per year of age, given every 4 hours. Thus a 5-year-old child may be given 5 grains of aspirin every 4 hours as an antipyretic. Liquid medications containing salicylates are commercially available and easily administered. It is my clinical impression, however, that they are less effective than tablet forms and that they are more easily used to excess. Aspirin can be given to even the

214

smallest infant by crushing the tablet between spoons and adding any desired kind of liquid vehicle.

Overdosage of salicylate may result in, among other things, renal damage. Salicylates should therefore be avoided in any condition in which improper or decreased renal function may be present, especially in newborn and premature infants, the vomiting patient, and the dehydrated patient.

Bathing the child for 15 to 30 minutes in lukewarm water may be effective as a substitutive or adjunctive measure. Properly executed alcohol sponging is very effective in reducing fever. The naked child should lie on a towel and an alcohol-soaked towel should be placed on his body for a few seconds. The towel should be removed and the skin allowed to dry before the child is turned over and the process repeated for as long as deemed necessary. Cold water enemas are cruel, generally ineffective, and potentially dangerous.

UNCONSCIOUSNESS

Perhaps it is appropriate to list a broad etiologic classification of the conditions that might render a pediatric patient unconscious. Primary intracranial disorders include convulsive disorders, infections, tumors, vascular conditions, and trauma. Systemic conditions affecting the central nervous system are metabolic disorders such as diabetes mellitus, hemorrhagic and cardiovascular conditions, infections, and intoxication. The discussion here will be limited to the emergency management of a convulsion and a discussion of intoxication caused by the ingestion of poisonous material.

All major seizures are recognized and managed, at least acutely, in essentially an identical manner, irrespective of whether the etiology is fever, poison, or unknown. The seizure is usually preceded by some sort of warning or aura, of which many older children are aware and can describe as peculiar visual disturbances, auditory hallucinations, or simply a sort of "premonition." The seizure then begins with spasm of the larynx followed quickly by generalized muscle tonicity and subsequent clonic movements. There usually follows fecal or urinary incontinence and, finally, sleep.

Once a convulsion has started, it can in no way be halted. If the seizure is prolonged beyond the usual 3 to 5 minutes, termination may be assisted by giving valium, 0.5 mg every 2 or 3 minutes, directly into a smoothly running intravenous tube. Because the process cannot be abruptly halted, management is aimed at prevention of bodily injury, particularly holding the patient so that he does not fall or bump his head. The time-honored method of inserting something between the teeth serves no purpose once the seizure has begun and may possibly harm the patient and the operator. The postseizure sleep state is often misinterpreted as coma. Distinguishing between the two requires an experienced clinician.

If the seizure does not respond to valium or other drug therapy and is prolonged beyond 20 to 30 minutes, the diagnosis of status epilepticus is made. Then additional management may include special attention to prolonged anoxia, dehydration, and aspiration pneumonia. Adequate oxygenation and administration of intravenous fluids will usually be necessary, and antibiotics may be required to combat pneumonia.

In this prolonged state of seizure, drug therapy is of utmost importance. We advocate the use of valium titrate, 0.5 mg every 2 to 3 minutes, as outlined above. The patient must be observed very closely for respiratory depression during this therapy.

POISONING

Despite complete coverage of poisoning in Chapter 28, certain pediatric aspects of the subject will be treated briefly here.

Children who have ingested hydrocarbons or corrosive agents should not be induced to vomit because of two factors: the danger of aspiration and the reexposure of the epithelial surfaces to corrosive action. For other poisons, and again contrary to common practice, spontaneous or induced vomiting is a much more effective procedure in emptying the stomach than is gastric lavage.

Drugs may be used to induce vomiting. Syrup of ipecac has stood the test of time, although the results are not consistently predictable. A dose of 15 cc given orally is usually followed by vomiting in 15 to 20 minutes. Extreme caution must be exercised to avoid the use of other forms of ipecac, since this agent may in itself be damaging to the central nervous system. More recently, intramuscular apomorphine, 0.06 mg/kg of body weight, has been advocated. The results very predictably result in violent vomiting a few minutes after injection.

Should lavage be required, the following points should be kept in mind. A large-caliber rubber tube should be passed into the stomach, usually through the nose of a pediatric patient. Water is always a safe lavaging agent, although if the specific neutralizing agent is known and available, it should be used. The patient's head should always be kept down in order to prevent aspiration. At the conclusion of the procedure, a neutralizing agent or a cathartic such as mineral oil may be instilled. The universal antidote—which contains activated charcoal, tannic acid, and magnesium oxide—may be used if specific agents are not available.

Accidental overdosage of aspirin is probably the most common poisoning in pediatric patients. As stated earlier, the maximum amount that can be tolerated in a 24-hour period is about 2 grains/kg of body weight; therefore, 1 grain/kg can usually be tolerated in one ingestion. Fortunately, most instances of aspirin poisoning are relatively mild and consequently require very little therapy. If an excessive amount has been ingested, the stomach should be emptied promptly. Alkalinizing fluids should be given, because an alkaline urine facilitates the excretion of salicylate. In mild situations carbonated beverages or baking soda may be given orally. In more severe instances, bicarbonate must be given intravenously. Intramuscular vitamin K is usually given to prevent hypoprothrombinemia. Very severe cases may require exchange transfusion or dialysis.

The major hydrocarbons accidentally ingested by children today are power mower gasoline and cigarette lighter fluid. Their ingestion in even small amounts is often followed by a chemical pneumonitis, while central nervous system depression may follow ingestion of large amounts. Emptying the stomach is crucial only when apparently more than 4 ounces was taken. Vomiting should be avoided because of the likelihood that aspiration may increase the severity of the pneumonitis. The patient must be observed very closely for pneumonitis and most often should have a chest x-ray a few hours after ingestion.

RESPIRATORY OBSTRUCTION

Although respiratory obstruction may occur with many infections, it may be complete or nearly complete in two particular situations: severe epiglottitis and foreign body aspiration.

In epiglottitis, if the obstruction is nearly complete, a tracheostomy must be done. In the absence of a skilled operator, insertion of several 13- to 15-gauge needles into the trachea may be lifesaving. Insertion is made into the trachea above the suprasternal notch, posteriorly in a caudad direction.

Children may aspirate any type of foreign body. Under 15 months of age, the object is usually a safety pin; over 15 months it is usually a vegetable particle, especially a peanut. Less than 2% of these objects are ejected spontaneously; this may occur immediately after aspiration. If the object is visible in the larynx or throat, one may try to retrieve it while the patient is placed in an *inverted* position in order to lessen the likelihood that the object may enter the lower respiratory tract.

Objects that pass the larynx will usually pass the trachea and will enter a bronchus. Such movement of the particle decreases the urgency but also makes diagnosis more difficult. Inspiration and expiration films and fluoroscopy are usually diagnostic. Diagnostic and removal bronchoscopy should be performed early.

ALLERGIC ASTHMA

The only promptly effective method of therapy for an *acute* asthmatic attack is prevention. This of course is not possible with the first attack. By the same token, anxiety generated in parents who observe their child's acute respiratory embarrassment, coughing, and wheezing makes them especially cooperative in attempting to prevent further attacks.

The recognition of an acute asthmatic attack is aided by knowing that the patient has a positive allergic history, especially a family history, and by noting that in the absence of obvious infection he suddenly begins to wheeze. Attacks are often precipitated by fatigue, apprehension, or (obviously) exposure to allergens. In many patients the attack is preceded by a type of aura that the parents and the patient quickly learn to recognize from such symptoms as sneezing, slight coughing, or throat clearing.

Once an attack seems imminent or the warning signs have appeared, the patient is put to bed in a room that is as free as possible of common allergens such as house dust, feathers, wool, or animals. The room should also be free of odors such as paint and tobacco smoke. The child is then given three medications on a 4-hour basis: nose drops or spray, an antihistamine cough preparation, and a specific bronchodilator. Every physician develops his favorite set of drugs; mine vary from time to time. When Tedral is used as a bronchodilator, parents must be warned about the potentiating effect of ephedrine and theophylline, which occasionally results in agitation and central nervous system stimulation of the patient.

If these procedures do not abort or modify the attack, the physician should be contacted. Epinephrine may then be given by injection. Some parents can be taught to administer epinephrine when indicated, but they often overdose the patient. Isoproterenol is the most acceptable inhalator. This is most effectively done with a nebulizing apparatus.

If the patient does not respond after epinephrine, he is said to be in status asthmaticus and he must then be hospitalized. As in all situations involving pulmonary disorders, asthmatic or otherwise, the importance of adequate hydration cannot be overemphasized. Water may be given orally if possible, otherwise intravenously. Other nonspecific measures include administration of oxygen, steam, iodides, and usually antibiotics.

Specific therapy usually consists of corticosteroids and aminophylline. It is rarely necessary, and usually not advisable, to prescribe corticosteroids in asthma of childhood except in status asthmaticus.

MENINGITIS

A patient with meningitis always produces anxiety, not only in his immediate family but in the school and community as well. The method of transmission from one individual to another is not clearly understood. With our present knowledge it seems advisable to prophylactically treat all persons who have been in contact with cases of meningitis caused by *Neisseria meningitides*. Such therapy should consist of rifampin, 10-20 mg/kg of body weight per day, one dose for 7 days.

In the infant the symptoms of meningitis appear quite different than those seen in the older child or adult. Not observed in the infant is the picture of high fever, headache, and stiff neck commonly seen in the patient who has reached a degree of neurologic maturity (closure of fontanels and sutures). With deceptive frequency, the infant may be hypothermic rather than febrile. Classic signs include bulging of the fontanel and projectile vomiting (manifested by headache in the adult and caused by increased intracranial pressure). Both of these findings may be very difficult to assess by an untrained person.

Anyone even remotely suspected of having meningitis should immediately seek expert attention. No illness of a medical nature is a greater emergency than meningitis. When the physician is able to identify the organism, specific antimicrobial agents are prescribed. In the absence of specific diagnosis, "therapy of unknown" is directed toward treating simultaneously all of the usually incriminated organisms. This consists of ampicillin, 300-400 mg/kg of body weight per day, in divided doses every 4 hours until the culture reports are available.

VOMITING AND DIARRHEA

Infants and small children are very prone to develop gastroenteritis, and they dehydrate very easily. Vomiting is especially common with any febrile illness and is, in fact, often the first symptom of such illness. Both vomiting and diarrhea are often caused by acute viral enteritis, and occasionally by food poisoning.

An adequate history will often reveal the cause of vomiting or diarrhea. A very ill child with bloody and mucoid stools usually has a bacterial enteritis. A child who has eaten spoiled food is rarely the only one who partook. If primary bacterial enteritis or that secondary to food poisoning can be excluded, the situation is generally less alarming.

Many individuals have an erroneous concept of what constitutes vomiting and diarrhea. The simple regurgitation or "spitting" so common in small infants is usually of little clinical significance and must not be confused with vomiting. Diarrhea is not related primarily to the number of stools in a period of time. Of greater importance is the character of the stools, particularly as to the amount of liquid present, since loss of water and electrolytes produces the dehydration. Often a mother changes the diaper several times during a single bowel movement and erroneously reports this as diarrhea.

When excessive loss of water and electrolytes from the body leads to severe dehydration, equilibrium must be reestablished by giving intravenous fluids. The majority of children, however, can be successfully treated with oral solutions. Ordinary carbonated beverages, fruit juices, and tea are satisfactory and safe.

How can dehydration be recognized? Several physical findings appear, related more to the patient's age than to the degree of dehydration. Failure to tear with crying, dry mucous membranes, decreased or absent urinary output, depressed fontanel, and dry skin with loss of turgor all indicate dehydration.

Vomiting can often be controlled by a short (1- to 2-hour) period of complete abstinence followed by small frequent sips of clear liquids such as tea, water, or 7-Up. Bland solid foods may be given after 8 hours (banana, cereal, toast and the like), followed by dilute, boiled skimmed milk after 24 hours. Diarrhea also will usually respond to these procedures. There is very little benefit from the use of kaolin, pectin, or opium medications for their intestinal coating action, and they may cause recurrence of vomiting. Very few children fail to respond to this regimen. If they do fail, medical attention should be sought promptly.

A large number of pediatric emergencies have been omitted from this discussion, partially because they are discussed elsewhere in this volume (cardiovascular and metabolic emergencies and care of the premature infant), and partially because they are types of emergencies not often encountered.

part seven

Preventive measures

chapter 38

Preventive aspects of tetanus

Wesley Furste

Tetanus or lockjaw is a severe and dreaded infectious complication of wounds and is caused by the toxin-producing *Clostridium tetani.* This disease is characterized by tonic spasms of the voluntary muscles and by a tendency toward episodes of respiratory arrest. Over the entire world it has a mortality rate of about 50%.

Tetanus has been recognized as a terrifying disease for 2,300 years. Hippocrates referred as follows to the master of a large ship who smashed the index finger of his right hand with the anchor: "Seven days later a somewhat foul discharge appeared; then trouble with his tongue . . . on the third day opisthotonos occurred with sweating . . . 6 days later he died." In the second century, Aretaeus, the Cappadocian, called the disease an inhuman calamity, an unseemly sight, a spectacle painful even to the beholder. He wrote: "The wish of the physician that the patient should expire, otherwise irreverent and objectionable, is, in this case well taken."

Tetanus continues to occur as a complication of lacerations, open fractures, burns, abrasions, hypodermic injections, operations on the gastrointestinal tract, and birth (infection of the umbilical stump in the newborn).

The introduction of tetanus toxoid about three decades ago, which was followed in many parts of the world by programs of immunization of the population, contributed greatly to the control of tetanus. Nevertheless, during the decade 1951-1960, tetanus remained an unsolved problem in many areas of the world. A 1966 report showed on the basis of the available literature and World Health Organization statistics that tetanus was causing more than 50,000 deaths each year all over the world. Indeed, this figure should be regarded as an underestimate, since it only partially reflected the actual situation.

Relatively few cases of tetanus occur in the Unites States. In fact, in 1971, only 120 cases were reported for the entire United States.

PROPHYLAXIS

The four bases upon which the pyramid of tetanus prophylaxis for the wounded is founded are: (1) tetanus toxoid, (2) surgical care, (3) antitoxin, and (4) emergency medical identification devices.

While every injury presents its own problems to the physician called on to treat it, active immunization with tetanus toxoid—as far as the risk of tetanus is concerned—has almost oversimplified tetanus prophylaxis in the majority of injured persons in that a small booster dose is usually given to those previously immunized and is most efficacious in preventing tetanus.

Sometimes a major problem, however, is the fact that neither the patient nor his

223

physician can be completely certain of prior protection by toxoid unless the patient carries an emergency medical identification device indicating protection or sensitivity to toxoid.

In association with the ever-increasing use of tetanus toxoid and the steadily declining incidence of tetanus, there has possibly developed a decreasing awareness by physicians that tetanus can occur. The possibility of tetanus should at least be thought of in the individual with unexplained irritability or convulsions.

That tetanus can be prevented is amply documented. The incidence of tetanus in a group of wounded Manila civilians without tetanus toxoid immunization during World War II was 900,000% greater than in wounded United States Army personnel with such immunization (Table 38-1).

Wound prevention

For tetanus to occur, *C. tetani* must gain entrance to the body by a wound, even though the wound may be so small that it is not recognized, and tetanus toxin, which is actually responsible for tetanus, must be produced. If wound prevention programs were completely efficacious everywhere, tetanus would not occur.

Individualization of wounded patients

Wounded patients are individuals. Some may not have had all the indicated tetanus toxoid injections, others may have had too many toxoid injections, and a small number may be hypersensitive to tetanus toxoid. A few may have insignificant wounds, others may have almost lethal wounds. Many may not have with them an up-to-date emergency medical identification device with significant tetanus toxoid injection information. Hence individualization of each patient for tetanus prophylaxis must be considered.

Toxoid

Prophylactic measures rendered at the time of injury to nonactively immunized persons cannot be guaranteed to offer protection, but, with prior active immunization, a booster dose at the time of injury offers effective and prolonged protection. In the previously immunized person, a very small booster dose of toxoid will produce antibody levels in 3 weeks, which can be interpreted as equivalent to a 1,000 to 100,000 unit dose of heterologous or homologous passive antibody. In addition, it has been demonstrated in animal studies with toxin that an active booster response appears earlier than can be estimated by blood antitoxin levels. To give greater protection against severe, slight, and unrecognized wounds, to maintain this protection, and to avoid the extra care and cost entailed in active-passive immunization, every practicing physician, regardless of his specialty, should make every effort to actively immunize with tetanus toxoid—and to keep actively immunized—his patients, their families, his family, and himself.

United States Army experiences with tetanus toxoid. During World War II the almost 100% efficiency and safety of tetanus toxoid as a prophylactic agent were proved by the experience of the United States Army. Only twelve cases of tetanus occurred in a series of 2,734,819 hospital admissions for wounds and injuries. The mortality in these twelve cases was 41.7%. As to immunization status, only four of these twelve patients had had both an initial immunization of fluid toxoid and a booster dose (Table 38-2).

Duration of effect of tetanus toxoid. The human body does not "forget" a dose of

Table 38-1 Incidence of tetanus in the United States Army

	Admissions for wounds and injuries	Cases of tetanus	Cases per 100,000 wounds and injuries
Civil War	280,040	505	18.03
World War I	523,158	70	13.4
1920-1941*	580,283	14	2.4
World War II	2,734,819	12	0.44
Korean War		6-8	
1956-November 1971 (including Vietnam conflict)		0	

*Inclusive.

Table 38-2 Tetanus toxoid immunization status of twelve cases of tetanus in 2,734,819 United States Army hospital admissions during World War II

	Fatal cases	Total cases
No active immunization	2	6
Initial immunization (three injections of fluid toxoid) accomplished but no emergency stimulating injection given	1	2
Initial immunization plus emergency stimulating injection given	2	4
Total	5	12

tetanus toxoid. The first injection sensitizes or triggers the body so that it responds to the second and reinforcing or booster doses of tetanus toxoid by producing circulation serum tetanus antitoxin and probably other protective mechanisms. As yet, there has not been determined a maximum period of time after which there is not an anamnestic response; antitoxin titers are frequently being determined for World War II veterans to determine whether or not there is such an interval.

A number of investigators have already shown an unexpectedly high incidence of long-lasting immunity; in their studies, 85% to 95% of individuals immunized against tetanus during World War II still carried protective antibody levels 15 to 21 years later. Furthermore, with practically no exceptions, these individuals responded well to a booster dose of toxoid.

No antitoxin if adequate tetanus toxoid immunization. It should be noted that in the United States armed forces in World War II protection against tetanus by booster toxoid after wounding was achieved without the simultaneous use of antitoxin when there was adequate prior tetanus toxoid immunization. Credit is given to the United States military forces consultants who recommended that antitoxin was not necessary with adequate toxoid prophylaxis.

Reactions to tetanus toxoid. Significant reactions to tetanus toxoid continue to be rare but are occurring more frequently (Table 38-3).

From 1951 until 1970 more than 2.5 million injections of adsorbed tetanus toxoid had

Table 38-3 Reactions of a male to tetanus toxoid with repeated doses

Date of age	Type of toxoid given	Reason	Reaction
1949; 2	DTP	Initial series	—
1949; 2	DTP	Initial series	—
1951; 4	Adsorbed T	Injury	—
1952; 5	DTP	Booster	—
1953; 6	Adsorbed T	Injury	—
1955; 8	Adsorbed T	Injury	Redness and induration greater than anticipated
1963; 16	Adsorbed T	Injury	Redness and induration of half of upper arm
1964; 17	Adsorbed T	Injury	Redness and induration from elbow to shoulder; "almost double in size"

September 1965: serum tetanus antitoxin titer: 3 units/ml. The protective level is 0.01 units/ml.

been given in Denmark with no reports of death and only a single case of neurologic complications with sequelae.

Because some individuals may be sensitive or become sensitive to tetanus toxoid, one main principle of active tetanus immunization must be to balance the dosage and administration of toxoid against the side reactions so as to obtain optimal protection with a minimal risk of complications.

Basic immunization; frequency of periodic nonwound tetanus toxoid boosters and of wound boosters. Since tetanus toxoid is a most effective antigen that may produce undesirable reactions, recommendations continue to be made for less frequent use and for smaller dosage of tetanus toxoid.

For *primary immunization* of children 2 months through 6 years, the manufacturer's recommended dose of diphtheria and tetanus toxoids and pertussis vaccine (DTP) is given intramuscularly on four occasions, three doses at 4- to 6-week intervals with a fourth dose approximately 1 year after the third injection. Ideally, immunization should begin at 2 to 3 months of age or at the time of a 6-week checkup if that is an established routine. For schoolchildren and adults, a series of three doses of tetanus and diphtheria toxoids, adult type (Td), are given intramuscularly, with the second dose 4 to 6 weeks after the first and the third dose 6 months to 1 year after the second.

For *routine nonwound booster doses* for children 3 through 6 years (preferably at time of school entrance, kindergarten or elementary school), one injection of the recommended dose of DTP is administered intramuscularly. Thereafter and for all other persons, the recommended dose of Td (adult) is given intramuscularly every 10 years. If a dose is administered sooner as part of wound management (see specific recommendations below), the next booster is not needed for another 10 years. More frequent booster doses are not indicated and may be associated with increased incidence and severity of reactions.

If an individual is wounded, the possibility of administration of a wound tetanus toxoid booster must be considered. Certain general principles that should be observed are given on p. 228 and then specific recommendations are made. This conservative guide to prophylaxis against tetanus in wound management has been developed in an endeavor to simultaneously eliminate unnecessary reactions to tetanus toxoid and absolutely prevent tetanus in the injured individual. A basic aspect of this guide is that for those with adequate prior active immunization, for the great majority of wounds no booster dose of tetanus toxoid is needed unless more than 5 years has elapsed since the last tetanus toxoid injection. For severe, neglected, or old (more than 24 hours) wounds no booster dose is necessary unless more than 1 year has elapsed since the last booster dose. Such a conservative attitude is based on these concepts:

1. In general, surgeons see a more severe and a more unusual wound than the nonsurgical physician. The long intervals between wound boosters are for the "usual types" of wounds.

2. Tetanus may occur in individuals who have no demonstrable wound or who have very minor wounds; hence, all individuals should have adequate serum tetanus antitoxin titers at all times.

3. Physicians want none of their patients—whether they have special problems or not—to develop tetanus.

4. The United States Army and Navy statistics are impressive: no cases of tetanus have been reported among active duty Army personnel from 1956 to November 1971 and among active duty Navy and Marine Corps personnel from 1946 to April 1972 (Table 38-4). In contrast to such statistics there were reported 120 civilian cases of tetanus in 1971 in the United States.

5. Patients do not have an immediately available emergency medical identification device with reliable tetanus data on it. In a survey of patients and their friends during parts of 1970, 1971, and 1972, only 22 of 428 (5.1%) had such data immediately available (Table 38-5). The recommendations of the U. S. Public Health Service are based on immediately available and accurate records with tetanus data.

6. For the particularly severe or contaminated, so-called tetanus-prone or unusual injuries, it has been stated that there is a need for additional booster doses.

Table 38-4 Voluntary versus controlled tetanus prophylaxis

Category of cases	Number of cases
United States civilians: 1971	120
United States Army personnel: 1956–November 1971	0
United States Navy and Marine Corps personnel: 1946–April 1972	0

Table 38-5 Survey of use of emergency medical identification device (EMID)

Category	July–August 1970	July 1, 1971 to Jan. 14, 1972	Total
Number of individuals	121	307	428
Number with EMID	7	15	22
Percent with EMID	5.8%	4.9%	5.1%

7. In general, reactions to tetanus toxoid are minimal, in contrast to the grim picture of a person with tetanus and to the average mortality rate of about 50%.

8. The drugstore cost of a booster dose of tetanus toxoid is small compared to the hospital cost of a case of tetanus ($9,773.80 for a recent case).

9. There are still a number of individuals who do not have adequate tetanus toxoid immunization but who may erroneously be considered to have such immunization when they are seen as wounded patients. In 1970 it was stated that one third of a random group of children of all ages in Hamburg, Germany, did not have tetanus toxoid immunization. More recently, the lagging immunity of our children in the United States has been emphasized.

10. Cases of failure of booster tetanus toxoid injections to prevent tetanus many years after injections or cases of modified tetanus after such injections have been reported.

11. The professional liability responsibilities of the surgeon are greater than those of the nonsurgeon physician.

12. Surgeons—in respect to the prevention of tetanus—do not want to be like the poet, Ovid, who wrote: "Too late I grasp my shield after my wounds."

Rapid, active, basic immunization at the time of injury. Rapid active immunization, that is, three to five doses of tetanus toxoid approximately every other day, will not produce active immunity rapidly enough to protect an individual in whom such immunization is started just after a wound has been inflicted.

Prophylaxis against tetanus by the first injection of toxoid given at the time of injury. The initial injection of toxoid at the time of an injury does not provide immunity for tetanus from the injury. If an injured patient who has not previously been given tetanus toxoid is given it immediately after an injury, this first dose does not provide immunity for the injury.

No active immunity from tetanus. The amount of the very potent tetanus toxin necessary to produce clinical tetanus is so small that it will not incite an active antibody level high enough to prevent a second attack of tetanus. Consequently, tetanus is a nonimmunizing disease; hence, a history of tetanus does not rule out the possibility of a second attack of tetanus.

To prevent such a second attack, when a patient is recovering from tetanus and is about 4 weeks past the onset of tetanus, his attending physician should begin active immunization with tetanus toxoid.

Surgical wound care

Surgical prophylaxis consists of the removal of *C. tetani* and nonviable tissues from wounds and of the best possible reconstruction of aerobic wounds. Meticulous surgical care of wounds is performed when the following are carried out:

1. The wounds are taken care of at the earliest possible moment.
2. Aseptic technique is observed with the use of gloves, gowns, masks, and sterile instruments and the application of proper solutions to prepare the skin before the necessary operative procedures at the injured site.
3. During skin preparation, the wound is covered with gauze to prevent further contamination.
4. Proper lighting is employed so that the surgeon can exactly identify and protect vital structures such as nerves and vessels.

A GUIDE TO PROPHYLAXIS AGAINST TETANUS IN WOUND MANAGEMENT

General principles

1. The attending physician must determine for each patient with a wound what is required for adequate prophylaxis against tetanus.
2. Regardless of the active immunization status of the patient, meticulous surgical care, including removal of all devitalized tissue and foreign bodies, should be provided immediately for all wounds. Such care is essential as part of the prophylaxis against tetanus.
3. Each patient with a wound should receive adsorbed tetanus toxoid* intramuscularly at the time of injury, either as an initial immunizing dose or as a booster for previous immunization, unless he has received a booster or has completed his initial immunization series within the past 5 years. As the antigen concentration varies in different products, specific information on the volume of a single dose is provided on the label of the package.
4. Whether or not to provide passive immunization with homologous tetanus immune globulin (human) must be decided individually for each patient. The characteristics of the wound, conditions under which it was incurred, its treatment, its age, and the previous active immunization status of the patient must be considered.
5. Every wounded patient should be given a written record of the immunization provided. He should be instructed to carry the record at all times and, if indicated, to complete active immunization. For precise tetanus prophylaxis, an accurate and immediately available history regarding previous active immunization against tetanus is required.
6. Basic immunization with adsorbed toxoid requires 3 injections. A booster of adsorbed toxoid is indicated 10 years after the third injection or 10 years after an intervening wound booster.† All individuals, including pregnant women, should have basic immunization and indicated booster injections.

Specific measures for patients with wounds

I.   Previously immunized individuals
  A.   When the patient has been actively immunized within the past 10† years
    1. To the great majority, give 0.5 ml of adsorbed toxoid* as a booster *unless it is certain that the patient has received a booster within the previous 5 years.*
    2. To those with severe, neglected, or old (more than 24 hours) tetanus-prone wounds, give 0.5 ml of adsorbed toxoid* *unless it is certain that the patient has received a booster within the previous year.*

---

*The Public Health Service Advisory Committee on Immunization Practices in 1969 recommended diphtheria and tetanus toxoids combined with pertussis vaccine (DTP) for basic immunization in infants and children from 2 months through the sixth year of age and combined tetanus and diphtheria toxoids, adult type (Td) for basic immunization of those over 6 years of age. For the latter group, Td toxoid was recommended for routine or wound boosters; but, if there is any reason to suspect hypersensitivity to the diphtheria component, tetanus toxoid (T) should be substituted for Td.

Continued.

A GUIDE TO PROPHYLAXIS AGAINST TETANUS
IN WOUND MANAGEMENT–CONT'D

 B. When the patient has been actively immunized more than 10† years previously
   1. To the great majority, give 0.5 ml of adsorbed tetanus* toxoid
   2. To those with severe, neglected, or old (more than 24 hours) tetanus-prone wounds
    a. Give 0.5 ml of adsorbed tetanus toxoid*‡
    b. Give 250 units§ of tetanus immune globulin (human)‡
    c. Consider providing oxytetracycline or penicillin
 II. Individuals *not* previously immunized
  A. With clean minor wounds in which tetanus is most unlikely, give 0.5 ml of adsorbed tetanus toxoid* (initial immunizing dose)
  B. With all other wounds
   1. Give 0.5 ml of adsorbed tetanus toxoid* (initial immunizing dose)‡
   2. Give 250 units§ of tetanus immune globulin (human)‡
   3. Consider providing oxytetracycline or penicillin

---

*The Public Health Service Advisory Committee on Immunization Practices in 1969 recommended diphtheria and tetanus toxoids combined with pertussis vaccine (DTP) for basic immunization in infants and children from 2 months through the sixth year of age and combined tetanus and diphtheria toxoids, adult type (Td) for basic immunization of those over 6 years of age. For the latter group, Td toxoid was recommended for routine or wound boosters; but, if there is any reason to suspect hypersensitivity to the diphtheria component, tetanus toxoid (T) should be substituted for Td.

†Some authorities advise 6 rather than 10 years, particularly for patients with severe, neglected, or old (more than 24 hours) tetanus-prone wounds such as may be sustained by military personnel in combat.

‡Use different syringes needles, and sites of injection.

§In very severe, very neglected, or very old wounds, 500 units of tetanus immune globulin (human) is advisable.

5. Adequate instruments and adequate help are at the surgeon's call so that there is the best possible and gentle retraction of structures in wounds.
6. Hemostasis is obtained with delicate instruments and with fine suture material so that there is a minimum of necrotic tissue left in wounds.
7. Gentle handling of tissues at all times is emphasized so that necrotic tissue is not produced.
8. Complete debridement with scalpel excision of necrotic tissue and with removal of foreign bodies is performed so that no pabulum is left on which any unremoved bacteria can propagate.
9. The wound is copiously irrigated with large amounts of physiologic salt solution to wash out minute avascular fragments of tissue and to eliminate foreign bodies.
10. If there is any doubt about producing anaerobic conditions so that the tetanus bacillus can grow and produce its lethal toxin in it, the wound is left wide open and drainage is instituted when necessary.

Antitoxins

Heterologous antitoxins. In 1890, von Behring and Kitasato demonstrated the formation of tetanus antitoxin, which was formed in the blood of mice and rabbits following active immunization. This antitoxin, injected into unvaccinated mice and rabbits, protected them against a subsequent tetanus infection. Other animals could also be treated with these sera with good results. Thus the practical value of both homologous and heterologous antisera was proved.

Few discoveries in the history of medicine have excited scientists and laymen alike as much as this one did, for the ever-present threat of tetanus could now be banished. By the end of the nineteenth century, in spite of some skepticism, antitoxin therapy and particularly prophylaxis were widely adopted and approved.

Homologous antitoxin: tetanus immune globulin (human). Tetanus immune globulin (human) or TIG(H) has been referred to by numerous scientific and trade names (Table 38-6).

TIG(H), a sterile solution containing 165 ±15 mg of gamma globulin per milliliter is prepared from human blood plasma having a high titer of tetanus antitoxin. Such plasma is obtained from blood of hyperimmunized volunteers, from blood for gamma globulin manufacture that has been screened for tetanus antitoxin titers, or from placentas from mothers who received tetanus toxoid booster inoculations a few weeks preceding delivery.

TIG(H) is effective prophylactically in patients with wounds that may be contaminated with *C. tetani*. Because it is of human origin, it is virtually free from the risk of inducing hypersensitivity. Its use is advised particularly when a history of active immunization with tetanus toxoid cannot be established with reasonable certainty and when the risk of immediate or delayed reactions to equine antitoxin must be avoided (patients known to be sensitive to horse serum, those who have had prior injections of horse serum, or those who have a history of allergy). When a history of previous active immunization can be established, the administration of a booster dose of tetanus toxoid is preferable.

Passive immunization with TIG(H) is no substitute for active immunization with tetanus toxoid, nor is it a substitute for adequate surgical care of contaminated or potentially contaminated wounds. The half-life of passively acquired TIG(H) is thought to be at least 3 weeks and possibly more than 4 weeks. By contrast, tetanus toxin

Table 38-6 Trade, commercial, or proprietary names for tetanus immune globulin (human)

United States	Europe
Hyper-Tet	Tetabullin (Austria)
Hu-Tet	Tetagam (West Germany)
Homo-Tet	Tetuman Berna (Switzerland)
Gamatet	Tetaglobuline (France)
Immu-Tetanus	
T-I-Gammagee	
Pro-Tet	
Gamulin-T	

antibodies from heterologous sources (equine or bovine antitoxins) have a relatively brief half-life, which may be as short as 2 or 3 days.

Studies on the absorption and persistence of TIG(H) indicate that about one half of an intramuscular dose appears in the plasma. The injection of 4 to 5 units/kg of body weight ensures a plasma level of 0.02 units/ml for as long as 4 weeks; this level probably is adequate to protect against any but a fulminating tetanus infection.

Unless extraneous contamination occurs, there is virtually no likelihood of transmitting viral hepatitis by the administration of this agent. The possibility that allergic reactions may occur is very remote. As with other gamma globulin preparations, however, pain and redness at the site of injection may rarely occur.

At the time of intramuscular administration, skin sensitivity testing need not be done, but care should be taken to draw back on the plunger of the syringe in order to be certain that the needle is not in a blood vessel. Under no circumstances should the globulin be given intravenously.

When TIG(H) is given, adsorbed tetanus toxoid should also be administered. A different sterile syringe and needle are used to inject the toxoid to lessen the possibility that some of the antitoxin and some of the toxoid may neutralize each other. Doses of 250 to 400 units of TIG(H) for adults and 75 to 250 units for infants and children do not appear to interfere appreciably with primary active immunization (Table 38-7). Thus simultaneous active-passive immunization, in which the adsorbed toxoid is injected into one deltoid muscle and the TIG(H) is injected into the contralateral gluteal muscles, can be accomplished. By such simultaneous immunization, immediate passive protection is conferred and active protection is initiated.

Antibiotics

Antibiotics such as penicillin have been shown to be effective against vegetative tetanus bacilli both in vitro and in experimental animals. They have no effect against toxin. The effectiveness of antibiotics for prophylaxis remains unproved; if used, they should be given over a period of at least 5 days.

Antibiotics should not be used as a substitute for active or passive immunization and/or as a substitute for proper surgical care of the wound, and antibiotics are not necessary to prevent tetanus in the actively immunized.

Emergency medical identification devices

In the United States, where now more and more individuals are actively immunized for tetanus, emergency medical identification devices (EMID) are becoming increasingly important. Clinicians in active practice are constantly faced with these questions in the management of the wounded persons:

Table 38-7 Prophylactic doses of tetanus immune globulin (human) for infants and children

Age	Dose
10 years or older	250 units
5 to 10 years	125 units
Under 5 years	75 units

1. Has the patient been actively immunized for tetanus?
2. If he is actively immunized for tetanus, when was it done?
3. Have there been reactions to tetanus toxoid?
4. Should TIG(H) be given?

Such questions can be immediately answered if each individual had on his person an up-to-date EMID.

Physicians have had patients tell them they have been given tetanus toxoid injections, but, on closer search of the history, they have learned that tetanus antitoxin, or diphtheria toxoid, or perhaps typhoid vaccine had been given, but not tetanus toxoid. If the history is vague and poorly documented, the patient should be given tetanus toxoid as though the dose or doses of toxoid in question had not been given.

In the United States at the present time, very few people have in their immediate possession an emergency medical identification device with tetanus data (Table 38-5).

The American Medical Association has prepared for physicians at low cost an emergency medical identification card. On this card, there is reproduced the American Medical Association identification symbol, which was adopted by the World Medical Association through an action by its Assembly in 1964 and which was recommended for use in the countries represented by the World Medical Association members. Similar cards or records are also available from the World Health Organization, the U. S. Government Printing Office, the American Academy of Pediatrics, the American Academy of General Practice, and the Michigan State Medical Society.

A button may be attached to underclothing, to a billfold, or to a purse.

Metal tags are available in attractive configurations, such as a heart.

In view of the cost of tetanus toxoid and the cost of the treatment of tetanus, need any more be said about tetanus toxoid prophylaxis being an economic triumph?

chapter 39

Rabies and its prevention

Jean-René Dupont

TREATMENT

All treatment of rabies encephalitis is broken down into two phases: prophylactic and supportive treatment. The current presentation is based on the recommendations of the U.S. Public Health Service dated October 19, 1969. These guidelines for prophylactic treatment are revised periodically and are therefore not absolute (Table 39-1).

Management of the wound is important. The wound should be carefully flushed under running water and scrubbed with a brush and a cleansing compound such as soap. It is unnecessary to use silver nitrate or electrocautery of these wounds. The mechanical cleansing is thought to be most salutary. Depending on the severity of the wound and the history of the offending animal, antirabies serum and vaccine or both may be administered. Tetanus prophylaxis is also given, and if the wound is large with a considerable amount of soft tissue destruction, antibiotics can be added to the regimen.

If the offending animal is a domestic animal and if no lesions are present, no antirabies serum or vaccine need be administered. In cases of severe exposure both serum and vaccine should be given. It is generally thought of value to begin the administration of vaccine 24 hours following the initial dose of the antirabies serum. The recommended dose for passive immunization utilizing hyperimmune serum is 1,000 units/40 kg of body weight. At least 5 ml of this serum should be injected locally into the edges of the wound around the area of the bite. With the use of hyperimmune rabies serum it may not be necessary in some cases to administer the vaccine. However, when dealing with skunk, fox, raccoon, or bat exposure the hyperimmune serum as well as the rabies vaccine should invariably be administered. With severe exposure the dose of vaccine may be doubled and given in 7 instead of 14 days. It is safe to modify the treatment rendered according to knowledge of wildlife rabies in the area and the status of the offending animal.

The dose of serum may be doubled if indicated. An animal with clinical rabies will be dead from 5 to 7 days following the onset of symptoms. If a biting dog is observed for this period of time and remains well, he is quite unlikely to be shedding rabies virus in the saliva. Today the emphasis is on the use of hyperimmune serum, which more and more replaces the blind and sometimes emotional administration of rabies vaccine. Whenever a

Table 39-1 Management of rabies

Animal bite treatment checklist

1. Flush wound immediately (first aid).
2. Cleanse wound thoroughly under medical supervision.
3. Give antirabies serum and/or vaccine as indicated.
4. Give tetanus prophylaxis and antibacterial regimen when required.

Postexposure Antirabies Prophylaxis Guide

Animal bite		Treatment per degree of exposure*		
Species	Status at time of attack	No lesion	Mild	Severe
Dog	Healthy	None	None	Serum
or	Signs suggestive of rabies	None	Vaccine	Serum/vaccine
cat	Escaped or unknown	None	Vaccine	Serum/vaccine
	Rabid	None	Serum/vaccine	Serum/vaccine
Skunk, fox, raccoon, coyote, bat	Regard as rabid in unprovoked attack	None	Serum/vaccine	Serum/vaccine

*Vaccine refers to duck embryo high egg passage vaccine. serum used for hyperimmune antirabies serum. The vaccine is given in fourteen injections of 1 ml of a 10% tissue emulsion or 2 ml of a 5% emulsion, depending upon the manufacturing process. Hyperimmune serum may be administered in doses from 40 to 100 IU/body weight, depending upon the severity of exposure.

physician treats a possible rabies victim, he should bear in mind that less than 10% of exposed patients will contract encephalitis if no treatment at all is given.

It is not unlikely that the future will see the development of a potent rabies vaccine based on the use of virus grown in human tissue culture. At the present time the duck embryo (DEV) high egg passage (HEP) vaccine has very largely replaced the older spinal cord vaccine of Semple, Pasteur, and Fermi.* The low egg passage vaccine (LEP) is generally used for immunization of animals but may at times prove virulent to cats.

Vaccination has been found to be helpful only when the incubation period of rabies is shorter than 30 days. All persons receiving vaccine for rabies exposure should also be given a booster injection 10, 20, and 30 days after the series has been completed. If central nervous system symptoms should appear during the course of vaccination, the injections should be stopped immediately for fear of precipitating an irreversible demyelinating disease. The common side effects caused by the duck embryo vaccine are pruritus, pain, and erythema at the site of innoculation. Adrenocortical steroids and epinephrine are helpful in combating the immediate reactions.

A number of treatment failures have been observed. However, in recent years, with the use of hyperimmune serum and modern vaccines, the incidence of treatment failures has

---

*The following are the more common spinal cord or brain vaccines: Pasteur, Hogyes, Fermi, and Semple. Avian vaccines include the duck embryo or the chick embryo HEP or LEP (high, 180, and low, 40 to 50 egg passages). The names Flury and Kelev imply a certain strain of the virus, the former being named after a young rabies victim from whom it was isolated in 1939.

been reduced to an absolute minmum whenever treatment with the serum commenced within 24 hours after exposure.

Once clinical rabies appears, supportive measures similar to those employed in tetanus may be efficacious. This entails prevention of fatal complications such as seizures, cardiac arrythmias, aspiration, or asphyxiation. It is of some comfort to the physician attending a rabies victim to know that transmission from man to man has not been described in the modern literature.

PREVENTION

Prevention, of course, is of paramount importance in a disease such as rabies, which has no cure for the clinical illness. The following measures are effective and reasonable.

1. Wild animal reservoirs should be reduced or exterminated if the risk of infection outweighs economic and ecologic considerations. It appears that the rabies virus has an epizootic cycle of about 100 years.

2. Stray dogs ought to be quarantined, vaccinated, and domesticated. If this is impossible, they should be eradicated.

3. Domestic dogs, cats, and other animals must be vaccinated if exposure to rabies is possible or probable.

4. Man should avoid wild animals that appear to have lost their natural shyness when approached (skunks, coyotes, foxes, and so on). All animals displaying an abnormal behavior or odd patterns of movements are best left alone (bats flying in daytime or biting, groggy canines).

5. Domestic dogs and cats biting without cause or provocation should be suspected of having rabies and should be quarantined for no less than 7 days, at which time they may be returned to the owner if showing no symptoms of rabies.

6. Animal handlers and high-risk personnel should be vaccinated against rabies and should receive a booster injection every year. Booster injections administered every 6 months induce antibody formation earlier.

7. Animals entering a country should be kept in quarantine for at least 45 days and should receive vaccination upon entry.

8. While the virus does not penetrate intact skin but may enter through mucous membranes, postexposure prophylactic vaccination should be undertaken when any person is bitten by wild animals, including bats, or domestic animals showing signs of rabies.

PHYSICAL EXAMINATION

During the prodromal phase of the disease the physical examination is often unremarkable. One may find a healed scar from a previous bite or scratch, or there may be no history of previous animal exposure. Neuritic pain referred to the site of the original bite is a frequent complaint. The patient is agitated, excitable, and restless. He has a mild coryza. Bradycardia out of proportion to the fever has been stressed as an important physical finding, but it is not invariably present. These vague findings during the early stages of the disease have often resulted in an initial diagnosis of "psychoneurotic disorder."

During the late stages of the illness paralysis appears, but most victims die before total paralysis has time to set in. It is during this time that the classic autonomic manifestations of pharyngeal spasms, hydrophobia, vomiting, retching, convulsions, tremor, cutis anserina, and excessive salivation are seen. As far as can be ascertained at this writing, there are no certain human survivors on record once the clinical signs of rabies appear.*

LABORATORY DIAGNOSIS

The laboratory diagnosis of rabies centers around two avenues of approach: (1) the histopathologic examination of the rabies victim at postmortem and (2) the serologic diagnosis of the disease.

Neutralizing antibodies to rabies can be demonstrated in the serum; and, with the advent of the fluorescent antibody technique, a sensitive tool has been furnished the clinician. These same two methods of diagnosis are available to the public health officer. It must be borne in mind that tissue examination of the brain of rabies victims should be carried out on fixed tissue, whereas serologic testing is limited to the fresh frozen specimen.

The routine laboratory tests are normal, including the spinal fluid. Albuminuria and a relative polymorphonuclear neutrophilia occur with regularity.

HISTOPATHOLOGY

Rabies encephalitis is an acute viral infection of the central nervous system predominantly affecting the gray matter of the brainstem. It is therefore a viral polioencephalitis. Present-day knowledge holds that the disease is caused by a single serologically distinct, rather large virus (100 to 150 mµ by filtration) that has some of the characteristics of a myxovirus.

PUBLIC HEALTH DATA

Rabies is a disease that may occur from Greenland to Cape Horn. South Central Asia and Southeast Asia, with 50% of the cases in recent years, appear to harbor the largest source of human exposures. New Zealand, Australia, and the Scandinavian countries reportedly have been free of rabies for several decades.

Because of the rapid transportation of today, unsuspected cases of rabies may crop up in the western hemisphere at odd times. Rabies has been diagnosed in patients visiting London and Western Europe from the Orient. In the United States the largest reservoir seems to be in the South and Southwest, as far as human case material is concerned. However, wildlife rabies is rampant throughout most of the central United States as far east as Maryland, as far north as the Dakotas, and south to the Mexican border and the Florida peninsula. A definite concentration of rabies in skunks and foxes appears to be found in Kentucky, Tennessee, and the neighboring states.

Prior to 1940 the domestic dog was by far the most important carrier as far as human exposure was concerned. Over the past two decades this has changed. The important carrier today is the wild animal, particularly the skunk, fox, and bat. It has furthermore been demonstrated that the skunk sheds the virus in extremely high concentrations in the saliva. Skunk bites should therefore always be considered dangerous.

---

*A child surviving probable rabies encephalitis has been reported from the Center of Disease Control, Atlanta, Georgia, December, 1970.

INCIDENCE

As with any viral encephalitis, the very young have an affinity for rabies. The female of the species seems to be more resistant to the virus than is the male, and the black individual is overwhelmingly more resistant to rabies infection than is the white one. In most series the ratio of male to female is generally three to one. In experimental animals it may go as high as seven males to one female.

TRANSMISSION

Rabies encephalitis is generally thought to be transmitted by the bite of a rabid animal. The virus is harbored in quantity in the saliva of clinically rabid animals, but it may be demonstrated in other parts of the body of these animals by special methods such as fluorescent antibody technique. Apparently, a certain number of wild animals can develop serum neutralizing antibodies to rabies without showing the clinically apparent disease. Today well over 50% of human cases are accounted for by wildlife exposure. In any study of rabies it is important to note that a fourth to a third of the patients yield no history of an actual animal bite or scratch. It has been believed that droplet and fomite transmission may be important. At the same time, however, one must consider that rabies virus does not appear to be an extremely infectious agent. It has been estimated that less than 10% of human exposures to actually known rabid animals will result in encephalitis and death. Most bites are on the hand; it is believed by some that bites on the extremities are less apt to result in clinical rabies than are bites on the face.

The average incubation period is around 57 days, with a range of 20 to 150 days. After the prodrome appears, the clinical course usually averages 7 to 8 days. If a very short clinical course is encountered in a patient who has received rabies vaccination, the physician should suspect an allergic reaction to the rabies vaccine rather than rabies encephalitis itself. It is an accepted fact that the incubation period is entirely unpredictable and has no relationship to the virulence of the clinical course. However, it is our belief that the most virulent form of the disease is encountered when the amount of local tissue destruction is great and the size of the innoculum large, such as is seen in facial bites from rabid wolves. The overt manifestations of the disease are completely unrelated to the site of the initial bite.

chapter 40

Immediate medicolegal facets of care and first aid

Elwyn L. Cady, Jr.

Lawsuits against physicians who gratuitously render immediate aid are extremely rare. Medicolegal interest is heightened, nevertheless, by passage of "Good Samaritan" legislation in a number of states and by reexamination of legal rules of conduct imposed in emergency situations.

EMERGENCY DEFINED

Although the law does not slavishly follow lexicographers in defining words, *Webster's Third New International Dictionary,* Unabridged (1961), notes three shades of meaning for "emergency":

1. An unforeseen combination of circumstances or the resulting state that calls for immediate action.
2. A sudden bodily illness such as is likely to require immediate medical attention.
3. A distressing event or condition that can often be anticipated or prepared for but that is seldom foreseen.

Likewise, the definition of "first aid" is helpful: emergency and sometimes makeshift treatment given to someone (as the victim of an accident) requiring immediate attention where regular medical or surgical care is not available.

With these generalizations as background, we should consider the obligations of a physician to undertake immediate care, the measure of his proper conduct toward the patient, and, finally, special medicolegal problems in which the concept of "emergency" figures.

ETHICAL DUTY

Although it is true that a physician is ordinarily under no legal obligation to undertake immediate care, Section 5 of the *Principles of Medical Ethics* (1957 edition of the American Medical Association) places a rather strict moral burden on the AMA-guided practitioner: "In an emergency . . . he should undertake to render service to the best of his ability."

The 1955 edition of the *Principles,* still used as an authoritative source by the AMA Judicial Council, was more detailed:

He should . . . respond to any request for his assistance in an emergency or whenever temperate public opinion expects the service . . . (Sec. 4). When a physician is called in an emergency because the personal or family physician is not at hand, he should provide only for the patient's immediate need and should withdraw from the case on arrival of the personal or family physician. However, he should first report to the personal or family physician the condition found and treatment administered (Sec. 5).

Thus the ethical practitioner is bound to engage in emergency treatment from time to time.

LEGAL STANDARDS OF CONDUCT

Once the physician undertakes to treat a victim of an accident, he then becomes subject to legal rules that measure the quality of his conduct. The basic rules are comprehended in the concept of "legal duty," the breach of which amounts to negligence in the basic liability formula (see Fig. 1).

Specifically, a physician is required to exercise the following qualities in order to avoid liability:

Knowledge or learning based on advanced training, degree, and license. Whether undertaking treatment without "paper qualifications" constitutes negligence has been debated in law reports. In emergency care and first aid, however, the necessity for immediate action is intrinsic. "The emergency begets the man"; he is not selected on the basis of prior qualifications or training. Consequently, the law is not inclined to penalize him for proceeding even though his background is deficient. He would not be relieved from the obligation of exercising ordinary care, the proper inquiry being whether he acted prudently in the context of the facts of the emergency.

Reasonable skill. This duty is the possession and exercise of that reasonable degree of skill ordinarily possessed by others of his profession practicing in similar circumstances.

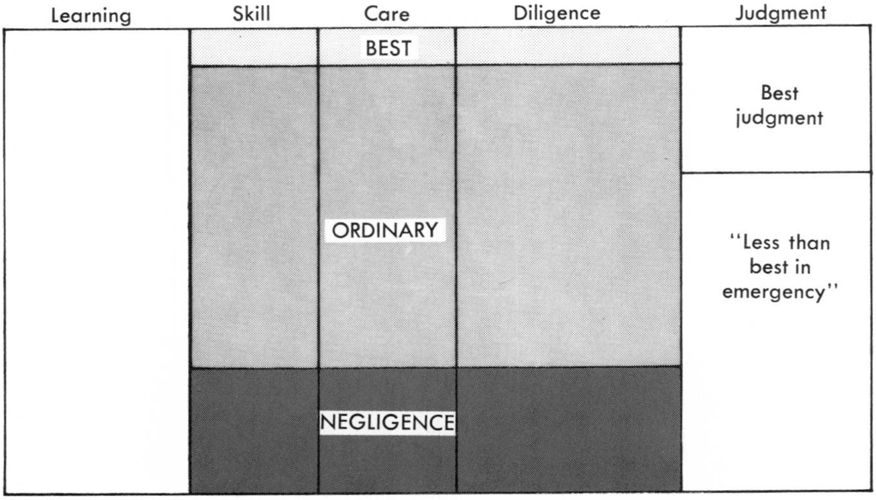

Fig. 1. Elements of legal duty.

Though a direct test in court as to requisite skill in an emergency has not been denoted, the cases justify certain generalizations:

1. A specialist in fact, who also holds himself out as a specialist, would be held to the skill of the up-to-date specialist in his particular field.

2. A general practitioner would be held to the standard of a general practitioner. Perhaps a specialist in fact who did not hold himself out as anything but "a doctor" when responding to an emergency call would need only meet this standard.

3. Residents, interns, externs, medical students, nurses, and nursing students would all be held to the standard commensurate with their particular level of training and experience.

4. Persons having particular training in first aid would presumably have this considered when a judge or jury weighed their conduct. A myocardial infarction case turned upon the negligence of a purser, also serving as pharmacist's mate, aboard a ship docked in London who permitted the patient to walk about the ship and go ashore to a hospital.

Ordinary care. This represents a minimum objective standard. Although referred to as "average care," this does not mean that one half of the professional group is automatically "below standard." Variability of this standard is illustrated by (1) the "proportionate to the character of injury" instruction and by (2) the "keeping abreast" rule:

1. Under a jury instruction that care and diligence used in attending an injured person should be proportionate to the character of the injury, an advocate can argue that actual performance in a life-threatening emergency should be superior to that expected in "minor emergencies." It is recognized, however, that to include the item or "skill" in such an instruction is wrong. "It can hardly be said that his skill should increase in proportion to the severity of the injury. One's skill is a matter of slow growth and cannot be increased on short notice." Judge Sturgis in Fowler v. Burris, 180 Mo. App. 347, 171 S.W. 620 (1914). A Kentucky court phrased it: "The duty performed is according to the exigencies of the case and proportionate to the dangers to be apprehended and guarded against." Johnson v. Vaughan, 370 S.W. 2d 591 (1963).

2. Ordinary care must reflect action consistent with technical advances. Thus Judge Choate included the following findings of fact in a cardiac arrest case, Kolessar v. United States, 198 F. Supp. 517 (1961):

A deprivation of an adequate supply of oxygen to the brain of a human being will most likely cause irreversible damage to the higher centers of the brain tissue and result in a neurologic deficiency in a human being. The extent of brain damage has a direct relation to the passage of time. This period was generally accepted by the medical profession on January 21, 1958.

Acceptable medical practice at Key West Naval Hospital on January 21, 1958, dictated a diagnosis of cardiac arrest and circulatory insufficiency as to Marrian Kolessar. At the time her abdominal incision did not bleed and she had no obtainable pulse. No notice was taken, or record kept, of the passage of time during either the various resuscitative procedures adopted or in connection with the initiation of a thoracotomy so as to manually restore circulation within the 4-minute period.

A period materially in excess of 4 minutes occurred between the time Marrian Kolessar's abdominal incision failed to bleed and her pulse became unobtainable until the time when resuscitative procedures were effective in that manual cardiac massage restored the flow of blood to the patient's brain. This constituted a departure from acceptable medical practice at Key West Naval Hospital on January 21, 1958.

Ordinary diligence. Emphasis on persistence characterizes this requirement. In evaluating a cardiac arrest situation, this diligence would imply a continuation of artificial respiration and massage through an extended period of time.

Best judgment. This element has particular application in emergency situations. It comprehends a subjective standard in contrast to the objective criteria for diligence and care. Thus presumably one could use his best judgment and, though it was far inferior to the judgment used by the average practitioner, he would still "pass muster." On the other hand, a particular physician actually possessing superior judgment would be bound to use it. So long as the physician used his best judgment at the particular time and under the particular circumstances, an error in his decision as to the proper course is excused.

Courts do not impose liability for "mere error of judgment" in this context. Furthermore, some negligence cases involving the "emergency doctorine" suggest that something less than "best judgment" is the requirement (see Fig. 1.):

> (T)he emergency doctrine . . . is that where one is confronted with a sudden emergency, without sufficient time to determine with certainty the best course to pursue, he is not held to the same accuracy of judgment as would be required of him if he had time for deliberation. Justice Anderson in Mississippi Cent. R. Co. v. Aultman, 173 Miss. 622, 160 So. 737, 940 (1935).
> (E)mergency does not lessen the obligation to use care, but merely excuses errors of judgment due to the excitement and necessity for haste produced by the emergency. Judge Dobie in Lachman v. Pennsylvania Greyhound Lines, 160 F. 2d 496, 502 (4th Cir. 1947).

It must be emphasized that the "emergency doctrine" is applied primarily to automobile accident cases in the law reports. Its use was tried unsuccessfully in the defense of a surgeon who "left" a hemostat. Long v. Sledge, 209 So. 2d 814 (Mississippi, 1968). One might well argue that all practitioners, or even students, should be prepared to meet a medical or surgical emergency with their best judgment. This, of course, is on the basis that an integral part of medical education is training in proper handling of emergency situations "with a cool head."

GOOD SAMARITAN LEGISLATION

California, in 1959, and other states since then have enacted statutes that purport to exempt physicians from negligence liability in emergency cases.

Under the common law system, conclusions as to the validity of such legislation must await court tests. Serious doubts on the constitutionality of such legislation have been voiced.

The only significant case to date construing such legislation found a passing motorist, Mrs. Turner, giving a ride to a man who had wrecked his car on the highway. Judge Wood interpreted the statute as applied to the facts in these words (Dahl v. Turner, 80 N. Mex. 608, 458 P. 2d 860 [1969]).

> The pertinent part of (the statute) reads: "No person who shall administer emergency care in good faith at or near the scene of an emergency, as defined herein, shall be held liable for any civil damages as a result of any action or omission by such person in administering said care, except for gross negligence; . . ."

(The statute) defines emergency to mean: " . . . an unexpected occurrence involving injury or illness to persons, including motor vehicle accidents and collisions, disasters, and other accidents and events of similar nature occurring in public or private places." . . .

If Mrs. Turner was administering "care" in providing transportation to plaintiff, such care was not emergency care within the meaning of the statute. There are no facts indicating a pressing necessity for such transportation; no facts indicating that the transportation was immediately called for.

After plaintiff wrecked his car he had a cut on his arm and appeared in a confused state. In such a situation, the State Police Officer would have tried to get plaintiff to go to the hospital but wouldn't have forced him to go. Plaintiff didn't want to go to a doctor. Plaintiff wanted to be taken to a friend at a motel in Silver City. That's what Mrs. Turner was doing . . . .

CONSENT IMPLIED

Any touching of the person without consent ordinarily constitutes an unlawful battery so that civil and perhaps criminal liability can attach. Bona fide immediate care, including heroic surgery, is permitted without the usual legal consent, however. As stated by Chief Justice Chavez: "It would indeed be most unusual for a doctor, with his patient who had just been bitten by a venomous snake, to calmly sit down and first fully discuss the various available methods of treating snakebite and the possible consequences, while the venom was being pumped through the patient's body." Crouch v. Most, 78 N. Mex. 406, 432 P. 2d 250 (1967).

Legal theorists say that consent is implied in fact or as a matter of law. Regardless of theory, the law does give a definite privilege for immediate care to proceed even though no actual consent is obtained. I will stand on this proposition even though contrary dictum is stated in some of the books authored by nurses or physicians who, it is submitted, fail to heed a basic view that the law represents "crystallized common sense." There has even been discussion as to whether or not there should be efforts made to gain consent from a victim's legal representative (such as parents, spouse, or guardian) before undertaking emergency surgery. The immediacy of surgery under principles of good practice as well as the impracticability of consulting such representatives should justify such surgery.

A related matter has been deviation from an original nonemergency procedure to one classed as an emergency based upon "newly discovered evidence." The trend of decision has been toward the doctrine enunciated by Judge Clayton of the Municipal Court of Appeals for the District of Columbia in Barnett v. Bachrach, 34 A. 2d 626 (1943):

We hold the law to be that in case of emergency a surgeon may lawfully perform, and it is his duty to perform, such operations as good surgery demands even when it means extending the operation further than was originally contemplated.

Emergency involuntary hospitalization. The old common law evolved a doctrine permitting anyone to restrain a person who became dangerous to himself or to others because of mental disorder. The doctrine was designed for instances where the urgency of the situation demands immediate intervention, that is, an emergency. Today, this doctrine has been supplemented in many states by mental health acts that authorize an emergency hospitalization for a limited period upon medical certification.

Duty of hospital to provide immediate care. It has become commonplace for hospitals to establish and maintain emergency rooms. A strong concurrent development in today's jurisprudence is a recognition that such hospitals have a positive duty to render immediate care.

TOWARD PREVENTION

In order to forestall medicolegal complications, several prophylactic avenues have been championed:

Detailed advance instructions should be given for the handling of emergency situations. As an example, the Medical Defense Union in England has issued the following memorandum in hope that "the wrong patient or part" cases may be minimized:

The Medical Defense Union and the Royal College of Nursing have given consideration to the steps that might be taken to obviate the risk of an operation being performed on:

(a) the wrong patient,

(b) the wrong side,

(c) the wrong digit.

During the period October, 1959, to September, 1961, the Medical Defense Union dealt with no fewer than *twenty-eight such cases* and it is hardly necessary to say that *these avoidable mistakes are quite indefensible.*

The Councils of the Medical Defense Union and the Royal College of Nursing are firmly of the opinion that in order to minimize the risk of such occurrences it is eminently desirable that wherever practicable the suggested safeguards as outlined below should be taken. It is appreciated that in certain out-lying or "cottage" hospitals there is no resident medical staff and that in some hospitals it may not always be possible to adopt these safeguards in their entirety.

(a) Operating on the wrong patient

Causes predisposing to error.

(i) In hospitals which undertake a vast amount of casualty work where *emergency patients* are being admitted in quick succession, some of them unconscious, there is the possibility of the notes becoming attached to the wrong patient. Where it is the practice to attach the patient's name to the clothing which has been removed in the casualty department, this does not always provide an adequate check because the clothes may be detached from the patient before or on admission to the ward.

(ii) In respect of patients for non-emergency operations who have been in the ward for a day or two prior to operation, mistakes may arise if on the day of operation the beds are changed round. This situation is exacerbated if the day of operation coincides with a change in several of the nursing staff and could lead to the wrong patient being sent to the theatre if the routine did not provide adequate safeguards against error.

(iii) Mistakes may occur when changes are made in theatre lists following the commencement of the operating session, particularly if such changes have not been notified to the ward immediately they have been made.

Suggested safeguards.

(1) All unconscious patients admitted through the casualty department should be labelled before they are taken to the wards. The identity disc or label should bear the patient's name, initials and hospital number where possible. *The labelling of the patient* should be the responsibility of the casualty sister or her deputy, or by night, the nurse-in-charge or her deputy.

(2) Following the admission to the hospital of a patient who is to undergo an operation, he *should be seen in the ward by the surgeon* who is to perform the operation. Prior to the operation the surgeon should examine the patient's records and make sure that the notes do in fact relate to that particular patient and that the entries contained therein are correct.

(3) All patients going to the operating theatre should be labelled by means of an *identity disc or label attached to the wrist or ankle.* The identity disc or label should bear the patient's name, initials and hospital number. The labelling should be carried out in the ward at the time the patient is prepared for the operating theatre and should be the responsibility of the ward sister or her deputy.

In rare cases where the patient goes direct from the casualty department to the operating theatre, the onus of correct labelling should rest on the casualty sister or her deputy. In either instance the labelling would constitute an additional check that the correct patient received the prescribed premedication and that the correct patient was sent to the theatre.

(4) In addition to the nature of the operation, the patient's name, initials and hospital number

should also appear on the operation list. A copy of the *operation list should be displayed in the anaesthetic room as well as in the operating theatre, thus enabling both the anaesthetist and the surgeon to check and ensure that the right patient is presented for operation.* A copy of the operation list should also be made available to wards in which the patients who are to undergo operation are accommodated.

(5) Patients should be sent for from the operating theatre by name and number and never as "the patient from such and such a ward." Where it is the practice for a porter from the theatre to collect the patients from the ward he should bring with him a slip bearing the name of the patient and his hospital number. In hospitals where the procedure is to telephone the ward to ask that the patient concerned be sent to the theatre, the patient's hospital number, as well as the name, should be quoted. The *ward sister* or her deputy should be responsible for seeing that:

(a)   the correct patient is sent to the operating theatre;
(b)   the patient has already signed the appropriate consent to operation form;
(c)   the patient has received the prescribed pre-operative preparation including premedication;
(d)   where appropriate the side of operation has been marked (see Section [b] Clause [1]);
(e)   the correct case papers, X-rays, etc., accompany the patient to the theatre.

(6) In the operating theatre one person should be made responsible for sending for patients. This should be the responsibility of the theatre superintendent but in large operating theatre suites it may be necessary for her to delegate this responsibility to some other person, e.g., the sister-in-charge of a particular theatre or the nurse taking the list in a particular theatre.

(7) When out-patients are admitted to the wards for the day for a minor operation, they should be labelled in the same way as the in-patients before they are taken to the operating theatre.

(8) Patients who are to be operated on in the out-patient theatre under a general anaesthetic should be labelled in the same way as the in-patients.

(9) Patients should have one hospital number which should be quoted on all papers concerning the patient. Where it is the practice to have departmental numbers these may be used additionally on the appropriate papers but never exclusively.

(10) In so far as children are concerned, the labelling should be carried out when they are admitted to the ward. As the case histories must be taken from the patient's relatives (who may not be present immediately prior to the operation) it is vital that no error should occur in these notes in reference to the side, limb or digit on which the operation is to be performed.

(b) Operating on the wrong side or limb

Causes predisposing to error.

(i) Wrong information on the case papers of the patient, i.e., "right" instead of "left."
(ii) Abbreviation of the words "right" and "left."
(iii) Illegible writing on the case papers.
(iv) Failure to check immediately prior to commencing to operate the entry on the operation list with the notes taken to the operating theatre.
(v) The wrong case papers accompanying the patient, combined with (iv) above.
(vi) The preparation of the wrong side or limb, combined with (iv) above.
(vii) No routine procedure for marking the operation side.

Suggested safeguards.

(1) The side on which the operation is to be performed should be indelibly marked before the patient reaches the theatre, and in order to denote the side a mark should be made with *an indelible skin pencil on the forehead* of the patient. This should normally be made the responsibility of the house surgeon. In the case of "listed" patients already in the ward, it is usual for the house surgeon or a house officer to see the patient on the evening before the operation and this would give the practitioner concerned an opportunity of marking the operation side. In the case of emergency operations the surgeon generally sees the patient in the ward before he is taken to the operating theatre, thus providing him with an opportunity for marking the operation side. In the rare instance of a patient who is taken direct from the casualty department to the operating theatre, the practitioner who decides upon an immediate operation should be made responsible for marking the operation side.

In the event of the ward sister or her deputy, or exceptionally the casualty sister or her deputy, finding that the side of operation has not been marked when the patient is due to be sent to the operating theatre, she should see that the surgeon who is to operate is informed accordingly, but she should not herself undertake the marking.

(2) The words "right" and "left" should be written in full in the patient's notes and in the operation list.

(c) Operating on the wrong digit

Causes predisposing to error.

  (i) Fingers referred to by numbers instead of by name.

  (ii) Wrong information on the case papers of the patient, i.e., "right" instead of "left."

  (iii) Illegible writing on the case papers.

  (iv) Failure to check immediately prior to commencing to operate the entry on the operation list with the notes taken to the operating theatre.

  (v) The wrong case papers accompanying the patient, combined with (iv) above.

  (vi) The preparation of the wrong digit combined with (iv) above.

  (vii) No routine procedure for marking the side on which the operation is to be performed.

Suggested safeguards.

(1) In order to avoid the possibility of any ambiguity concerning the finger(s) on which the operation is to be performed, the finger(s) should always be described as thumb, index, middle, ring and little fingers and not as first, second, third, fourth and fifth. In so far as the toes are concerned, the accepted practice is to describe them as hallux (big), second, third, fourth and fifth (little) toes and this should always be adhered to.

(2) The words "right" and "left" should be written in full in the patient's notes and on the operation list.

In order to reach agreement on a routine procedure, incorporating as far as possible the safeguards put forward in this memorandum, to be adopted in a particular hospital or group of hospitals, it is suggested that joint committees of medical and nursing staff should be set up on a local basis. The committees should include, inter alios, the matron and a representative of the consultant surgical staff.

Competent medicolegal consultation services should be made immediately available. Unusual situations may necessitate sound medicolegal guidance for the practitioner. As a rule, such advice should be secured promptly so that "hindsight headaches" can be avoided.

Above all, the practitioner should keep the anxiety-relieving thought in mind, grasping a few fundamentals mentioned here, that "pitching in" with first aid and immediate care is *not* legally hazardous. Statistically speaking, true Good Samaritans rarely lose lawsuits!

part eight

Postscript

John H. Henzel

Not long ago a marine who survived a through-and-through high-velocity missile wound of his chest in Vietnam attended the funeral of his youngest brother, the victim of a near-identical but accidental gunshot wound. The macabre irony of the incident was not that two brothers received anatomically identical left chest gunshot wounds at the same age but rather that the emergency transportation and acute resuscitative care that the younger brother received in a major midwestern city was found lacking in comparison to that available under combat conditions halfway around the globe.

Along this same line, the vital signs, cardiac output, and respiratory dynamics of a space program environmental stress volunteer were recently being monitored by sophisticated and expensive biosensor equipment when the experiment volunteer was notified that his child had been struck by an automobile and rushed to a local hospital. While visiting his son during the critical hours immediately following injury, the father experienced a feeling of resigned exasperation as he observed the archaic intensive care unit monitoring equipment, realizing that valuable equipment was available but unused in a research laboratory a few miles from the hospital.

During another era, a different generation would have paid little heed to the events described. Fortunately, this generation has seen through the imperfections of a technologic society that has the wherewithal to lower mortality of acutely treated battlefield casualities below 5% and to monitor vital processes of men exploring the moon, while fellow citizens want for stateside emphasis on related health care technology. In 1972 almost 50,000 victims died as a result of highway accidents in the United States and thousands more incurred potentially preventable morbidity in association with their injury. When statistics clearly reveal that paramedical personnel, field hospitals, and physicians can provide war casualties halfway around the world with a better chance for survival than ambulance crews and emergency room teams can currently provide in the richest of nations, and when aerospace laboratory programs of 5 years ago had biomedical monitoring equipment that only selected major hospitals can afford to implement today, it is time for society, medical educators, and medical students to delegate trauma a priority rating equivalent to those other issues of the health care delivery system about which society is presently concerned. The relevancy of trauma education lies within the significance and implications of these facts and figures.

The 1970's is a difficult time in which to implement trauma education. The educational system is currently pressed by advocated innovations originating from socioeconomic health care problems; many would-be innovators are nonphysician health planners who are unfamiliar with the trauma problem. Today highway accident victims arrive at hospitals daily with seatbelt injury, fat embolism, and a myriad of increasingly challenging therapeutic problems. Only 10 years ago seatbelt trauma was unknown, and few victims of major trauma survived long enough to require treatment for fat embolism. The assessment and management of the 1980 high-speed traffic victim will need the background knowledge to diagnose and manage cardiac contusion, shock lung, fractured liver, and a whole host of simultaneously occurring injuries that will be encountered with increased frequency as shoulder harnesses, collapsible steering columns, and padded dashboards allow passengers to survive increasingly severe impact trauma.

Too long has trauma education occupied a void, been ignored, or been delegated a low priority in medical education. Once comprehensive socioeconomic efforts have provided health-equalizing employment, immunization, sanitation, and nutrition to inner city ghettos and rural Appalachia, society will awaken to the magnitude of the trauma problem and the low priority that trauma education currently occupies. Acquisition of the capability and expertise needed to provide safe and effective care is not an impossibly complex goal. However, since the trauma victim usually is thrust upon the physician quite unexpectedly, success (productive survival) or failure (preventable death or disability) depend upon information, decisions, and therapeutic maneuvers that have to be known. There is no time for textbook reading or literature review, little room for uncertainty, and none for indecision or error. Needed information and skills must have been previously made available through education. Herein lies the reason for this textbook and for that stimulus which motivated its authors.

chapter 41

Accidents as a disease

Charles F. Frey

Accidents are the fourth leading cause of death in the United States, after heart disease, cancer, and stroke. One would think that, because of the magnitude of the problem, accidents would deserve attention by the public and by the medical profession. Yet accidents have not been called the neglected disease of modern society by the National Research Council without reason.

Why do government and the private sector give millions of dollars for medical research and clinical care for the study of diseases much less lethal or disabling and affecting far fewer people than do motor vehicle accidents alone? Why are funds available for care of patients who are often old and who have chronic, malignant, and often incurable diseases when in the same institution there is not an intensive care or shock unit for victims of trauma, for patients who are usually young, with their future still before them? In contrast to many diseases upon which funds are lavished, the etiology of accidents, methods for prevention, and technology to improve the treatment of the injured and effect a reduction in mortality are all known and available. Why is it that an occasional homicide arouses a community to a frenzy? Newspaper and television editorials are felt necessary, police leaves are canceled, and the public is aroused. On the other hand, deaths from motor vehicle accidents are most likely to occur in young people and are far more frequent than homicides, yet they evoke no more than a mention from the newspapers, are seldom mentioned on television, and stir no break in routine for the police. Why is there widespread legislative and student protest about the killing in Vietnam and none about the slaughter on our highways, which in total far exceeds that of all our wars combined? Apparently, the manner in which one is killed is crucially important to arousing the sensibilities of vocal, seemingly pavlovian-reflexed groups in our society.

Perhaps some cultural anthropologist from another planet might have the objectivity to understand why customs and taboos inhibit members of our society from examining the problem of accidents in order that measures can be taken to protect society from the accident epidemic.

Unfortunately, medical school curricular planners are subject to the same taboos, fads, and foibles of the remainder of society. For the most part they have not chosen to include the study of accidents in their curricula, although in the United States in 1969 accidents claimed 115,000 lives, disabled 11 million persons, were the leading cause of death between ages 1 and 39, cost the nation $22 billion, and took up 22 million bed days a year or 12% of the total general hospital space. Past neglect of the accident problem by medical school curricular planners might be understandable if the etiology of the disease were unknown or if treatment were impossible, but this is not the case.

There are many paradoxes and inconsistencies in the public attitude toward accidents and their sequelae. Perhaps it is understandable that the public believes accidents to be "inevitable" or resulting from carelessness that is an "inevitable trait of human nature." Then why does the public, having seemingly accepted the "inevitability of accidents," not also accept the need and responsibility for good emergency medical services to care for the accident victim? Why do they not accept the definition of emergency medical services as including the care the patient receives at the scene of the accident and in transit to the hospital, as well as the care received after hospital arrival? Unfortunately, the public has accepted no more responsibility for emergency medical services than it has for accident prevention. Both the medical community and the public would be shocked if a child in the community died from diphtheria or smallpox. Because of the availability of immunization, these diseases are preventable. Yet it is estimated that over half the deaths resulting from motor vehicle accidents are preventable if people always wore their shoulder and lap belts. Perhaps the public feels that those careless enough to cause accidents are not deserving of good emergency medical service. However, this hardly seems a satisfactory solution for those innocent victims of someone else's carelessness.

There is now much talk about the need to reestablish the priorities of society. Medical school curricula are no exception. Subjects and diseases to be included in the curriculum should be reexamined. How can the medical schools any longer ignore accidents, a disease that is the fourth cause of death and the leading cause of death between ages 1 and 37 years in the United States? The medical schools must help future physicians and health care leaders understand the causes and prognosis of the accident epidemic, not just the treatment of specific injuries. Let us then look at the major causes of accident epidemic.

During the 5-year period from 1964 through 1968, in spite of increases in population, there has been little change in the total number of deaths from work or home accidents.

	Work	Home
1964	14,200	28,000
1968	14,300	28,500

However, in spite of efforts by motor companies, road designers, and law enforcement agencies to prevent accidents and reduce injury occurring during accidents, the deaths from motor vehicle accidents have risen from 47,700 in 1965 to 56,600 in 1972 in the United States. It now seems probable that death and injury from motor vehicle accidents will continue to be an appreciable problem for some time.

Therefore, the medical profession must prepare itself and the public to treat, rehabilitate, and return to society large numbers of injured patients. In order to meet this responsibility, the medical profession must actively participate in and initiate training programs for emergency medical technicians, establish ordinances, support efforts for a communications network between hospital and ambulance, and see that hospital emergency departments are adequately staffed and equipped to meet the contingencies of acutely ill and injured individuals. The medical profession, through advance planning on an areawide basis, must make provisions so that the injured patient is always delivered to an emergency department equipped to cope with his injuries.

For the physician to fulfill these responsibilities, he will have to step outside the ivory tower of his hospital and deal with police, firemen, ambulance drivers, hospital administrators, public health officials, businessmen, labor unions, and politicians in his community. Establishment of emergency services health councils with wide representation in the community is one technique physicians may employ to influence community action to improve emergency medical services. If the medical profession does not provide leadership in the effort to improve emergency medical service, it is my conviction that the government, because of the seriousness of the problem, may eventually tell the medical profession what it must do.

The medical profession needs to arouse the social conscience of medical school curricular planners to the necessity of exposing medical students to the accident epidemic. The accident problem should be presented to the students in a wide, overall view that will include its etiology in terms of human factors and road or vehicle design, the pattern of injury, the physiologic and metabolic responses of the body and its tissues to injury, heart-lung resuscitation, and the physical and emotional reactions of the patient and his family to injury and economic loss.

It is the medical schools' duty to help medical students recognize their responsibility for improving emergency medical services in the local community, in the state, and in the nation. It is also the medical schools' responsibility to help the medical student realize that implementation of improved emergency medical service will require him to step outside the hospital to communicate and work with nonmedical groups and politicians within his community. Accidents are more than just another disease; they are an epidemic.

Index